VETERINARY CLINICAL PATHOLOGY

Veterinary Clinical Pathology

Editor:

Stephen Rego, Ph.D.

Delve Publishing
www.delvepublishing.com

Veterinary Clinical Pathology
Editor: **Stephen Rego, Ph.D.**

708 3rd Avenue, 6th Floor
New York, NY 10017
United States of America
www.delvepublishing.com

ISBN: 978-1-68095-870-6

Library of Congress Control Number: 2016951621

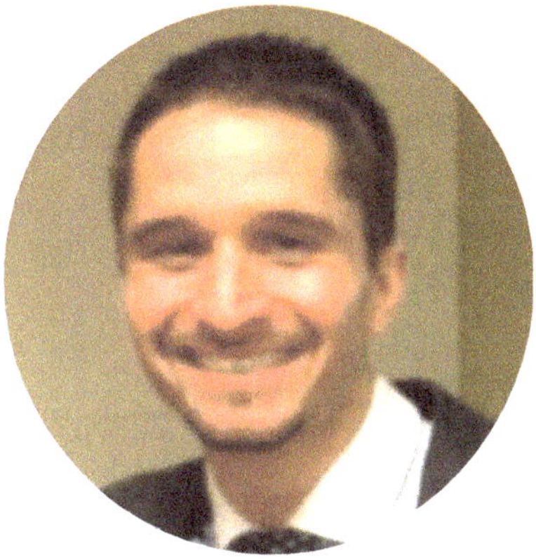

About the Editor

Stephen Rego, Ph.D.

Stephen obtained his PhD from the University of North Carolina at Charlotte in 2013 where his graduate research focused on cancer immunology and the tumor microenvironment. He received postdoctoral training in regenerative and translational medicine, specifically gastrointestinal tissue engineering, at the Wake Forest Institute of Regenerative Medicine. Currently, Stephen is an instructor for anatomy and physiology and biology at Forsyth Technical Community College.

Contents

List of Contributors....................xiii
Preface....................*xvii*
Introduction....................*xix*

Chapter 1 Past, Present and Future: Overview on Histology and Histopathology...... 1

1. Editorial 1
2. Histology 2
3. Histopathology.................... 3

Conclusion.................... 4
Acknowledgement 4
Publication History 4
References 5

Chapter 2 Characterization of Adult Male Albino Rat Mammary Gland: A Histological and Serological Study.................... 7

1. Introduction 7
2. Materials and Methods.................... 8
3. Results 11
4. Discussion 18

Conclusion.................... 20
Authors' Contributions 20
Acknowledgement 20
References 21

Chapter 3 Seven Common Mistakes to Avoid in Achieving Long-Term Success with Dermatology Patients.................... 25

1. Not Appreciating Appropriate Clinical Timelines.................... 25
2. Not Appropriately Framing Client Expectations 27
3. Not Viewing the Situation in Terms of Quality of Life.................... 28
4. Not Following Evidence-Based Standards of Care.................... 29
5. Underestimating the Role of Compliance.................... 31
6. Lacking Realistic Product and Pricing Models 32
7. Considering Dermatology Clients a Nuisance 32

References 32

Chapter 4 Efficacy of Glucocorticoid Monotherapy for Treatment of Canine Meningoencephalomyelitis of Unknown Etiology: a Prospective Study In 16 Dogs.................... 35

1. Introduction 35

	2.	Materials and Methods	36
	3.	Results	38
	4.	Discussion	40
		Conclusions	41
		References	42
Chapter 5	**Grapiprant: An Ep4 Prostaglandin Receptor Antagonist and Novel Therapy for Pain and Inflammation**		**45**
	1.	Introduction	45
	2.	The Piprant Class: Pra	48
		Conclusion	50
		Acknowledgement	51
		Conflicts of Interest	51
		References	51
Chapter 6	**Comparative Aspects of Canine Melanoma**		**55**
	1.	Introduction	55
	2.	Canine Melanoma Epidemiology	56
	3.	Canine Malignant Melanoma Etiology	58
	4.	Canine Melanoma Pathological Aspects and Prognosis	58
	5.	Canine Melanoma: Molecular Aspects	60
	6.	Canine Oral Melanomas	62
	7.	Canine Ocular Melanomas	65
	8.	Canine Digital Melanomas	66
	9.	Treatment Modalities for Canine Melanomas	67
		Conclusions	73
		Acknowledgments	73
		Author Contributions	73
		References	73
Chapter 7	**Understanding the Osteosarcoma Pathobiology: A Comparative Oncology Approach**		**83**
	1.	Introduction	83
	2.	Human Osteosarcoma	85
	3.	Canine Osteosarcoma	87
	4.	Mouse Models of Osteosarcoma	88
	5.	Conserved Drivers of Osteosarcoma	89
	6.	Advantages of a Multi-Species, Comparative Osteosarcoma Study Approach	93
		Conclusions	93
		Acknowledgments	94
		Author Contributions	94
		References	94

Chapter 8 **Kidney Ischaemia Reperfusion Injury in the Rat: The EGTI Scoring System as a Valid and Reliable Tool for Histological Assessment** **103**

1. Introduction 103
2. Methods 105
3. Results 107
Discussion 111
Conclusion 112
Authors' Contributions 112
Acknowledgement and Funding 113
References 113

Chapter 9 **Effect of Homocysteine on the Histological Structure of Femur in Young Male Albino Rats and the Possible Protective Role of Folic Acid** **115**

1. Introduction 115
2. Materials And Methods 117
3. Results 120
4. Discussion 126
Conclusion 128
Authors' Contributions 129
Acknowledgement 129
References 129

Chapter 10 **Effect of Topical Aloe Vera on the Process of Healing of Full-Thickness Skin Burn: A Histological and Immunohistochemical Study** **135**

1. Introduction 135
2. Material and Methods 136
3. Results 138
4. Discussion 145
Conclusion 147
Authors' Contributions 147
References 148

Chapter 11 **Cytogenomics of Feline Cancers: Advances and Opportunities** **153**

1. Introduction 153
2. Gross Karyotypic Organization in the Domestic Cat 154
3. Generation of a Reference Cat Genome Sequence Assembly 154
4. Fundamentals of Cancer Cytogenomics 155
5. Injection-Site Sarcoma 155
6. Lymphoma 158
7. Mammary Carcinoma 159

Conclusions 160
References 161

Chapter 12 From "One Health" To "One Communication": The Contribution of Communication in Veterinary Medicine to Public Health........ 167
1. Introduction 167
2. Veterinary Medicine And Public Health 169
Conclusions 175
Author Contributions........ 175
References 175

Chapter 13 A Review on the Public Health Importance of Bovine Salmonellosis 183
1. Introduction 183
2. General Overview of Bovine Salmonellosis........ 184
3. Disease in Human........ 191
4. Public Health Aspect of Bovine Salmonellosis........ 193
5. Diagnosis of Salmonellosis........ 194
6. Culture Methods 194
7. Prevention and Control 196
Conclusion and Recommendation 198
References 199

Chapter 14 Laboratory Manual and Review on Clinical Pathology........ 203
1. Introduction 203
2. Objectives of Clinical Pathology Practical Course 204
3. Part One: Hematology 204
4. Blood Collection 205
5. Staining Dyes 208
6. Methods of Staining (Staining Procedure) 209
7. Smear Preparation........ 211
8. Hemoglobin Determination 213
9. Hematocrit Determination (PCV) 214
10. Total Count of RBC 214
11. Total Count of WBC (White Blood Cells) 216
12. Differential Leukocyte Count 217
13. Determination of Erythrocyte Sedimentation Rate (ESR) 221
14. Coagulation Time Determination (Whole Blood Clotting Time) 222
15. Bleeding Time 224
16. Calculating Red Blood Cell Indices 225
17. Part Two: Function Tests 228
18. Determination of Alkaline Phosphatase (ALP) 229
19. Determination of Creatinine 230

20. Total Protein Determination 231
21. Urea Determination 232
22. Total and Direct Bilirubin Determination 234
23. Enzymatic Kinetic Colorimeter Test (God – Pap) 235
24. Liver Function Test 236
25. Wallace-Diamond Test 237
26. Kidney Function Test 238
27. Microscopic Examination of Urine Sample 240
28. Protein Test 242
29. Glucose Test 242
30. Acetone (Ketone Body) 243
31. Rumen Function Test 244
32. Sedimentation Activity Time 245
33. Bacteria Examination 246
34. Microscopic Examination of Rumen Content Protozoan's 246
35. Cellulose Digestion Test 247
36. Pancreatic Function Test 247
37. Trypsin 248
38. Gelatin Test Method 248
References 249

Index **251**

List of Contributors

Giuseppe Musumeci
Department of Bio-medical Sciences, Anatomy and Histology Section, School of Medicine, University of Catania, Italy

Zienab A. Gouda
Department of Histology and Cell Biology, Faculty of Medicine, Zagazig University, Zagazig 44519, Egypt

Samah M. Ahmed
Department of Histology and Cell Biology, Faculty of Medicine, Zagazig University, Zagazig 44519, Egypt

Nabila M. Elghonaimy
Department of Histology and Cell Biology, Faculty of Medicine, Zagazig University, Zagazig 44519, Egypt

Lowell Ackerman
DVM DACVD MBA MPA Westborough, Boston, Massachusetts, USA

Miyu Mercier
VCA Aurora Animal Hospital, 2600 West Galena Blvd, Aurora, Illinois, 60506, USA

Heidi L. Barnes Heller
VCA Aurora Animal Hospital, 2600 West Galena Blvd, Aurora, Illinois, 60506, USA

Kristin Kirkby Shaw
Animal Surgical Clinic of Seattle, Seattle, Washington, USA

Lesley C. Rausch-Derra
Aratana Therapeutics, Inc., Kansas City, Kansas, USA

Linda Rhodes
Aratana Therapeutics, Inc., Kansas City, Kansas, USA

Adriana Tomoko Nishiya
Department of Pathology, School of Veterinary Medicine and Animal Science, University of São Paulo, Av. Prof. Dr. Orlando Marques de Paiva, 87, CEP 05508-270, São Paulo, Brazil

Cristina Oliveira Massoco
Department of Pathology, School of Veterinary Medicine and Animal Science, University of São Paulo, Av. Prof. Dr. Orlando Marques de Paiva, 87, CEP 05508-270, São Paulo, Brazil

Claudia Ronca Felizzola
Department of Pathology, School of Veterinary Medicine and Animal Science, University of São Paulo, Av. Prof. Dr. Orlando Marques de Paiva, 87, CEP 05508-270, São Paulo, Brazil
Surgical Oncology Rua Antônio Alves Magan, 124, CEP 01251-150, São Paulo, Brazil

Eduardo Perlmann
Department of Surgery, School of Veterinary Medicine and Animal Science, University of São Paulo, CEP 05508-270, São Paulo, Brazil

Karen Batschinski
Department of Pathology, School of Veterinary Medicine and Animal Science, University of São Paulo, Av. Prof. Dr. Orlando Marques de Paiva, 87, CEP 05508-270, São Paulo, Brazil

Marcello Vannucci Tedardi
Department of Pathology, School of Veterinary Medicine and Animal Science, University of São Paulo, Av. Prof. Dr. Orlando Marques de Paiva, 87, CEP 05508-270, São Paulo, Brazil

Jéssica Soares Garcia
Department of Pathology, School of Veterinary Medicine and Animal Science, University of São Paulo, Av. Prof. Dr. Orlando Marques de Paiva, 87, CEP 05508-270, São Paulo, Brazil

Priscila Pedra Mendonça
Department of Surgery, School of Veterinary Medicine and Animal Science, University of São Paulo, CEP 05508-270, São Paulo, Brazil

Tarso Felipe Teixeira
Pathology Veterinary Medicine, FEPI Itajubá University Center, Dr. Antonio Braga Filho Street, 687, Itajubá, 37.501-002 Minas Gerais, Brazil

Maria Lucia Zaidan Dagli
Department of Pathology, School of Veterinary Medicine and Animal Science, University of São Paulo, Av. Prof. Dr. Orlando Marques de Paiva, 87, CEP 05508-270, São Paulo, Brazil

Jyotika Varshney
Masonic Cancer Center, University of Minnesota, Minneapolis, MN 55455, USA
Department of Surgery, University of Minnesota Medical School, Moos Tower, 11-212420 Delaware Street, S.E.; MMC 195, Minneapolis, MN 55455, USA

Milcah C. Scott
Masonic Cancer Center, University of Minnesota, Minneapolis, MN 55455, USA
Animal Cancer Care and Research Program, University of Minnesota, St. Paul, MN 55455, USA
Department of Veterinary Clinical Sciences, College of Veterinary Medicine, University of Minnesota, St. Paul, MN 55108, USA

David A. Largaespada
Masonic Cancer Center, University of Minnesota, Minneapolis, MN 55455, USA
Department of Pediatrics, University of Minnesota, Minneapolis, MN 55455, USA

Subbaya Subramanian
Masonic Cancer Center, University of Minnesota, Minneapolis, MN 55455, USA
Department of Surgery, University of Minnesota Medical School, Moos Tower, 11-212420 Delaware Street, S.E.; MMC 195, Minneapolis, MN 55455, USA

Usman Khalid
Cardiff Transplant Unit, Department of Nephrology and Transplant Surgery, University Hospital of Wales, Heath Park, Cardiff, UK
Institute of Nephrology, Cardiff University, Cardiff, UK

Gilda Pino-Chavez
Institute of Nephrology, Cardiff University, Cardiff, UK

Prabhu Nesargikar
Cardiff Transplant Unit, Department of Nephrology and Transplant Surgery, University Hospital of Wales, Heath Park, Cardiff, UK
Institute of Nephrology, Cardiff University, Cardiff, UK

Robert H. Jenkins
Institute of Nephrology, Cardiff University, Cardiff, UK

Timothy Bowen
Institute of Nephrology, Cardiff University, Cardiff, UK

Donald J. Fraser
Institute of Nephrology, Cardiff University, Cardiff, UK

Rafael Chavez
Cardiff Transplant Unit, Department of Nephrology and Transplant Surgery, University Hospital of Wales, Heath Park, Cardiff, UK
Institute of Nephrology, Cardiff University, Cardiff, UK

Rania A. Zidan
Department of Histology and Cell Biology, Faculty of Medicine, Zagazig University, Egypt

Heba M. Elnegris
Department of Histology and Cell Biology, Faculty of Medicine, Zagazig University, Egypt

Ahmed A.M. Abdel Hamid
Department of Histology and Cell Biology, Faculty of Medicine, Mansoura University, Egypt

Mona FM Soliman
Department of Histology and Cell Biology, Faculty of Medicine, Mansoura University, Egypt

Rachael Thomas
Department of Molecular Biomedical Sciences, College of Veterinary Medicine & Center for Comparative Medicine and Translational Research, North Carolina State University, Raleigh NC 27607, USA

Micaela Cipolla,
Department of Veterinary Science and Public Health (DIVET), Università degli Studi di Milano, via Celoria 10, 20133 Milano, Italy

Luigi Bonizzi
Department of Veterinary Science and Public Health (DIVET), Università degli Studi di Milano, via Celoria 10, 20133 Milano, Italy

Alfonso Zecconi
Department of Veterinary Science and Public Health (DIVET), Università degli Studi di Milano, via Celoria 10, 20133 Milano, Italy

Jelalu Kemal
College of Veterinary Medicine, Haramaya University, Ethiopia

Preface

Clinical pathology is important for the general and emergency care of both humans and animals. This practice is a commonly utilized tool in every veterinary clinic. Veterinary clinical pathology is the bedrock on which animal health welfare rests and veterinary pathologists throughout the world have made valuable contributions in the understanding in animal disease and their diagnosis and also in the teaching. Veterinary clinical pathology has made great strides in recent years. The advances may prove to be a great asset in the new millennium in research, disease investigation and differential diagnosis of animal diseases. With the advancement of knowledge most sensitive, quick, reliable and specific methods for diagnosis have been evolved. These methods are proving invaluable to the disease investigators. Moreover, modern techniques and tools are able to differentiate diseases at a molecular level. Recent advances in veterinary pathology, narrated in this review should be taken as complementary to the conventional methods of clinical pathology, histopathology and various cultural and serological tests. Most conventional methods have stood the test of time and would undoubtedly work in tandem with the newer molecular tools in veterinary pathology. Strong inputs of modern technology have to go into the various aspects of health care, viz. disease surveillance, prevention and effective therapeutic measures. The field of clinical pathology involves the laboratory analysis of bodily fluids, such as blood and urine, to study and diagnose diseases in animals. One of the primary techniques used in clinical pathology is histology, which involves the study of microscopic anatomy of the cells in the blood to determine their phenotype, function and relative abundance. Histology is a major focus of this book and a number of articles reviewing this specialty are given. Aside from histology this book also provides numerous examples of specific diseases and their diagnosis using techniques in clinical pathology. Some of the diseases, conditions and treatments discussed in this book include dermatological diseases, meningoencephalomyelitis, pain and inflammation, Monensin Toxicosis infection, Kidney ischaemia reperfusion injury, hormone replacement therapies, endosulfan, tadalafil and ochratoxin-A therapies, hepatitis, burns and cancer which is discussed in detail. Along with veterinary professionals, animal owners may gain valuable insights into clinical pathology through reviewing these materials. This book is intended to help prospective and active pathology trainees, their mentors, and educational administrators optimize opportunities to ensure the future vitality of veterinary pathologists, and their contributions, in basic and applied research.

Editor

Stephen Rego, Ph.D.

INTRODUCTION

Veterinary pathologists are doctors of veterinary medicine who specialize in the diagnosis of diseases through the examination of animal tissue and body fluids. Like medical pathology, veterinary pathology is divided into two branches, anatomical pathology and clinical pathology. Other than the diagnosis of disease in food-producing animals, companion animals, zoo animals and wildlife, veterinary pathologists also have an important role in drug discovery and safety as well as scientific research.

Veterinary Pathologists recognize major health hazards before almost anyone else; for example, the West Nile Virus. When diseases attack or kill animals, they can be potentially dangerous for humans as well, as animals interact with humans in many positive ways, including companionship, providing therapy, and preparation of food, among others. Veterinary Pathologists are responsible for studying disease and its effect on animals, which, in turn, helps cure and prevent both animal and human disease.

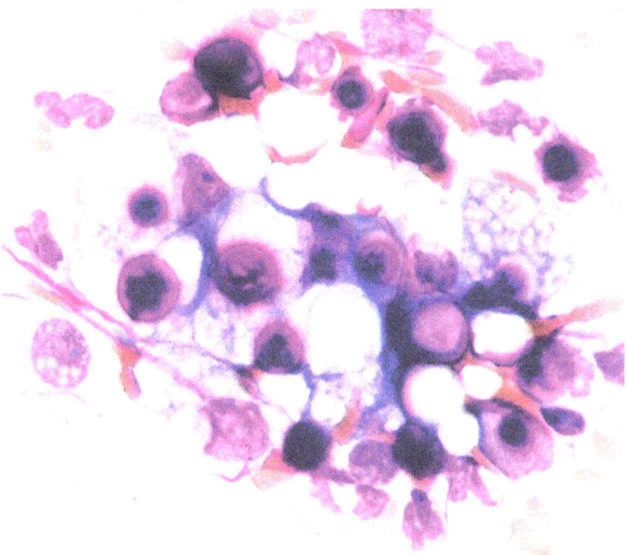

Clinical pathology is the study and diagnosis of diseases by analyzing body fluids. Clinical pathologists study fluids such as blood and urine to diagnose diseases. A clinical pathologist may choose to specialize in one type of pathology, such as chemistry, hematology or microbiology.

Clinical pathologists are certified through the American Board of Pathology. This board licenses physicians in a variety of specialties. In some countries, it is not necessary to be a doctor to specialize in clinical pathology. Some countries allow other medical professionals, such as pharmacists, to receive licensing.

Each area of specialization in clinical pathology has its own unique set of standards. Clinical chemistry, for example, focuses on the study and analysis of body fluids. Clinical chemistry is also known as chemical pathology. Laboratories that focus on chemical pathology run tests to measure hormone function, the immune system and antibody function and the function of drugs on the system, or pharmacology.

Blood that will be used for transfusions will not have the components separated out, but will have a preservative added. Some collected blood is spun in a centrifuge. This causes the heavier components to settle to the bottom, separating the red blood cells and plasma. Proper handling of blood after collection is vital for the safety of the patient as well as to prevent valuable blood from being wasted.

A final specialization in clinical pathology is medical microbiology. Medical microbiology is the study of bacteria, viruses and parasites. This type of pathology is closely related to the study of immunology and the study of infectious diseases.

Clinical pathology is one medical career path that has many branches. Some clinical pathologists will work closely with others, while others will spend a great deal of time alone in a laboratory. When deciding on what area to specialize in, you should take into consideration how much solitary time you want as part of your work load. Regardless of the specialty, few clinical pathologists work directly with patients.

Another clinical pathology specialty is in hematology. These clinical pathologists work with blood banks to process donated blood so that it can best be used. While the majority of blood that is donated is donated as whole blood, it is often broken down into various components before it is used.

Clinical pathology is one of the two major divisions of pathology, the other being anatomical pathology. Clinical pathology is itself divided in to subspecialties, the main ones being clinical hematology/blood banking, clinical chemistry, hematopathology and clinical microbiology and emerging subspecialties such as molecular diagnostics. Hematology studies the blood and blood-forming tissues to evaluate presence of disease and assist in therapeutic interventions as clinically indicated. Clinical chemistry (also known as chemical pathology and clinical biochemistry) is the area of clinical pathology that is generally concerned with analysis of bodily fluids. Blood parameters play a critical role in diagnosis, assessing progression, and in the characterization of disease and phenotypes in clinical and research situations. The accuracy and reliability of the whole blood parameter analysis depends on identification and control or elimination of variables that may affect these results. Different blood collection and handling strategies represent source of variability that can be controlled in many instances. Basic hematological procedures such as the complete blood count are frequently conducted to help physicians and veterinarians arrive at a diagnosis and prognosis, also to evaluate treatment. Hematology testing includes, but is not limited to: Hematology Sample Processing, Hematology Research Services, Hematology Automated Testing, Lamellar Body Counts, Microscopic Cellular Analysis, Body Fluid Analysis and Specialized Stains. The outline of this laboratory manual deals with the basic hematological procedures and clinical chemistry analysis which is meant for students use. The study of hematology begins with proper sample collection and handling. Part one deals with hematology containing different sections. Part two covers clinical chemistry including functional tests. All of the procedures described in this manual are classical methods that are routinely performed in a standard clinical pathology laboratory. Detail procedures including preparation of reagents, solutions, stains and buffers are given. Calculations of blood indices and chemical analysis are also discussed in part one and part two respectively.

A clinical pathologist looks at blood, urine, and other body fluid specimens under a microscope, or with other diagnostic tools, to observe levels of certain chemicals and/or other substances in the body.

Types of Specimens used in Clinical Pathology

Blood

- Blood is used in many tests. Blood can either be examined as a "whole," as plasma (the fluid left when red and white blood cells are removed), or as serum (a clear fluid that separates from blood when it clots).
- Blood is usually drawn with a needle from a vein, usually in the forearm. (This is also called venipuncture). Sometimes, the tip of the finger is pricked and then squeezed to draw blood (called a finger stick).

Urine

Urine is also used for a wide range of tests. Urine specimens can be obtained by:

- Random method. The patient urinates in a cup.
- Clean catch specimen. The outer genital area has been cleaned before urinating in a cup.
- Sterile urine test. This requires catheterization (a tube is put into the urethra and goes to the bladder to obtain urine).

Sometimes, a doctor will require the patient to do a timed test to measure substances excreted into the urine over several hours.

Sputum

Sputum can be coughed into a clean container.

Feces

Feces or stool is usually collected by the patient in a clean cardboard or plastic container.

Other body fluids

Other body fluids collected for testing may include the following:

- Spinal fluid
- Pleural fluids. These fluids are around the lungs and/or in the pleural cavity (the space between the two membranes that surround the lungs).
- Abdominal (belly) fluids
- Joint fluids
- Bone marrow

Other branches of pathology include:

- Anatomic pathology. The study of tissues, organs, and tumors.
- Cytopathology. The study of cellular changes and everything related to cells.
- Forensic pathology. Performance of autopsies and legal pathology tests.
- Molecular pathology. The study of DNA and RNA sequencing, genes, and genetics.

Some pathologists specialize in these different areas.

Blood Collection

- *Site*: The following lists of veins are the most appropriate blood collection sites from different species of veterinary importance
- *Jagular vein*: the most commonly used site in the horse, cattle, sheep, goat, camel and large wild mammals: used occasionally in small animals. Vacutainer tube, vacutainer needle, syringe, needle, needle holder, and disinfectant should be used for blood sample.

Procedure

- Placement of the thumb of the left hand in the jagular furrow to occlude and anchor the jagular vein, while manipulating the syringe and needle with the right hand
- Clipping the site of sampling especially in long haired animals is recommended

- The veins are more clearly out lined when the site is rubbed with alcohol

- *Cephalic vein*: The most commonly used site for collection of small amount of blood in the dog. By constricting the area on the dorsal aspects of the fore limb at the level of the elbow which can be raised beginning just above the carpal vein.
- *Ear vein*: can be used in small dog, pig, cat and small lab animals (small dog, rabbit, guinea pig, and monkey).
  - A marginal vein on the dorsal side of the ear is selected
  - Remove the hair by shaving, clipping, or other method
  - Swab the skin with alcohol or other
  - Place the left index finger under the ear at the point of applying stylet or syringe
  - Gentle aspiration is used when using a syringe in small animals like rabbit, to avoid collapse of the vein

Toe or Toe nail: can be used in small dog, puppy, guinea pig etc

- Clip the hair away
- Disinfect the capillary bed of the nail
- Cut in to just short of the base of the nail
- Take 20-40 drops as well as 80 drops (4ml) of blood

Tail: can be used in pig, cattle, sheep, rat, and mouse

- Venipuncture –of the coccygeal vein on the ventral side
- Amputation – commonest method used in the rat and mouse. A small transverse incision with a razor blade produce drops of blood

Heart: may be used in animals like bird, fish, and others

Femoral or Tibial vessels: used in dog, cat, small mammals, rat etc

Mammary vein: used for dairy cattle. The vein appears at the anterior border of the mammary gland lateral from the linea Alba and runs forward passing through a foramen in the abdominal wall posterior to ribs.

Anterior vena cava: used for the pig. A needle (4½ – 6 in. and 17 to 20 gauge needle) is inserted just anterior and slightly lateral to the cariniform cartilage and a line from the cartilage to the base of the ear.

Retro orbital Venus plexus: used for the rat, mouse, guinea pig

- A best method for obtaining a large quantity of blood (1ml) in mouse
- This technique is reported to be less traumatic than others

Wing vein or comb: used for birds

- After the feathers in the axillary region are plucked, the alar vein is seen running from beneath the pectoral muscle then along the ventral surface of the humerus

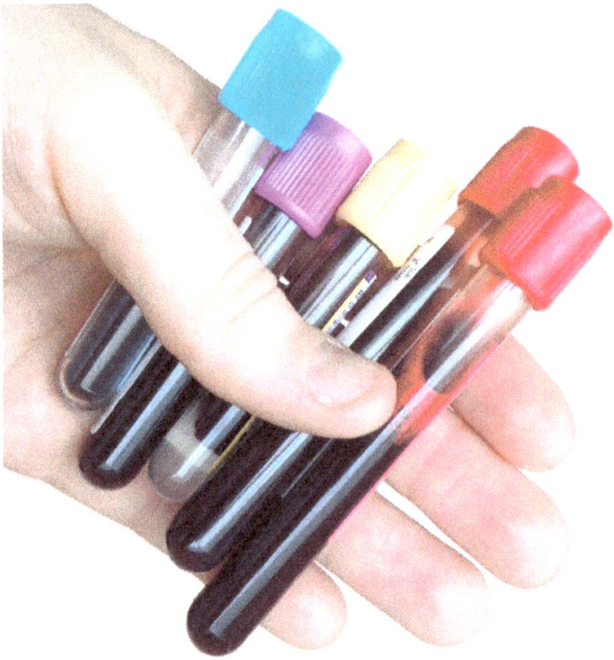

Conventional Diagnostic Methods in Pathology

A tissue sample from a patient by any of the above-mentioned methods, it is necessary to fix it. Fixation is a way of treating a tissue using specific kinds of chemicals, usually in the form of fluids. The process of tissue decay and organ destruction begins as soon as the tissue is detached from the body and has lost its source of blood supply. It is a self-destruction and autolytic process that can continue up to the complete destruction of the sample. In the case of inappropriate and untimely fixation, the tissue consistency will be lost and it will not be possible to examine the tissue at both the macroscopic and microscopic levels. In some cases, it is very important that the pathologist provides the clinicians with some information about the characteristics and composition of the constituting cells at the molecular level. Such molecular evaluations are exceedingly difficult if not impossible to carry out on improperly fixed samples.

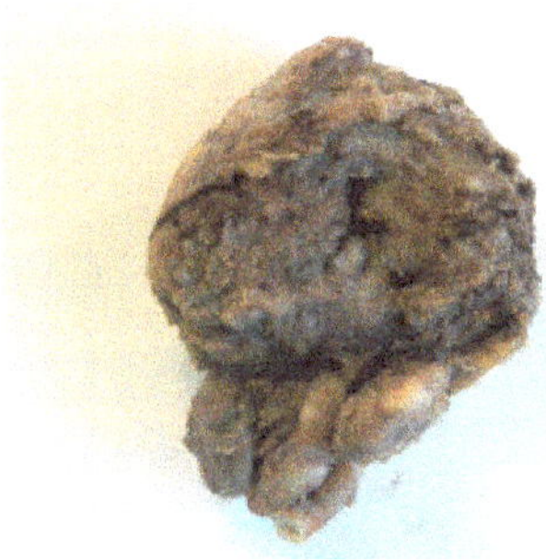

(a)

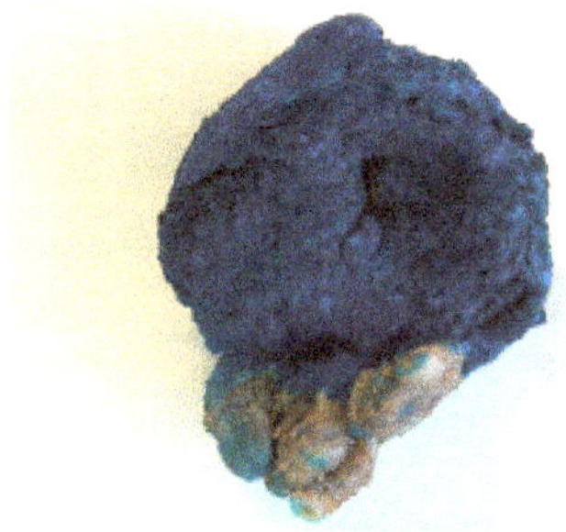

(b)

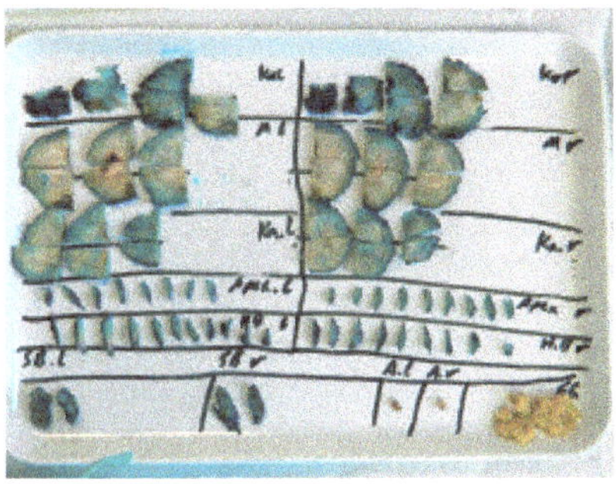

(c)

The most universally used fixative solution in most of the pathology laboratories around the world is buffered 4% formalin solution. There are many other fixatives that can be used in specific situations. Most of them suffer from one or more drawbacks such as high costs, problems with disposal, need for specific methods of tissue processing after fixation, too long a fixation time, and effects on the results of immunohistochemical or molecular examinations.

Cytology

The specimens that are received for cytologic examinations are usually in the form of an aspirated, expectorated, or washed fluid. One or more smears are usually prepared from the sediment of a centrifuged fluid. Depending on the desired staining method, these smears can be fixed by chemicals or are air-dried. The rest of the sediment can be processed similarly as for a tissue sample by transferring the cells into a network of protein material, for example, protein glycerin or plasma, followed by coagulation with thrombin.

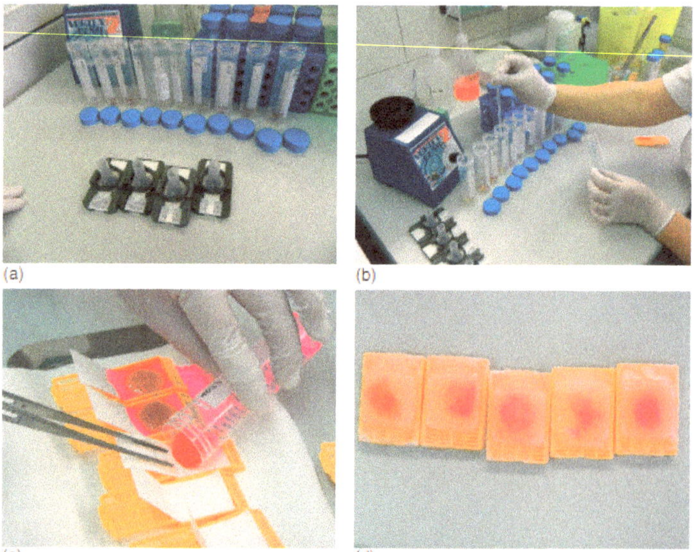

(a) (b) (c) (d)

The cells are then fixed in formalin followed by paraffin embedding just like a tissue sample. If these cell blocks contain a sufficient number of cells, they serve as a very helpful reserve for further examinations such as immunohistochemical or sometimes molecular genetic tests.

Histology

Immediately after submission to a pathology laboratory, every tissue sample is given a numerical code. Different methods of labeling, such as bar coding, can be used for coding the samples. The process of tissue examination by a pathologist begins by naked eye examination. A lot of information can be obtained after a careful macroscopic tissue examination or grossing. For small biopsy samples, these pieces of information are usually limited to the dimensions, as well as the number, color, and amount of the sample. It provides basic information regarding the adequacy of the specimen for further evaluations. In the case of some specific types of specimens, it is the duty of the pathologist to examine the small specimens by a hand lens or by a low-power microscope before subjecting it to complete formalin fixation and ordinary tissue processing. The best example is the renal needle biopsy. By low-power microscopic examination, the pathologist can tell the clinician whether he or she was successful in obtaining an adequate amount of renal tissue. On the other hand, the pathologist may need to divide the sample appropriately into three portions. Each portion is then handled differently for different methods of examination, that is, fresh tissue for immunofluorescent examination, fixation in glutaraldehyde for electron microscopy, and fixation in buffered formalin for conventional tissue microscopy and specific chemical staining. The last option represents the standard procedure that is applicable in all cases.

The most important role of grossing is in the evaluation of large resection samples. It is evident that microscopic evaluation of a whole resection sample, for example, the complete removal of an organ or extremity, is neither possible nor necessary. There are specific guidelines from which a pathologist can obtain information on how a resection specimen should be sampled and examined for microscopy. In most cases, these resection samples are those that contain a malignant tumor. In this situation, the clinicians might want to know the extent of the tumor and the completeness of its removal. The macroscopic examination defines the exact location, size, shape, and configuration of the tumor, the depth of local invasion (in tumors of luminal structures such as intestinal tract), the relationship with adjacent normal tissue, and the distance from surgical resection margins. It is also necessary to look for lymph nodes to examine them for possible metastatic foci. According to the guidelines, a pathologist takes small tissue fragments from the tumor, resection margins, and lymph nodes, which should not be less than a minimum recommended number. In some types of specimens, for example, radical prostatectomy specimens, it is recommended to completely embed the specimen in thin sections. To maintain the orientation during the microscopic examination, it is sometimes necessary to paint the specific areas such as resection margins by the different colors of specific dyes.

The prepared tissue slices are then placed in a plastic cassette. On this cassette, the code number of the specimen and if necessary the specific code of the area of sampling are written or typed. Now the tissue slices are ready to be processed. Tissue processing is a vital step for preparing the tissue slices for microscopic examinations. This task is performed automatically by a "tissue processor." The device consists of vessels containing specific chemical compounds (mainly alcohol and xylene) at a previously determined and graded concentration. The processing of tissue is enhanced and accelerated in new-generation tissue processors by the application of microwave energy or vacuum. The tissue processing ends with embedding the tissue in a paraffin block. Now the tissue is ready to be cut to obtain thin slices for microscopic examinations. Using specific sharp blades and a precisely designed device, it is possible to cut the paraffin blocks into very thin sections (preferably 3–5 μm in thickness). The sections are placed on a glass slide, stained, and finally cover by a cover slip. They are now ready for microscopic examination by a pathologist.

Microscopy

A physician collects the necessary information by examining a patient and observing the signs and symptoms of the disease. Then he or she makes a list of differential diagnoses and tries to reduce the size of this table by the application of specific laboratory tests. The final target is to reach an accurate diagnosis. Pathology as a practice has similar components. By careful examination of the microscopic changes on a slide, a pathologist tries to gather specific morphologic signs and symptoms (in this situation the key morphologic findings) in order to have a list of differential diagnoses. The basic forms of pathologic changes (with few exceptions) more and less resemble each other in the different organs and body tissues. For example, an acute or a chronic inflammatory reaction is accompanied almost always by a predominantly neutrophilic or lympho-plasmacytic inflammatory cell infiltration, respectively. The basic microscopic examinations are performed almost always in the first step on H&E stained slides. By using two different acidic (eosin) and basic (hematoxylin) stains, the basophilic components of the cell structure (mainly RNA and DNA) gain a deep blue color and the acidophilic components (cell cytoplasm and interstitial stromal materials) gain a pale to deep pink appearance. Some specific cell components or specific cell types can be amphophilic (neither eosinophilic nor basophilic). Although the basic structure of the tissue and basic forms of pathologic processes are in most cases easily appreciable during this primary microscopic evaluation, it is sometimes necessary to stain new tissue sections to answer specific questions. Some examples of chemical-specific tissue stains are as follows:

Periodic acid-Schiff (PAS): Using this stain, we can see a better reaction of chemicals or structures with a high content of carbohydrates or glycoproteins. It shows better intracytoplasmic or interstitial accumulations of mucinous secretions (for example, in mucin-secreting adenocarcinomas). Some specific forms of microorganisms, for example, fungi, are better recognizable by this type of staining. A pathologist can find more easily the megakaryocytes in a closely packed and hypercellular bone marrow tissue. It is also a very good staining of the basement membrane in different epithelial coverings, and its application plays a crucial role in the microscopic investigation of glomerular diseases in the field of renal pathology.

Giemsa: It is one of the basic special stains and is regularly used in the microscopic examination of lymphoid and hematopoietic tissues (lymph node or bone marrow biopsies). In addition to providing better nuclear morphology, application of this staining is a single histologic method for the evaluation of tissue infiltration by mast cells. Most of the microorganisms, particularly bacteria, are better recognizable by this method of staining. A modified Giemsa staining is routinely used in gastric mucosa biopsies for the evaluation of Helicobacter pylori infection.

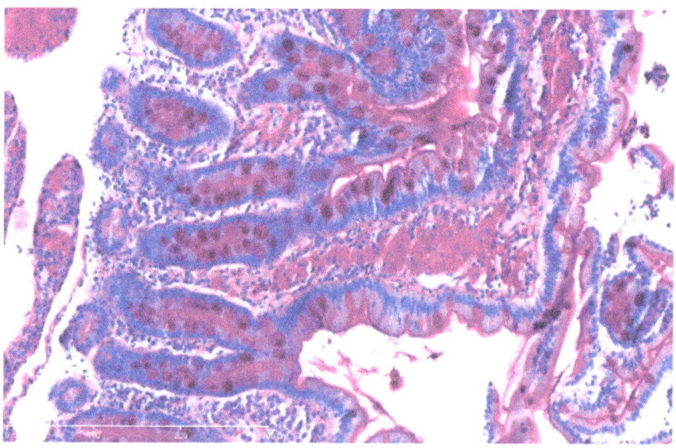

Masson trichrome: It provides a better evaluation of the extent and severity of tissue fibrosis. In liver pathology, its routine application is one of the bases of diagnosis of advanced liver fibrosis or liver cirrhosis. Its application in medical renal biopsies as adjunct to other specific chemical stains (such as Jones staining) is extremely useful in judging the presence of fibrinoid necrosis, glomerulosclerosis, and abnormal depositions in the mesangial spaces and basement membrane.

Iron staining: Iron depositions in tissue are recognized in routine H&E staining as coarse dark-brown crystalloid materials. Although an experienced pathologist can recognize iron deposition by noticing the background histologic features and morphologic characteristics, in the liver tissue, for instance, it can be often mistaken for the intracellular bilirubin (a product of hepatocytes) or lipofuscin (a final metabolite of fat in senescent or hypoxic injured cells). In one of the specific iron staining methods (Prussian blue), the iron crystals gain a deep blue stain, while the other two remain unstained. The same staining can help a pathologist to differentiate between iron-laden intra-alveolar macrophages (i.e., heart failure cells) from pigment-laden macrophages with ingested coal particles. The estimation of iron stores in bone marrow specimens is important to differentiate pathologic situations with increased iron stores (for example, myelodysplastic syndromes, sideroblastic anemia, and anemia of chronic disease) from situations with low iron stores (such as iron deficiency or chronic hemorrhagic anemia).

1
CHAPTER

PAST, PRESENT AND FUTURE: OVERVIEW ON HISTOLOGY AND HISTOPATHOLOGY

Giuseppe Musumeci

EDITORIAL

With sincere satisfaction and pride, I present this first editorial of the Journal of Histology and Histopathology edited by myself. I know this is a very challenging task, assuming the editorial coordination of this journal, targeted to enhance the work of so many esteemed international experts as well as dear colleagues, who work on morphological research. A special thanks goes to our current editorial team (Sherif M Karam, Xueyong Zhu, Gjumrakch Aliev, Khin Thway, Han-Seung yoon, Paul Evans, George Perry and Khush Mittal) and the publishing group (Herbert Publications) that, day after day, thanks to their valuable contribution, make possible the growth of this journal. Reviewing a manuscript is time-consuming and unpaid, and often reviewers are bombarded with requests to review simultaneously from several journals. I hope to increase the number of editors of the editorial board members (with different geographical origin), to assure a rapid publication. My aim and that of all the other editors is that this journal will constitute a valuable tool, of both learning and research, to understand how modern histology and histopathology can be a fundamental bridge between molecular and anatomicalphysiological disciplines and how the structural organization of cells in tissues is inextricably linked to the functions that the pathological and normal tissues must perform. These concepts must constitute a significant part of imprinting training, necessary to help researchers to work in a more guided way, increasingly interested in a cellular approach to diseases and their related treatments. Finally, conscious of the fact that this journal can be considered a "system" subjected to the laws of evolution, we welcome criticism and suggestions for its improvement in the future. The purpose of this editorial was to explain my view on histology and histopathology of today, providing a brief overview from the past to the future.

Citation: Giuseppe Musumeci, Past, present and future: overview on histology and histopathology, DOI: http://dx.doi.org/10.7243/2055-091X-1-5.

HISTOLOGY

Histology and Histopathology are often discussed and described together. In fact, the concept of histopathology cannot be separated from that of histology since understanding of normal histology is essential for histo-pathological interpretation. It is indeed obvious and necessary to prepare histology slides of a sample or specimen and examine them first in order to find out if the cells or tissue are healthy or diseased. Moreover, expert histo-pathologists should also be able to inform histologists about normal variations of tissue morphology, improving in this way histo-pathological interpretations. We could state then, that histology and histopathology are inter-dependent. In the 19th century, histology was an eminent academic discipline in its own right and the first half of the 20th century was a very productive period for new staining techniques in histology and histopathology. Indeed the 1906 Nobel Prize in Physiology or Medicine was awarded to histologists Camillo Golgi and Santiago Ramon y Cajal. They had conflicting interpretations of the neural structure of the brain based on differing interpretations of the same images. Cajal was appreciated for his correct theory and Golgi for the staining technique that he invented. Many of the centenary staining techniques in cell biology and histopathology are still used and continue to provide valuable diagnostic information. Histology is the study of the microscopic details and structures of biological cells and tissues, using light, fluorescence or electron microscopes, examining a thin slice (called a «section») of tissues, that have been previously prepared using appropriate processes called «histological techniques». The first microscope had been constructed in 1591 but had several optical problems. In 1673 Anton van Leeuwenhoek developed a simple microscope with a single lense but with improved magnification and resolution. The first microtome suitable for sectioning animal tissues was constructed in 1848. During the 19th century paraffin wax was introduced for infiltration and support during sectioning. Over the years different laboratory substances were investigated for use as fixatives. Formalin was first used in 1893 and today is widely employed [1-3]. In order to better underline different biological structures, histological stains are often used to modify or enhance the colors of certain types of these biological structures differently from the others that may be located next to them or be in contact with them. There are many different histology stains selected according to the type of tissue to be observed. Some stains are more widely used, instead others are only used to study very specific types of biological tissues. One of the oldest stains was Prussian blue, introduced in 1774. Furthemore, Perl›s reaction, discovered in 1867, is still widely used to localize intracellular iron and uses just Prussian blue for the histochemical localization of hemosiderin in tissues. Hematoxylin and eosin (H&E stain) is the most commonly used histology stain for light microscopy. Hematoxylin stains the nuclei within cells blue and eosin stains the cytoplasm of cells pink. H&E is a permanent histology stain, as opposed to a temporary stain. The hematoxylin and eosin staining techniques were first described in 1875–1878, with later modifications. Hematology took advantage from the introduction in the 1890s of Romanovsky-type staining for blood smears, including Giemsa›s and May-Grunwald staining which are still fundamental in clinical practice. Louis B. Wilson was the first to develop a method using methylene dyes to stain fresh-frozen tissue of surgical specimens (1906). The periodic acid-Schiff (PAS) technique of McManus (1946) is still one of the most common diagnostic staining methods in histopathology, it superseded Best›s carmine (1906) to stain polysaccharides and is widely used in liver and muscle disease [4-6]. Oil Red (ORO), introduced by French in 1926 highlights the presence of fat or lipids in fresh, frozen tissue sections. ORO is a fat soluble diazo dye, and is classified as one of the Sudan dyes used since the late 1800s. Feulgen stain (1924) is a staining technique used in histology to identify chromosomal material or DNA in cell specimens and has been the basis of many subsequent applications in cell biology. The Ziehl–Nielsen stain for Mycobacterium tuberculosis (1883) and Gram›s stain for bacteria (1884) are examples of diagnostic bacteriological and pathological techniques, which are still used over a century since their discovery. Paul Ehrlich, who received the Nobel Prize in 1908 for his discovery and his work on «magic bullets», developed the use of dyes to combat disease i.e. methylene blue (1891) to fight malaria and trypan red (1904) against the trypanosomes. Trypan blue remains in widespread as a vital stain, particularly in highlighting cataracts during eye surgery [4-6]. These staining methods are generally inexpensive, reliable, fast, produce permanent preparations that are easy to interpret and archive, and deliver information for diagnoses that cannot be achieved by other means. For these reasons they remain useful and irreplaceable tools in the histology discipline.

HISTOPATHOLOGY

Histopathology regards biological tissues and cells with their microscopic changes or abnormalities that can be the causes or the result of diseases. The main application of histopathology in clinical medicine, is in the examination of a biopsy (i.e., a surgical sample or specimen taken from patients possibly for diagnosis and screening of various tumors) by a specialist physician called a pathologist. The pathologist may be more accurately referred to as a histopathologist. However, for some histopathologists the microscopic examination of diseased tissues may be only a relatively minor part of their overall professional responsibilities. A pathologist or histopathologist studies specimens of cells and tissue samples removed from the patients, processed using special histological techniques (histological slides and sections prepared and stained in order to make the sample ready for observation with a microscope). Either a light microscope or an electron microscope may be used to examine histology slides. The first book on the specialization of histopathology techniques, entitled, "On the Nature and Structural Characteristics of Cancer" was written in 1838 by Johannes Müller. Enzyme histochemistry, electron microscopy, and polarizing microscopy have all become diagnostic tools during the last 50 years. Actually, the use of electron microscopy is rare, except for specific contexts or disciplines such as renal pathology. The use of immunohistochemistry, still under development with new antibodies and biomarkers, began in the 1980s and has revolutionized cancer diagnosis [1-3]. The histology laboratory experienced several changes in the mid 20th century when cryostats, enclosed tissue processors, plastic cassettes, and disposable knives were introduced. The emergence of immunohistochemistry in the 1980s was a revolution among the histopathology methods [1-3] and made obsolete the necessity for the use of electron microscopy. New techniques include flow cytometry, fluorescence in situ hybridization

(FISH), DNA and genetics studies, proteomics, telepathology, and digital imaging. The field of proteomics will be widened by the discovery of new biomarkers and new immunohistochemical tests. These new tests must be accepted by the medical community, and therefore histology laboratories in various hospitals will have to work together to standardize their protocols. Telepathology will be implemented for consultation and diagnosis. However, technicians will have to be sure that a slide prepared in one laboratory when sent as a scan to another laboratory for diagnosis conforms to certain criteria. Thus, specimen collection, fixation, and processing will need to be consistent between laboratories. In less-developed countries these telepathology techniques and equipment will be of benefit to patients [1-3].

CONCLUSION

We can be proud that basic histological, histochemical and immuohistochemical methods have a very long and productive history and continue to give us useful information. We have an enormous debt to the pioneers who discovered stains for coloring tissues and combating disease together with subsequent techniques. These old methodologies still continue to play an important role in the histopathology laboratory and remain at the forefront of research in these disciplines with an enormous long-term impact in cell biology and molecular biology. Histology is the tool for accessing a specific knowledge of the microscopic organization of the organs, microscopic anatomy, which is essential to understand the histopathology for a possible diagnosis. Although today in the research field these disciplines may seem displaced by the *in vitro* study of cell biology, molecular biology, genetics studies and proteomics, in my opinion, remain a key to help and sustain, with the *in vivo* study of tissue and organs, an efficient clinical practice. In confirmation, it is known that histopathology is an essential tool in diagnosis and the experience of the histopathologist is prime and irreplaceable for the correct interpretation of the data obtained. Although immunohistochemical analyses and molecular biology are useful for diagnostic purposes, light microscopy remains preeminent in cytological and histological diagnosis on a daily basis. Hematoxylin and eosin stain is still the gold standard for diagnosis, also in malignancy diagnosis that is based on the interpretation of cytological and architectural features, while immunohistochemistry and molecular biology are ancillary tools which can provide useful information in confirming histologically-based diagnosis.

ACKNOWLEDGEMENT

I thank Prof. Gaetano Magro from Department G.F. Ingrassia, Anatomic Pathology Section, University of Catania, Catania, Italy, for his kind support.

PUBLICATION HISTORY

Editors: Sherif M Karam, UAE University, Al-Ain UAE.
Khush Mittal, New York University School of Medicine, USA.
Received: 24-May-2014 Final Revised: 26-Jun-2014
Accepted: 27-Jun-2014 Published: 05-Jul-2014

REFERENCES

1. Titford M. A Short History of Histopathology Technique. *J Histotechnol.* 2006;29:99-110.
2. Titford M. Progress in the development of microscopical techniques for diagnostic pathology. *J Histotechnol*. 2009; 32:9-19.
3. Titford M and Bowman B. What May the Future Hold for Histotechnologists? *LabMedicine*. 2012; 43:5-10.
4. Coleman R. The impact of histochemistry--a historical perspective. *Acta Histochem.* 2000; 102:5-14.
5. Coleman R. The long-term contribution of dyes and stains to histology and histopathology. *Acta Histochem.* 2006; 108:81-3.
6. Coleman R. Eponyms in histology and histochemistry: do they still serve a purpose, or should they be abandoned in favor of standard non-eponymous terminology? *Acta Histochem.* 2006; 108:241-2.

2

CHAPTER

CHARACTERIZATION OF ADULT MALE ALBINO RAT MAMMARY GLAND: A HISTOLOGICAL AND SEROLOGICAL STUDY

Zienab A. Gouda, Samah M. Ahmed and Nabila M. Elghonaimy

Keywords: Male rat, mammary gland, growth factors, prolactin, progesterone, whole mount carmine alum

INTRODUCTION

The MG has been of great interest to generations of biologists from many disciplines. The structure of the male and female MG can provide a sensitive indicator of endocrinal disturbance [1]. This gland is particularly suited for studying developmental processes as it is readily amenable to experimental manipulation and can be easily accessed. Furthermore in animals, MG tissue is abundant because there are 6 pairs in each animal [2].

In females, a major part of MG development occurs postnatal, with distinct periods of intensive morphogenesis taking place at puberty and during pregnancy and lactation [3]. A course of ductal development includes multiple stages of proliferation and morphogenesis that are largely directed by concurrent alterations in key hormones and growth factors. Estrogen hormone is responsible for ductal elongation and bifurcation of MG [4]. While, progesterone hormone is responsible for lateral branching and alveologenesis of MG [5]. Further alveologenesis and differentiation of the luminal mammary epithelial cells into milk producing cells during late pregnancy require prolactin hormone [3]. EGF, IGF I and TGFα factors are potent mitogenic factors for both normal and transformed (neoplastic) mammary epithelium either *in vivo* [6] or *in vitro* [7].

Citation: Zienab A. Gouda, Samah M. Ahmed and Nabila M. Elghonaimy, Characterization of adult male albino rat mammary gland: a histological and serological study, DOI : http://dx.doi.org/10.7243/2055-091X-2-5.

Histologically, in virgin female animal, MG tissue contains epithelium and stroma. The mammary epithelial cells forming lactiferous ducts are bi-layered epithelium, with the inner luminal cells facing a central cavity and surrounded by the outer basal, myoepithelial cells. It also harbors stem and progenitor cells, which are the source of both luminal and myoepithelial cells [8]. The stroma includes fibrous connective tissue, and a wide variety of cell types, including inter- and intralobular fibroblasts, adipocytes, endothelial cells, and innate immune cells [9].

In male of most mammals, a rudimentary mammary structure is encountered; however the male albino rat MG is unique in displaying marked development (physiological *gynecomastia*) and in showing great sexual dimorphism [10]. *Gynecomastia* is a female like enlargement of the male breast resulting from increased parenchyma, stroma or fat. It is a common problem in the male population, particularly in young adults. Enlarged man breast can cause functional problems, psychosocial discomfort and fear of malignancy. So; it is the most common cause for seeking medical advice for a breast condition in men [11]. Despite the fact that there are no great quantitative differences between men and women either in progesterone secretion or serum progesterone levels, a little is known about the physiology, endocrinology, and pharmacology of progesterone and progestins in male gender or men especially in mammary gland development [12].

Being an organ designed to deliver nourishment and passive immunity to mammal's infants, most discussions of the functional and developmental anatomy and histology of the mammary gland focused on the female and not on the male one [13].

The aim of the present study was to detect causes and importance of mammary gland development in adult male albino rat to relate this normal appearance to *gynecomastia* in human. We hypothesized that histological examination of mammary glands in both sexes via whole mount carmine alum technique; H&E and MT stains will clarify structural differences. Moreover, analysis of serum levels of estrogen, progestrone and prolactin hormones and EGF, IGF I and TGFα tissue proteins and immune-staining for ER and PR could explain the causes of male mammary gland proliferation. We expected that the levels of tested steroid hormones and growth factors of both sexes may be equal or show slight differences.

MATERIALS AND METHODS

In this study, 28 adult albino rats of average weight 200-220 gm were used. The animals were obtained from the animal house, Faculty of Medicine, Zagazig University, Zagazig, Egypt. The animals were kept under strict care and cleaning measures. They were housed in hygienic cages according to the guidelines for animal research issued by the National Institute of Health and approved by Animal Ethics Committee, Zagazig University.

Chemicals

For whole mount carmine alum staining

Carmine (Aldrich Chemical Co Ltd, Gillingham Dorset England) and aluminum potassium sulfate (BDH Chemicals, Ltd, Poole, England) were purchased from Algomhuria co (Mohafza st, Zagazig, Egypt).

For hematoxylin and eosin staining

Harris hematoxylin (Park Scientific Limited, Northampton, UK) and Eosin (Sigma-Aldrich chemie, Steinheim, Germany) were purchased from Algomhuria Co (Mohafza st, Zagazig, Egypt).

For immunohistochemical staining

Anti-progesterone and estrogen antibodies, (Novacastra Laboratories Ltd, UK) were purchased from Sigma office (Egyptian International Center for Import, Cairo, Egypt). Mayer's hematoxylin (Sigma-Aldrich chemie, Steinheim, Germany)were purchased from Algomhuria co (Mohafza st, Zagazig, Egypt).

Experimental procedure

The rats were separated into two groups: *Female group*: 14 rats. *Male group*: 14 rats. The female group was sacrificed at estrus stage under anesthesia by intraperitoneal injection of pentobarbitone sodium 60 mg/kg [14]. To determine the estrus stage in female rats, they were co-cycled for preparation of vaginal smears. The vaginal smears were taken via vaginal lavage with distilled water and were transferred to glass slides and allowed to dry at room temperature. Once dry, they were immediately stained with crystal violet stain. Microscopically, three types of cells could be recognized: epithelial cells, cornified cells and leukocytes. Prominence of cornified cells indicated the estrus stage [15].

Serological analysis of serum ERB, PRA and PRL hormones

Venous blood samples were withdrawn from the retro-orbital sinus by capillary tube and collected in clean glass centrifuge tubes. Blood samples were allowed to clot at room temperature for 30 minutes and then, the sera were stored at −20°C [16].

Histochemical analysis of EGF, IGF I and TGF tissue protein

Small biopsies of the right mammary glands were weighed, homogenized in 20 volumes (wt/vol) of PBS at 37°C and centrifuged at 15,000 X gm for 20 min at 4°C; then, the supernatants were stored at −20°C [16]. Both serological and histochemical analyses were done in (Biochemistry Department, Faculty of Medicine, Cairo University, Egypt).

Whole mount carmine alum staining technique

The left dissected mammary glands were immediately spread on large glass slides, fixed in Carnoy's fixative (25% glacial acetic acid, 75% absolute ethanol), at room temperature in fume hood for 2 days then, washed in 70% ethyl alcohol for 1 hour, rinsed in distilled water (DW) for 30 min, stained in carmine alum stain for 2 days, dehydrated in ascending grades of alcohol and cleared in xylene at least for 2 days. To prepare carmine alum stain; 1 gm carmine and 2.5 gm aluminum potassium sulfate in 450 ml distilled water was boiled for 20 min. Final volume was adjusted to 500 ml with DW [17].

Histological study

In both sexes, the remaining parts of right fourth, fifth and sixth inguinal mammary glands were fixed overnight in 10% neutral buffered formalin and processed into paraffin blocks. They were cut into 5μm sections and stained with H&E, MT [18] and immunohistochemical procedure [19].

Immunohistochemistry technique

To examine the distribution of Progesterone and Estrogen receptors, streptavidin-biotin immunoperoxidase system was used. In brief, deparaffinized sections 3 μm thick were rehydrated in a descending graded alcohol series and washed twice with distilled water for 5 min each time. Antigen retrieval was conducted for all sections using heat–induced epitope retrieval, through immersion of tissue sections in citrate buffer, pH 6.0, autoclaved at 105°C, for 20 min. Endogenous peroxidase was blocked by incubating sections in 3% H_2O_2 in absolute methanol for 30 min at 4°C, followed by flushing with water. After blocking solution treatment (biotinylated rabbit anti-mouse secondary antibody),the sections were incubated overnight at 4°C with the primary antibody for ER and PR (monoclonal antibodies of estrogen and progesterone) diluted in 0.01 M phosphate buffered saline (PBS). The sections for negative controls were incubated in 0.01 M PBS without primary antibody. Finally, the mammary glands were visualized with 3,3'- diaminobenzidine tetrahydrochloride H_2O_2 solution for 3 min. Sections were washed in distilled water, and finally counterstained slightly with Mayer's hematoxylin [19].

Morphometric analysis

The image analyzer computer system Leica Qwin 500 (Leica Imaging system, Ltd, Cambridge, England) was used to measure the terminal ductules thickness using whole mount carmine alum stained slides (Pathology Department, Faculty of Dentistry, Cairo University, Cairo, Egypt).

Statistical analysis

Serum levels of steroid hormones, tissue levels of growth factors and terminal ductules thickness were statistically analyzed. The obtained data were expressed as mean values

±standard deviation and analyzed using unpaired student's T-test. Difference was considered to be significant at $P<0.05$ between groups.

RESULTS

Serological results

The male group revealed a high statistically significant decrease of PRL hormone ($P<0.001$) and a statistically significant decrease of ERB hormone levels ($P<0.05$) in comparison to female group. Progesterone hormone serum level showed no statistically significant ($P>0.05$) difference between both groups (Table 1) and (Histogram 1). Statistically significant decreases regarding tissue EGF, IGF I and TGFα in male group were detected (Table 2) and (Histogram 2).

Table 1: Statistical analysis of serum levels of ERB, PRA and PRL hormones

Hormones	Female		Male		T test	P Value
	Mean±SD	Range	Mean±SD	Range		
Estradiol 17β (pg/ml)	40.2±10	19.2-55.8	8.9±2.3	4.6-11.1	9.9.65	0.013*
Progesterone (ng/ml)	32.4±16	14.8-64.4	29.7±9	11.4-39.8	8.18	0.554
Prolactin (pg/ml)	84.9±10	64.9-104.9	25.8±7	11.4-39.8	234.42	<0.001**

This table shows a highly significant difference of Prolactin level as $P<0.001$, and a significant difference of Estradiol 17β level as $P<0.05$. A non significant difference of Progesterone level between both groups is detected as $P>0.05$.

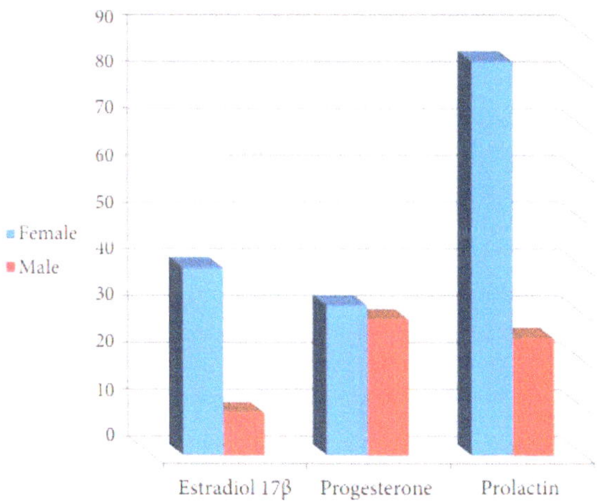

Histogram 1: Mean values of serum Estradiol 17β, Progesterone and Prolactin hormones in both groups.

Table 2: Statistical analysis of tissue EGF, IGF I and TGFα in both groups

Factors	Female		Male		T test	P Value
	Mean±SD	Range	Mean±SD	Range		
EGF	0.48±0.1	0.28-0.68	0.24±0.01	0.22-0.26	7.55	0.023*
IGF I	0.63±0.1	0.23-1.03	0.53±0.1	0.33-0.73	5.0	0.036*
TGFα	0.25±0.04	0.21-0.33	0.12±0.01	0.1-0.14	9.97	0.01*

This table shows significant differences regarding tissue EGF, IGF I and TGFα as P<0.05.

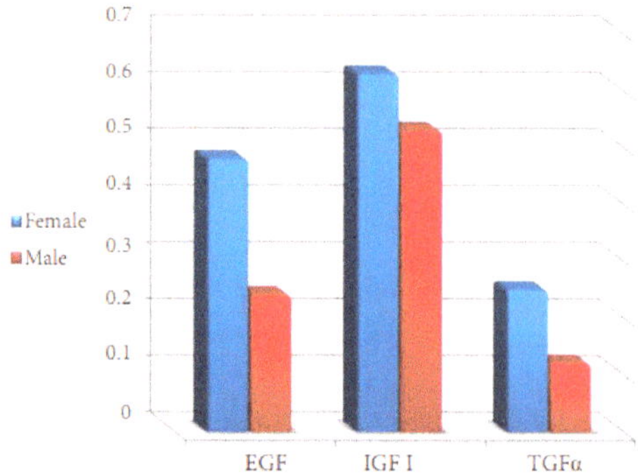

Histogram 2: Mean values of EGF, IGF I and TGFα in both groups.

Whole-mount results

The whole-mount carmine alum stained slides showed that the ductal tree of the female MG reached the edge of the fat pad (Figure 1a). The ductal tree of male MG nearly filled half of the fat pad (Figure 1b). In the female mammary gland, extensively branched lactiferous duct in an apparent mass of fat pad was detected. The primary ducts were slightly thick and relatively short. The secondary ducts were thinner and longer than the primary ducts. The tertiary ducts were numerous, long, very thin and nearly formed the ductal tree (Figure 2a). A thin long tertiary duct bifurcated at its end into subtending duct that further bifurcates into long thin terminal ducts interlacing with large amount of fat pad (Figure 2b). In the male mammary gland, less extensively branched ductal tree in a little mass of fat pad was nearly reached the edge. The primary, secondary and tertiary ducts were indistinct from each other and nearly had the same thickness and length while the terminal ducts were well defined (Figure 2c). Arborization of apparently thick subtending ducts into irregular outlined short ducts showed small lobules at their ends and their walls had irregular shaped tiny lateral lobulation (Figure 2d). Smooth outlined terminal ducts, terminal end buds and lateral buds had thin stalks and bifurcated smooth bulbous structure at its ends were seen in female rat mammary gland (Figure 3). Large irregularly outlined lobules at the end of terminal ductules were characteristic to male mammary gland (Figure 4).

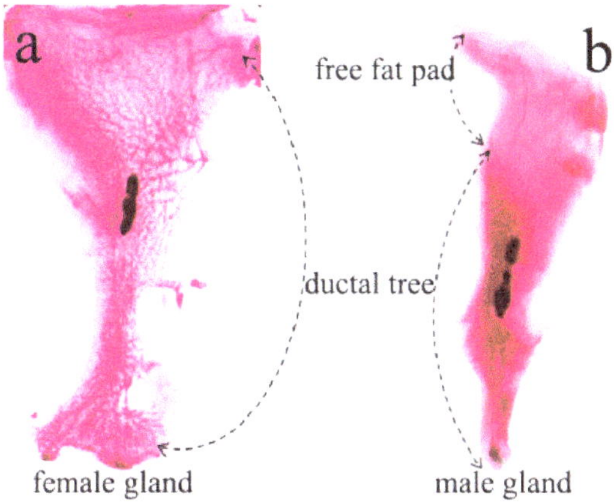

Figure 1: The ductal tree of female (a) and male (b) mammary glands according to whole-mount carmine alum stain. (a): The ductal tree nearly reaches the edge of the fat pad. [Carmine Alum stain]. (b): The ductal tree nearly fills half of the fat pad. [Carmine Alum stain].

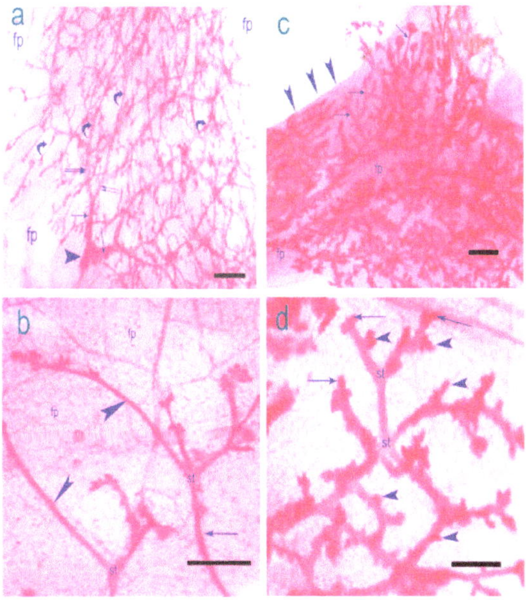

Figure 2: The female (a,b) and male (c,d) mammary glands according to whole mount Carmine alum stain. (a): Showing extensively branching lactiferous duct (arrow head) in an apparent mass of fat pad (fp). The primary ducts (arrows) are slightly thick and relatively short. The secondary ducts (double arrows) are thin and long. The tertiary ducts (curved arrows) are numerous, long, very thin and nearly formed the ductal tree. [Carmine Alum stain, X10. Bar, 1.2mm]. (b): Showing a thin long tertiary duct (arrow) bifurcating into subtending ducts (st) which bifurcates into long thin terminal ducts (arrow heads) interlacing with fat pad (fp). [Carmine Alum stain, X40. Bar, 2.4mm]. (c): Showing less branched ductal tree in a little mass of fat pad (fp) nearly reached

the edge(arrow heads). The primary, secondary and tertiary ducts are indistinct and nearly of the same thickness and length while the terminal ducts are well defined (arrows). [Carmine Alum stain, X10. Bar, 1.2mm]. (d): Showing thick subtending ducts (st) arborized into irregular outlined short ducts that end as small lobules (arrows). Their walls have irregular tiny lateral lobulation (arrow heads). [Carmine Alum stain, X40. Bar, 1.8mm].

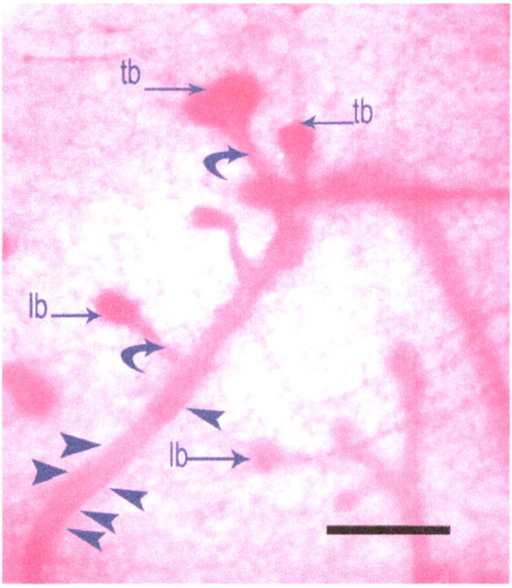

Figure 3: The mammary gland of female rat according to whole-mount carmine alum stain: Showing smooth outlined terminal ducts (arrow heads). The terminal bulbous end buds (tb) and lateral buds (lb) have thin stalks (curved arrows). [Carmine Alum stain, X80. Bar, 4.8mm].

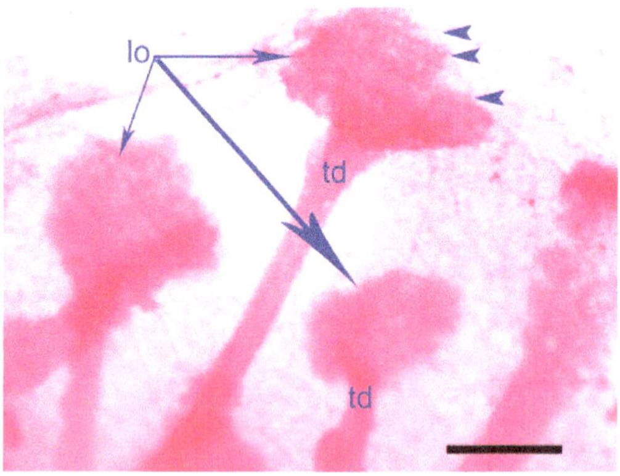

Figure 4: The mammary gland of male rat according to whole-mount carmine alum stain: Showing large irregularly outlined (arrow heads) lobules (lo) at the end of terminal ductules (td). [Carmine Alum stain, X80. Bar, 4.8mm].

Histological results

H&E

Examination H&E stained sections of female gland showed thick capsule and vascular adipose connective tissue stroma containing ducts (Figure 5a). Scattered tubular duct system was surrounded by thick dense eosinophilic fibrous stroma which was full of fibroblasts (Figure 5b). The male gland showed less developed stroma, thin capsule and thin periductal fibrous stroma. Many alveoli and inguinal lymph node were also seen (Figure 5c). Lobulo-alveolar structures were predominant in male gland (Figure 5d).

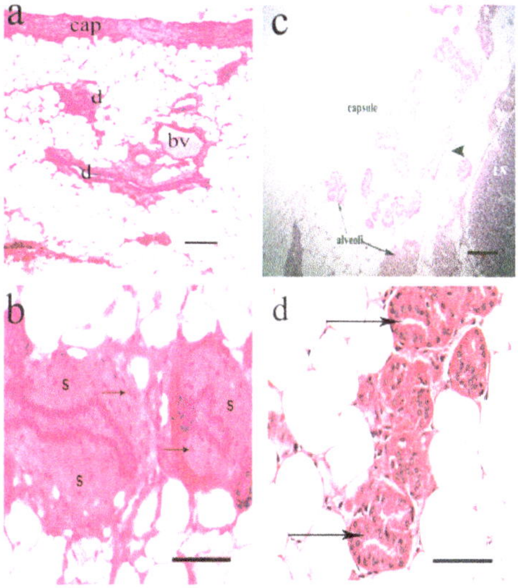

Figure 5: The structure of female (a,b) and male (c,d) mammary gland sections according to H&E stain. (a): Showing thick capsule (cap), vascular stroma (bv) and ducts (d). [H&E, X100. Bar, 100μm]. (b):Showing scattered duct system surrounded by dense eosinophilic stroma (s) which is full of fibroblasts (arrows) [H&E, X400. Bar, 100μm]. (c): Showing thin capsule, thin periductal fibrous stroma (arrow head), many alveoli and inguinal lymph node (LN). [H&E, X100. Bar,100μm]. (d): Showing lobulo-alveolar structure (arrows) predominant in male gland. [H&E, X400. Bar, 100μm].

The female mammary gland ducts were lined by stratified epithelium. The luminal cells were cuboidal and had large central rounded nuclei. The basal cells were flat with flat nuclei. Flat nuclei of fibroblasts were also seen in the fibrous stroma (Figure 6a). The male mammary gland large ducts were lined by multiple layers of large vacuolated luminal epithelial cells. Their nuclei were large and rounded. Luminal and ductal apoptotic cells and acidophilic secretion filling the lumen were detected. Thin layer of fibrous stroma around the ducts was seen. Thin outlined white unilocular adipocytes with large cytoplasmic fat droplets and peripheral nuclei surrounded the fibrous stroma (Figure 6b). Thick ductal fibrous stroma surrounded the small ducts and numerous small blood vessels were observed (Figure 6c). Very thin stroma and a few numbers of fibroblasts around the small ducts which were lined by two layers of vacuolated cells with rounded nuclei were seen. Deeply acidophilic secretion filling the lumen was also seen (Figure 6d).

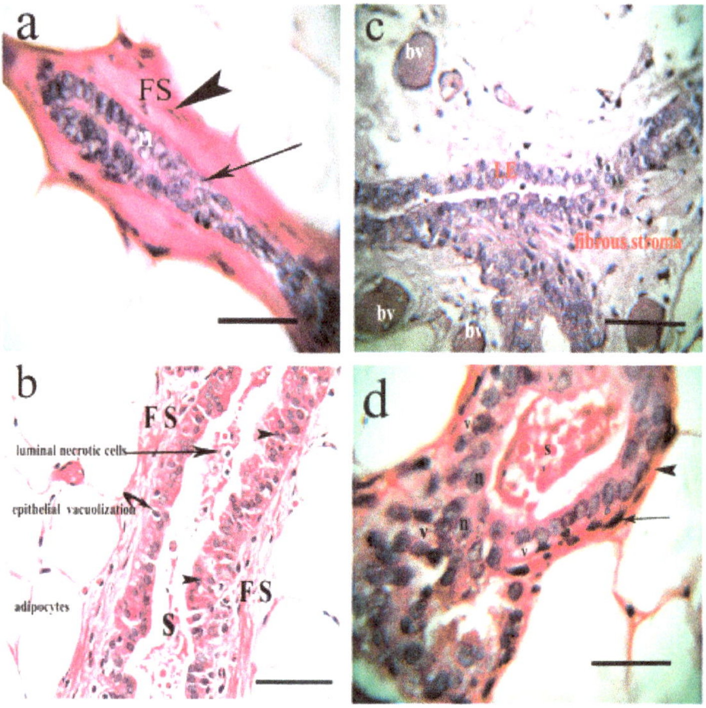

Figure 6: The structure of ducts of female (a) and male (b-d) mammary gland sections according to H&E stain. (a): Showing the duct is lined by stratified epithelium. The luminal cells are cuboidal with large central rounded nuclei (n). The basal cells are flat with flat nuclei (arrow). Flat nuclei of fibroblasts (arrow head) are seen in the fibrous stroma (FS). [H&E, X400. Bar, 100μm]. (b): Showing the large duct is lined by multiple layers of vacuolated large luminal epithelial cells (closed arrow) with large rounded nuclei (arrow heads). Luminal and ductal necrotic cells (arrows) and acidophilic secretion (S) are seen in the lumen. The fibrous stroma (FS) around the duct is thin. Large unilocular adipocytes surrounded the fibrous stroma are noted. [H&E, X400. Bar, 100μm]. (c): Showing the small duct (LE) is surrounded by thick fibrous vascularized stroma (bv). [H&E, X400. Bar, 100μm]. (d): Showing the subtending duct is lined by vacuolated cells (v) with rounded nuclei (n). Very thin stroma (arrow head), a few number of fibroblasts (arrow) and deeply acidophilic secretion (s) is seen. [H&E, X400. Bar, 100μm].

Masson's trichrome

The female mammary gland showed thick layer collagen fibers around the blood vessels and ducts (Figure 7a). In male group, the alveoli were devoid of connective tissue. The collagen fibers around the ducts were thin while, around blood vessels were thick (Figures 7b and 7c).

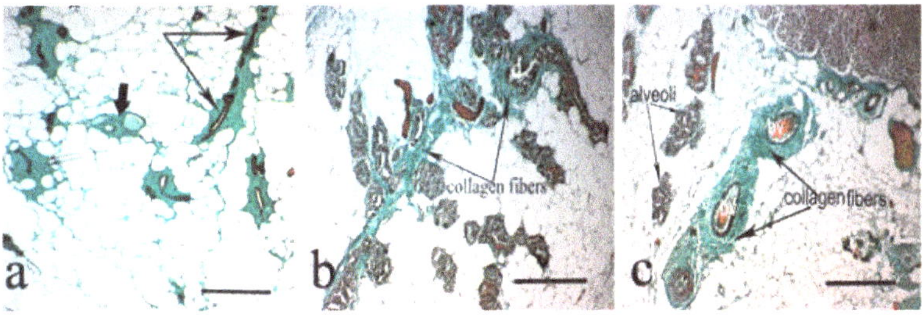

Figure 7: The female (a) and male (b,c) mammary gland sections according to MT stain. (a): Showing the fibrous stroma around the ducts (arrows) and the blood vessels (thick arrow) is thick collagenous. [Masson's trichrome, X100. Bar, 200μm]. (b): Showing a thin layer of collagen fibers around the ducts. [Masson's trichrome, X100. Bar, 200μm]. (c): Showing a thick layer of collagen fibers around blood vessels while, alveoli are devoid of connective tissue [Masson's trichrome, X100. Bar, 200μm].

Immunohistochemical results

The female mammary gland showed positive reaction for progesterone in some ductal cells (Figure 8a) and a dense positive reaction for estrogen in most of ductal cells (Figure 8b). In male group, patchy distributed pattern was seen for progesterone positive reaction in some ductal epithelial cells, in luminal secretion and in fibroblastic stromal cells. A negative reaction for estrogen in the ductal epithelium and a weak positive reaction in periductal stroma were observed (Figures 8c and 8d).

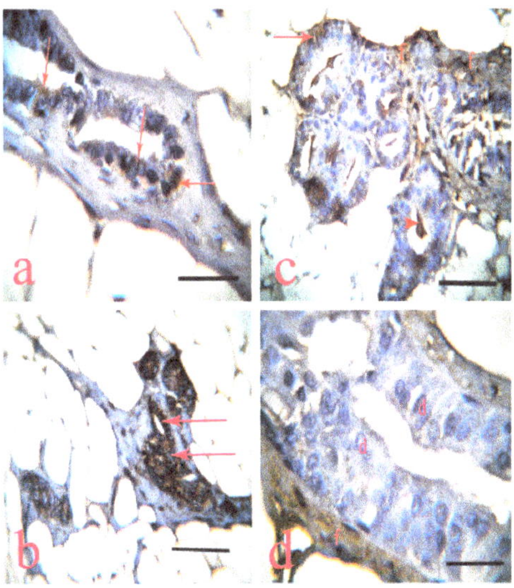

Figure 8: Immunodetection of progesterone and estrogen β receptors of female (a,b) and male (c,d) mammary gland sections. (a): A positive reaction for progesterone receptor in some ductal cells (arrows) is seen. [Progesterone receptor immunostaining, X400.

Bar, 100μm]. (b): A tense positive reaction for Estrogen β receptor in most of ductal cells (arrows) is seen. [Estrogen β receptor immunostaining, X400. Bar, 100μm]. (c): A patchy distributed pattern for progesterone receptor positive reaction in some ductal epithelial cells (arrow), in luminal secretion (arrow head) and in fibroblastic stromal cells (f) is noticed. [Progesterone receptor immunostaining, X400. Bar, 100μm]. (d): A negative reaction for estrogen β receptor immunostaining in the ductal epithelium (d) a weak positive in reaction in periductal stroma (f) is detected. [Estrogen β receptor immunostaining, X1000. Bar, 20μm].

DISCUSSION

In most mammals, the male mammary gland is regarded as a rudimentary organ without ascribed functions; as a result, research on the development and endocrine responses of male mammary glands has been limited [20]. In female, the MG is an important tool for examining some developmental, endocrinal and tumor biological aspects [21]. So, most discussions of the functional and developmental anatomy and histology of the mammary gland were focused on the female and not on the male [10].

Determination of estrous cycle stages is emerging as an important consideration when working on female animals in several research areas. In the present work, the time of sacrifice was at the estrus stage in the female group [15]. Unlike all other stages, during estrus stage, the rat serum prolactin was found to be the highest as determined by enzyme immunoassay. Additionally, it represents the most differentiated mammary gland state [21].

Necessity of Prolactin [22] and Progesterone [23] for lobuloalveolar development of female MG was reported. So, blood samples from both groups were collected to determine concentrations of hormones known to be involved in mammary gland growth and differentiation. Despite of a highly statistically significant decrease in Prolactin hormone and a non significant decrease in Progesterone serum levels in male rats, their mammary glands exhibited lobulo-alveolar secretory parenchyma. Knight and Peaker [24] referred this unique sex-specific morphology of rat male MG to tissue sensitivity that increases the susceptibility and responsiveness of mammary gland to various endogenous hormonal stimuli. Their explanation was confirmed by our data obtained from immunostained sections in male glands (intense positive immunoexpression to progesterone receptors in all parenchyma).

In the current study, EGF, IGF I and TGFα tissue protein, were measured as these factors were documented as potent mitogenic factors for both normal and neoplastic mammary epithelium either *in vivo* [7] or *in vitro* [8]. Interestingly, a significant increase in these factors was detected in female group in comparison to male group.

It is well known that both estrogen [25] and epidermal growth factor [26] are responsible for extensive branching and ductal elongation of the mammary glands. In addition, progesterone is responsible for lobulo-alveolar development [27]. In the current work, immuno-staining of PRA and ER β receptors were carried out aiming to reveal the exact causes of male mammary growth in rats. A striking observation was the strong positive expression of PR in male mammary luminal epithelial cells, luminal secretion and peri-alveolar stroma. Similar patterns of expression were observed for PRA in human female mammary gland [28]. The presence of PRA all over the mammary cells may provide a clue for lobuloalveolar predominance in male glands. In the male group of present work, the negative immunoexpression to ER in the luminal epithelium and the weak positive reaction to ER in periductal stroma can be correlated with the stunted ductal growth of the male mammary ductal tree [25].

Whole-mount technique is considered the most reliable technique used to visualize epithelial ductal and alveolar structures against a translucent fatty background as it readily reveals the extent of ductal elongation, branching, and alveolar development and allows strict quantitative measurements [17]. Based upon analysis of whole-mount slides, the male MG ducts were short, with irregular outline and nearly of the same thickness and length. The terminal ductules were well defined. These data were in accordance with Shyamala [23]. He recorded thick short ducts with extensive lateral branching and large numbers of terminal buds in transgenic mice with an excess PRA expression. Also, in knocked out estrogen receptor α animals, hypoplastic development of the epithelial tree was demonstrated [25]. The limited branching and length of male mammary ducts were related to decreased periductal collagenous connective tissue stroma [29]. Furthermore, estrogen drives extensive growth and branching of female mammary gland [25].

The development of the mammary ductal tree depends on stromal–epithelial interactions, and these interactions are important in embryonic and postnatal evolvement. The stromal compartment is composed of mesenchymal cells (fibroblasts and leukocytes) and extra-cellular matrix as laminin, fibronectin, collagen and proteoglycans [30]. In male albino rats, less developed stroma in the form of thin capsule and thin periductal stroma around the large ducts were in accordance with [1]. They suggested that extra-cellular matrix is involved in the interactions between the mammary cells and their environment.

The ducts of male mammary gland showed two different lining epithelium in relation to their size: the large ducts were lined by multiple layers of vacuolated luminal epithelial cells with large and rounded nuclei. The smaller ducts were lined by doubled layers of low epithelial cells. These features in male mammary gland structure were documented [31]. These features referred probably to a higher sensitivity of male rat mammary tissue to steroid hormones than other male mammals e.g., mice [32]. A completely different picture of male mammary glands in other male rodents was recorded. Their mammary glands were described as a rudimentary mammary glandular tissue [3].

The cells lined large male mammary ducts were characterized by abundant foamy eosinophilic cytoplasm containing distinct variable sized vacuoles. Their lumina were mostly contained evidence of secretory activity with apoptotic bodies and fragmented epithelial cells. These histological changes were identified in rats' female mammary gland after Dehydroepiandrosterone (DHEA) treatment [33]. They showed that, the potent stimulatory effects of androgens on lobuloalveolar as well as ductal development in the female rat mammary gland are due to intracrine conversion of DHEA into active sex steroids with predominant or even possibly exclusive androgenic activity in the mammary gland. They added that local formation of androgen and estrogen through intracrine activity in rats plays a major role in these histological features.

Masson's trichrome staining revealed that the male periductal stroma was much reduced relative to that in female, especially around small ducts and alveoli. The previous hypotheses proposed that the mammary gland development and branching is partially dependent on the amount of extracellular matrix [34,35].

Gynecomastia is a proliferation of the glandular component of the male breast. In most cases, it is a pathological condition in response to increased level of estrogen or decreased level of testosterone [36], drugs e.g., ethionamide [37], spironolactone, cimetidine and ketoconazole [38] or increased endogenous Prolactin [39]. In the current work, evaluated steriodal hormones were within normal levels in both groups.

CONCLUSION

The results of the present study concluded that proliferation of male albino rat MG occurred despite of normal levels of its serum steroid hormones and without drug supplementation or any endocrinal disturbance. This condition can provide fundamental information about a physiological type of *gynecomastia* that does not need hormonal correction and may need only cosmetic surgical intervention. We recommended immuno-staining of breast biopsy in diagnosed cases of *gynecomastia* in men. In addition, further serological and histological investigations of male rat mammary tissue are needed to strengthen our data.

AUTHORS' CONTRIBUTIONS

Authors' contributions	**ZAG**	**SMA**	**NME**
Research concept and design	√	--	--
Collection and/or assembly of data	√	--	--
Data analysis and interpretation	√	√	√
Writing the article	√	√	√
Design of figures	√	--	√
Critical revision of the article	√	√	√
Final approval of article	√	√	√
Statistical analysis	--	√	--

ACKNOWLEDGEMENT

We would like to thank Prof. Dr. Fadia Khalid Abdo for her English language editing and reviewing of the manuscript, Prof.Dr.Dalia Elrobi for morphometrical aid and Dr.Eman Elshahate for statistical aid.

REFERENCES

1. Lucas JN, Rudmann DG, Credille KM, Irizarry AR, Peter A and Snyder PW. The rat mammary gland: morphologic changes as an indicator of systemic hormonal perturbations induced by xenobiotics.*Toxicol Pathol.* 2007; 35:199-207.
2. Brisken C and O'Malley B. Hormone action in the mammary gland. *Cold Spring Harb Perspect Biol.* 2010;2:a003178.
3. Richert MM, Schwertfeger KL, Ryder JW and Anderson SM. An atlas of mouse mammary gland development. *J Mammary Gland Biol Neoplasia.* 2000; 5:227-41.
4. Forster C, Makela S, Warri A, Kietz S, Becker D, Hultenby K, Warner M and Gustafsson JA. Involvement of estrogen receptor beta in terminal differentiation of mammary gland epithelium. *Proc Natl Acad Sci U S A.* 2002; 99:15578-83.
5. Beleut M, Rajaram RD, Caikovski M, Ayyanan A, Germano D, Choi Y, Schneider P and Brisken C. Two distinct mechanisms underlie progesterone-induced proliferation in the mammary gland. *Proc Natl Acad Sci U S A.* 2010; 107:2989-94.
6. Vonderhaar BK. Local effects of EGF, alpha-TGF, and EGF-like growth factors on lobuloalveolar development of the mouse mammary gland in vivo. *J Cell Physiol.* 1987; 132:581-4.
7. Valverius EM, Bates SE, Stampfer MR, Clark R, McCormick F, Salomon DS, Lippman ME and Dickson RB.Transforming growth factor alpha production and epidermal growth factor receptor expression in normal and oncogene transformed human mammary epithelial cells. *Mol Endocrinol.* 1989; 3:203-14.
8. Visvader JE. Keeping abreast of the mammary epithelial hierarchy and breast tumorigenesis. *Genes Dev.* 2009; 23:2563-77.
9. Sternlicht MD. Key stages in mammary gland development: the cues that regulate ductal branching morphogenesis. *Breast Cancer Res.* 2006; 8:201.
10. Vandenberg LN, Schaeberle CM, Rubin BS, Sonnenschein C and Soto AM. The male mammary gland: a target for the xenoestrogen bisphenol A. *Reprod Toxicol.* 2013; 37:15-23. Abstract Full Text
11. Arvind A, Khan MA, Srinivasan K and Roberts J. Gynaecomastia correction: A review of our experience.*Indian J Plast Surg.* 2014; 47:56-60.
12. Oettel M and Mukhopadhyay AK. Progesterone: the forgotten hormone in men? *Aging Male.* 2004;7:236-57.
13. Masso-Welch PA, Darcy KM, Stangle-Castor NC and Ip MM. A developmental atlas of rat mammary gland histology. *J Mammary Gland Biol Neoplasia.* 2000; 5:165-85.
14. Ozmen J, Bobryshev YV, Lord RS and Ashwell KW. Identification of dendritic cells in aortic atherosclerotic lesions in rats with diet-induced hypercholesterolaemia. *Histol Histopathol.* 2002;17:223-37. Pdf
15. McLean AC, Valenzuela N, Fai S and Bennett SA. Performing vaginal lavage,

crystal violet staining, and vaginal cytological evaluation for mouse estrous cycle staging identification. *J Vis Exp.* 2012; e4389.

16. Ingman WV, Wyckoff J, Gouon-Evans V, Condeelis J and Pollard JW. Macrophages promote collagen fibrillogenesis around terminal end buds of the developing mammary gland. *Dev Dyn.* 2006;235:3222-9.
17. de Assis S, Warri A, Cruz MI and Hilakivi-Clarke L. Changes in mammary gland morphology and breast cancer risk in rats. *J Vis Exp.* 2010.
18. Bancroft JD and Layton C. The Hematoxylin and eosin. In: Suvarna SK, Layton C and Bancroft JD editors.Theory and Practice of histological techniques. 7th ed., ChurchillLivingstone of El Sevier. Philadelphia. Ch 10 and 11. 2013; 172–214.
19. Jackson P and Blythe D. Immunohistochemical techniques. In: Suvarna SK, Layton C and Bancroft JD editors.Theory & Practice of histological techniques. 7th ed., Churchill Livingstone of El Sevier. Philadelphia. Ch. 18. 2013; 381–434.
20. Wang XJ, Bartolucci-Page E, Fenton SE and You L. Altered mammary gland development in male rats exposed to genistein and methoxychlor. *Toxicol Sci.* 2006; 91:93-103.
21. Fata JE, Leco KJ, Voura EB, Yu HY, Waterhouse P, Murphy G, Moorehead RA and Khokha R. Accelerated apoptosis in the Timp-3-deficient mammary gland. *J Clin Invest.* 2001; 108:831-41.
22. Das R and Vonderhaar BK. Prolactin as a mitogen in mammary cells. *J Mammary Gland Biol Neoplasia.* 1997; 2:29-39.
23. Shyamala G. Progesterone signaling and mammary gland morphogenesis. *J Mammary Gland Biol Neoplasia.* 1999; 4:89-104.
24. Knight CH and Peaker M. Development of the mammary gland. *J Reprod Fertil.* 1982; 65:521-36. Article
25. Feng Y, Manka D, Wagner KU and Khan SA. Estrogen receptor-alpha expression in the mammary epithelium is required for ductal and alveolar morphogenesis in mice. *Proc Natl Acad Sci U S A.* 2007;104:14718-23.
26. Walczak M, Pawlus B, Kędzia A and Walkowiak J. Active synthesis of epidermal growth factor in human mammary glands. *Acta scientiarum polonorum technologia alimentaria.* 2010; 9:237-241.
27. Aupperlee MD and Haslam SZ. Differential hormonal regulation and function of progesterone receptor isoforms in normal adult mouse mammary gland. *Endocrinology.* 2007; 148:2290-300.
28. Li S, Han B, Liu G, Ouellet J, Labrie F and Pelletier G. Immunocytochemical localization of sex steroid hormone receptors in normal human mammary gland. *J Histochem Cytochem.* 2010; 58:509-15. Article
29. Kass L, Erler JT, Dembo M and Weaver VM. Mammary epithelial cell: influence of extracellular matrix composition and organization during development and tumorigenesis. *Int J Biochem Cell Biol.* 2007;39:1987-94.
30. Couldrey C, Moitra J, Vinson C, Anver M, Nagashima K and Green

J. Adipose tissue: a vital in vivo role in mammary gland development but not differentiation. *Dev Dyn.* 2002; 223:459-68.

31. Cardy RH. Sexual dimorphism of the normal rat mammary gland. *Vet Pathol.* 1991; 28:139-45. Article
32. Neumann F. Early indicators for carcinogenesis in sex-hormone-sensitive organs. *Mutat Res.* 1991;248:341-56.
33. Sourla A, Martel C, Labrie C and Labrie F. Almost exclusive androgenic action of dehydroepiandrosterone in the rat mammary gland. *Endocrinology.* 1998; 139:753-64.
34. Wiseman BS and Werb Z. Stromal effects on mammary gland development and breast cancer. *Science.*2002; 296:1046-9.
35. Muschler J and Streuli CH. Cell-matrix interactions in mammary gland development and breast cancer.*Cold Spring Harb Perspect Biol.* 2010; 2:a003202.
36. Nordt CA and DiVasta AD. Gynecomastia in adolescents. *Curr Opin Pediatr.* 2008; 20:375-82. Article
37. Dixit R, George J, Sharma AK, Chhabra N, Jangir SK and Mishra V. Ethionamide-induced gynecomastia.*J Pharmacol Pharmacother.* 2012; 3:196-9.
38. Deepinder F and Braunstein GD. Drug-induced gynecomastia: an evidence-based review. *Expert Opin Drug Saf.* 2012; 11:779-95.
39. Carlson HE. Approach to the patient with gynecomastia. *J Clin Endocrinol Metab.* 2011; 96:15-21.

3
CHAPTER

SEVEN COMMON MISTAKES TO AVOID IN ACHIEVING LONG-TERM SUCCESS WITH DERMATOLOGY PATIENTS

Lowell Ackerman

NOT APPRECIATING APPROPRIATE CLINICAL TIMELINES

While most veterinarians focus on the needs of the client and pet at the time of a specific office visit, it is important to realize that for many dermatologic conditions opportunities exist on a time continuum for intervention and client education. In some instances, the first discussions with the owner may take place long before there is even a skin problem to treat. So, for the owner of a breed at risk for atopic dermatitis, discussions should actually start during puppyhood, long before there might be any clinical evidence of allergies (Ackerman 2011). This is the best time to instruct owners to be vigilant looking for early signs of disease, such as licking and chewing at the feet, ear infections, or rashes in the axillary and inguinal areas. Perhaps more importantly, this provides an opportunity to discuss that if atopic dermatitis is eventually diagnosed in the pet that this is a lifelong condition without a cure, but early detection provides the most options for successful long-term management. This might also prompt a discussion of the likely costs associated with long-term management, so the owners might consider their options for risk management strategies, including pet insurance.

Appreciating appropriate timelines also helps in treatment selection. When a two-year-old atopic patient presents with pruritus, the first tendency might be to treat with glucocorticoids (corticosteroids) to achieve short-term relief. However, when you reflect on how that same patient might look at 8 or 10 years of age with such treatment, there is often a different perspective on what the long-term liabilities are for such short-term gains, and alternative more targeted treatments might be selected, given the need for sensible long-term solutions.

Citation: Lowell Ackerman, Seven common mistakes to avoid in achieving long-term success with dermatology patients, DOI: 10.1002/vms3.1.

It is also important to schedule effectively. No one can solve a complicated dermatology case in a single visit, regardless of the appointment's duration, or the clinician's expertise. You can address the client's primary concerns, but be clear with the client that the pet's problems will likely not be solved with that single visit. The key to successful dermatology management is scheduling frequent re-evaluation appointments. The success of this strategy is predicated on sharing the action plan with pet owners, so they can understand and appreciate what is expected to be accomplished, and according to what timeline.

For a young dog with localized juvenile demodectic mange, the owner should expect regular re-evaluations over a several-month period. They also need to realize that the underlying problem could be some form of immune dysfunction, which might be transitory or long-lasting. Regardless, the condition is characterized by the overpopulation of mites normally resident in the skin (these are not external invaders), which in turn typically causes bacterial infections in the hair follicles, and the sequel to that is inflammatory changes and hair loss. The initial goal might be to control the associated bacterial folliculitis, provide supportive care in terms of frequent shampooing with a follicular-flushing agent, ensure there is no evidence of other internal or external parasites, assess immune function, and put the pet on an improved plane of nutrition. Actually killing the mites might not even be necessary as a first treatment attempt. If the owner realizes that a cure without miticidal therapy is possible because many young animals 'self-cure' with appropriate supportive therapy, they are more likely to understand why you are approaching the problem in stages, rather than just reaching for the strongest mite-killing therapy on the shelf. Miticidal therapy can always be used if this otherwise healthy young animal fails to self-cure in a reasonable amount of time. The pathway to resolution might include supportive care, decreasing mite numbers, resolution of the secondary bacterial folliculitis and, finally hair regrowth. It is also important for owners to realize that clinical cure often precedes microscopic cure, so it is important to continue to monitor with recheck examinations and skin scrapings before stopping therapy prematurely; otherwise, recurrence is more likely. When owners understand the plan, they can also appreciate the timeline to achieve it.

There are many dynamics at work in the development and resolution of skin problems and they can either work for or against the clinician depending on how they are relayed to pet owners.

The skin is not a sterile surface and is home to a large population of resident organisms. There are also lots of occasions for the skin to be colonized by the opportunistic overgrowth of organisms typically present in small numbers, the most common of which are bacteria (such as*Staphylococcus pseudintermedius*) and yeasts (such as *Malassezia pachydermatis*). As it is neither possible nor desirable to try to sterilize the skin, the goal needs to be to address the underlying reason for the microbial overgrowth (allergies, hypothyroidism, immune dysfunction, skin folds, etc.), manage it effectively (possibly long term) and use sensible systemic and topical therapies to help curb the microbial populations. The population dynamics also dictates reasonable treatment intervals. If staphylococcal populations can double in number within minutes to hours on the skin surface, can an every-other-week bathing schedule ever have much of an impact? Probably not. If owners want to help control surface bacterial numbers with topical therapies, they need to realize that more frequent treatments are likely needed, at least initially.

Similarly, when it comes to epidermal turnover rates in keratinization disorders (e.g. seborrhea), we are at the mercy of those skin cell dynamics. Even if you could wave a magic wand and immediately correct the problem, it would still take weeks for the 'normal' skin to grow through the epidermal layers and replace the abnormal skin cells on the skin surface. Without a magic wand it takes many more weeks and even months for progress to be noted. When clients realize this, it helps them be more realistic with their expectations.

NOT APPROPRIATELY FRAMING CLIENT EXPECTATIONS

Many pet skin problems cannot be cured, regardless of the medication selected, so set realistic expectations with clients early in the process. Fortunately, control of the condition and a better quality of life for the pet can be attained with appropriate management. For the pet with atopic dermatitis, you might explain to clients that this is no different than addressing other incurable but manageable medical conditions such as diabetes mellitus or degenerative joint disease (osteoarthritis). We can often achieve excellent long-term control with ongoing treatment and close monitoring, but it is unlikely that we will be able to 'fix' the underlying problem. Usually once owners appreciate that the goal is control rather than cure, their expectations tend to be more reasonable and realistic.

Similarly, it is important to manage expectations around the metrics of treatment success and the timeframe in which such judgment can be anticipated. For example, in a dog with demodicosis and associated hair loss, the pet owner may judge success as hair regrowth, while the clinician will likely be more focused on controlling mite numbers initially. So, how long after treatment initiation should the client expect to see hair regrowth if the treatment is working? If the owners are told to expect the likely onset of hair regrowth eight weeks or so after the mite population has been satisfactorily reduced, they will not be expecting that hair growth shortly after starting treatment; hopefully they will appreciate that mite population control must happen first, before hair regrowth can start. They should also then be attentive at recheck visits and use progress on mite control reported by the clinician as a signpost for the path to eventual resolution (and hair regrowth).

For the dog with sarcoptic mange, it is important to notify the owner that the pruritus is likely to persist for another week or two even after successful treatment has been initiated. This occurs because mite faecal pellets that remain in the epidermal burrows still trigger hypersensitivity reactions, and because dead and decaying mite fragments in the skin tend to be irritating. Aggressive topical therapy and some pruritus-relieving medications will definitely help, but complete resolution requires the elimination of all mite-related remnants from the skin. With absolute adherence to veterinary recommendations regarding treatment of the pet and in-contact animals, the itching should start to substantially abate after two weeks, with complete resolution to be anticipated within 6–8 weeks if the pet is not reinfested from its environment. Setting realistic expectations with clients is critical because ultimate success and client satisfaction will be measured by the owner's perception. Similarly, if you perform a flawless surgery but discharge the animal soiled with faecal matter, the client's perception of the procedure's success may differ significantly from your own. As it is the client who is paying for the service and the one (by definition) who ultimately determines customer satisfaction, the client's interpretation takes precedence. Accordingly, take the time to understand those expectations so you can plan to meet and even exceed them, or be prepared to discuss more realistic expectations with the owner before starting treatment.

NOT VIEWING THE SITUATION IN TERMS OF QUALITY OF LIFE

Veterinarians might sometimes view dermatologic problems as minor medical issues because often the pet's life is not at risk, but pet owners may not share that same perspective. Pet owners may not know what a diseased liver looks like, but they are certainly aware when their pet keeps them awake at night while scratching, has bald patches in its fur, or harbours offensive odours, rashes, parasites, or skin colour changes associated with a variety of skin diseases. There might also be a certain amount of guilt associated with friends and relatives asking why they have not done a better job of treating their pet's skin ailments, even when the pet owner has done everything they have been instructed to do. Veterinarians and hospital staff would do well to consider what pet owners find stressful, in addition to what might be causing the pet discomfort.

Pet owners are often concerned with the responsibility of successfully managing their pet's problems at home. In many instances, it is stressful for clients to have to regularly administer medications, bathe their pets, apply parasite-control products on schedule, and other tasks often assigned by hospital staff. Even something as basic as applying ear drops can be a trying experience if the pet demonstrates discomfort, cries, or retreats from the owner, adversely affecting the human–animal bond. People own pets for the positive connection that develops between them and anything that interferes with that is likely to be stressful for both. Veterinary staff should do everything in their power to set clients up for success at home. This includes honestly assessing the recommendations being made and the likelihood that they can be successfully accomplished at home.

When medically prudent to do so, the use of injectable medications is often preferred because it frees the owner up from having to administer medication to their pet. Rather than asking the pet owner to do something at home that might cause their pet discomfort, such as applying ear drops to a painful inflamed ear, the pet might be admitted into the hospital, sedated and appropriately treated and administered anti-inflammatory therapy or pain management so that the owner is not required to contend with an objectionable experience at home. This might not be possible in all instances, but hospital staff should always strive to make the pet owner's tasks easier at home and to reinforce the human–animal bond at every opportunity by offering such services.

NOT FOLLOWING EVIDENCE-BASED STANDARDS OF CARE

Most pet owners do not want their pets to serve as learning tools, so they appreciate knowing that veterinarians know what they are treating, the chances of success, what problems might be encountered, and the alternatives available should the need arise. Pet owners also appreciate that such knowledge is evidence-based and reflects established expertise, even if not direct experience. They find comfort in consistent messaging from hospital staff, specialists, and even Internet resources.

Having an evidence-based action plan assures owners that their pet is not the first to experience this problem, and that there is collective wisdom and experience in how it is best managed (Ackerman 2014).

Standards of care should be created by hospitals to provide this assurance, and to guarantee the best care to all patients and all pet owners, regardless of the individual experience and expertise of the clinician currently treating that pet. Protocols are often used for standardized approaches to basic preventive and acute care (e.g. parasite control, treatment of sarcoptic mange) while care pathways represent a model for approaching problems that might require long-term or even lifelong care (e.g. atopic dermatitis, demodicosis, pemphigus foliaceus, etc.) (Ackerman *et al.* 2013).

One of the benefits of standards of care is that owners realize that even with a well-conceived plan, outcomes cannot be guaranteed, and contingency plans may be needed. For example, when treating a dog with bacterial pyoderma, you might select an antibiotic empirically based on the likelihood that the organism is *Staphylococcus pseudintermedius* and that there is a predictive rate of susceptibility and resistance to specific antibiotics. If the pet owner realizes that your plan is based on the likelihood that the organism will be sensitive to the antibiotic selected, but cannot be guaranteed, they can likely also appreciate the need to re-evaluate the pet at some point and for a bacterial culture and susceptibility test to be performed if there is no evidence of substantial improvement by that time. In fact, following a plan of action allows the owner to feel more engaged in the decision-making process. They might even participate more fully in the discussion, asking if it might be worthwhile to consider the culture even before starting empirical therapy. This is much more desirable than dispensing treatment, and if it does not seem to be working the owner just decides to get the opinion of another primary-care veterinarian. Sharing your action plan and thought processes with pet owners can make all the difference in client engagement, consent, and satisfaction.

As the majority of dermatologic cases have underlying disorders, it makes sense to perform tests to try to identify them, so they may be addressed, if possible. Utilizing the basic diagnostic tests, such as skin scrapings, cytology, and fungal cultures, is good medicine and good business. And, if you do have something such as sarcoptic mange on your list of differential diagnoses, it is reasonable to do a parasite-control trial – even if you do not find parasites on skin scrapings. A properly conducted dietary trial also yields a lot of useful information in the workup of a pruritic animal. However, it is important to have a clear diagnostic plan and to proceed logically. For example, the results from biopsies are more likely to be useful if a thorough history, clinical description and differential diagnoses are provided to the pathologist (images are a nice touch as well). Also, it is worth deciding how and if the test results will potentially change your treatment plan. If they will not alter your decisions, what is the purpose of running the tests?

Because most dermatologic presentations have underlying disorders, you should anticipate recurrence if that underlying problem cannot be permanently corrected. Reaching for a stronger medication just temporarily masks the underlying problem, and clients are quick to recognize this. The answer is to start looking more intently for the primary causes. So, tell clients that you will consider attempting symptomatic therapy at first with an appropriate product, but also tell them that if the problem recurs when the medication is discontinued, more investigation may be warranted before stronger medications are considered. In fact, it is possible that methicillin-resistant staphylococci might potentially arise in some cases from the unnecessary escalation of antibiotic therapy, among many other theoretical causes (Weese *et al.* 2012).

Dermatologists will tell you that many clients come to referral appointments with a plastic bag full of products that have been ineffective. Clients are often looking for the magic bullet, the one special drug that the dermatologist has access to, but the primary-care veterinarian does not. The reality is that dermatologists do not have any magic bullets, and rarely rely on one product to address all the needs of their patients. Dermatology patients often have multiple issues to contend with, and treating only one may not be enough to resolve the clinical problem.

For example, many pets with dermatologic issues also have secondary microbial overgrowth (bacterial and/or yeast dermatitis) that needs to be addressed. If those secondary infections are not properly managed, it may be difficult – or impossible – to assess the response to other treatments.

We must also be aware that even well-accepted theories of cause and effect can and do change over time, and our standards of care must be prepared to change with them. For example, we once thought of atopic dermatitis as a classic Type I hypersensitivity reaction primarily driven by mast-cell dynamics in response to inhaled allergens. We now know that the major allergen presentation occurs across the skin surface via Langerhans cells and that inflammatory mediators such as interleukin-31 (IL-31) and other pruritogenic cytokines are most responsible for the scratching that we see in our allergic patients (Marsella *et al.* 2012). This helps explain why antihistamines are often of limited benefit, and points the way to more targeted therapies that can and should be considered.

When creating standards of care for your hospital, remember to build into the model specific points at which referral to a specialist should take place. The best referral happens as part of a well-conceived plan, not as an afterthought. It helps to prepare clients early on that the first course of treatment may not resolve the problem, and if so, that you may try other options or recommend the assistance of a specialist. Clients will appreciate your efforts to inform them now, rather than when they are frustrated, upset, and depleted of funds.

For example, dogs with recurrent pyoderma may be controlled adequately with a combination of medications and topical therapies, but including a dermatologist in the decision-making process early in the course of the condition has many benefits, including helping to determine the underlying causes, and exploring long-term solutions before chronic changes have occurred in the skin, which might limit the benefits of some treatment options. This can also decrease reliance on medications over the long term, and perhaps stave off the development of antibiotic resistance, so has the potential of saving the owner money, health risks, and effort over time. It is much better for all concerned to have specialists involved early in the course of the disease, when they can play an invaluable role as part of the pet's health care team.

In addition to Standards of Care, Consistency of Care is important in multi-doctor hospitals. Consistent messaging to clients only occurs when the process of creating standards helps clinicians achieve consensus in their approaches to common clinical entities, so there can be alignment of hospital team members around an established evidence-based approach, whenever possible.

UNDERESTIMATING THE ROLE OF COMPLIANCE

When it comes to managing many skin conditions, client compliance is an issue that must be considered.

Before dispensing any medications to owners, be realistic in your expectations for what can be reasonably accomplished at home. Better yet, have that exact conversation with owners, including asking open-ended questions of their previous experiences, so you can plan your treatment accordingly. Owners are more likely to be compliant treating clinical signs they can judge (e.g. control of scratching or pain), and can be less compliant with things that are not as obvious, such as administering antibiotics orally at specific intervals or remembering to give parasite-control products on schedule when no parasites are seen.

Because compliance is such an important issue in the resolution of most dermatologic problems, clinicians must recognize this and create treatment plans accordingly. If it is medically prudent to do so, injectable medications should be first line therapy, if available, because they offer convenience to the owner and guaranteed compliance. The next preferred medications are ones that can be administered once daily, followed by those that can be administered every 12 h. It is unlikely that oral medications needing to be administered more often than twice daily will be given on schedule other than by the most dedicated of pet owners (Adams, *et al*, 2005). It is also important to remember that administering a medication twice daily is not the same as administering it every 12 h, so even clients that remember to give a medication twice in any given day might not give it at the appropriate interval consistent with the drug's pharmacokinetics. If so, the pet is not receiving the true intended benefit of that medication.

Finally, cost might be one consideration in medication selection, but if the goal is for the pet to actually receive all the benefit of any selected medication, compliance should be the main selection attribute. The most costly medication (in terms of time and medical outcomes) is actually the medication that fails to deliver the anticipated benefits because it was not administered appropriately.

LACKING REALISTIC PRODUCT AND PRICING MODELS

Veterinary hospitals benefit from carrying appropriate products in inventory, pricing them competitively, and tracking compliance to ensure that pets and owners are actually receiving the full benefit of products dispensed and administered.

While clients might want to browse retail store shelves for the best bargains, when it comes to treating their pets with medical issues, they typically want a firm recommendation made by the veterinarian, not a list of possible treatments that the owner can consider. Be prepared to make clear product recommendations, and be prepared to explain why this is the best option for a particular pet. Some clients will always want the least costly option, but veterinarians owe it to their clients to make firm recommendations, based on evidence-based criteria of what is in the pet's best interest.

Dermatology patients tend to be managed long-term, so consider which products and pricing models work best for you and your clients to keep that revenue in your practice. It pays to stock products that are priced appropriately for the value delivered, and that have been researched, safety tested, and labelled for use in the species to which they are being administered. However, inventory should be kept lean and there is little need to keep multiple products on the shelf that do essentially the same thing.

CONSIDERING DERMATOLOGY CLIENTS A NUISANCE

You are in business to serve the needs of your clients. Owing to the nature of dermatologic diseases, you will see most of your dermatologic patients and their owners many times during the year, for many years to come. That gives you a great opportunity to bond with these pet owners and help shape a positive and mutually beneficial veterinarian–client–patient relationship. These are exactly the clients that you should crave for your practice. The next time the pollen count rises and your telephone starts ringing frequently from clients with itchy pets – do not curse – give thanks! If properly counselled, these are probably the most dedicated clients you will have in your practice.

REFERENCES

1. Ackerman L. (2011) The Genetic Connection, 2nd edn: A Guide to Health Problems in Purebred Dogs & Cats. 329pp. AAHA Press: Lakewood, CO.
2. Ackerman L. (2014) Standards of care & care pathways. In: Five-Minute Veterinary Practice Management Consult (ed L.J. Ackerman), 2nd edn, pp 384–387. John Wiley & Sons, Inc.: Ames, Iowa.
3. Ackerman L., Ball E., Brunt J., Chmiel D., Felsted K., Glickman L. et al. (2013) The Zoetis Lifelong Care Initiative: Putting the Promise into Practice. Clinician's Update, pp 1–8. This is a stand-alone supplement to Clinician's Brief, published by the North American Veterinary Community.
4. Adams V.J., Campbell J.R., Waldner C.L., Dowling P.M. & Shmon C.L. (2005) Evaluation of client compliance with short-term administration of antimicrobials to dogs. J Am Vet Med Assoc 226(4), 567–574.
5. Marsella R., Sousa C.A., Gonzales A.J. & Fadok V.A. (2012) Current

understanding of the pathophysiologic mechanisms of canine atopic dermatitis. Journal of the American Veterinary Medical Association 241, 194–207.

6. Weese J.S., Faires M.C., Frank L.A. et al. (2012) Factors associated with methicillin-resistant versus methicillin-susceptible Staphylococcus pseudintermedius infection in dogs. Journal of the American Veterinary Medical Association 240, 1450–1455.

4
CHAPTER

EFFICACY OF GLUCOCORTICOID MONOTHERAPY FOR TREATMENT OF CANINE MENINGOENCEPHALO-MYELITIS OF UNKNOWN ETIOLOGY: A PROSPECTIVE STUDY IN 16 DOGS

Miyu Mercier and Heidi L. Barnes Heller

INTRODUCTION

Canine meningoencephalomyelitis is a heterogeneous collection of inflammatory and infectious diseases of the central nervous system (CNS). In the majority of dogs, meningoencephalomyelitis has an inflammatory non-infectious etiology. There are several non-infectious inflammatory forms of meningoencephalomyelitis, including granulomatous meningoencephalitis (GME), necrotizing meningoencephalitis (NME), necrotizing leukoencephalitis (NLE) and eosinophilic meningoencephalitis (EME). Due to the distinctive high eosinophil presence in CSF and on histopathology, EME can be readily distinguished from GME, NME, and NLE. Dogs with GME, NME, and NLE may be any age, breed, or sex. Many dogs diagnosed with GME, NME, or NLE are small-breed dogs, but the presence of the disease is not restricted to this population. (Granger *et al.* 2010) Diagnostic imaging for GME, NME, or NLE often involves magnetic resonance imaging (MRI) and may be normal or show focal or multifocal changes. Mononuclear pleocytosis is often present but this varies widely, and cerebrospinal (CSF) analysis may be normal in 12–22% of cases. (Granger *et al.* 2010) In the absence of histopathologic examination, GME, NME, and NLE are indistinguishable on the basis of clinical presentation, breed, sex, age, advanced imaging, and CSF analysis. When histopathologic examination is not available for a given dog, the term meningoencephalomyelitis of unknown etiology (MUE) is used to describe suspected GME, NME, or NLE. (Zarfoss *et al.* 2006; Granger*et al.* 2010;

Citation: Miyu Mercier and Heidi L. Barnes Heller, Efficacy of glucocorticoid monotherapy for treatment of canine meningoencephalomyelitis of unknown etiology: a prospective study in 16 dogs, DOI: 10.1002/vms3.4.

Talarico & Schatzberg 2010). Following a diagnosis of MUE, initial therapy consists of glucocorticoid (GC) drugs, with or without the addition of other immunosuppressant medications. (Adamo *et al.* 2007; Coates *et al.* 2007; Menaut *et al.* 2008; Pakozdy *et al.* 2009; Talarico & Schatzberg 2010; Wong *et al.* 2010; Flegel *et al.* 2011; Lowrie *et al.* 2013) Glucocorticoid monotherapy has been considered the standard therapy (Zarfoss *et al.* 2006; Adamo *et al.*2007; Jung *et al.* 2007; Pakozdy *et al.* 2009; Talarico & Schatzberg 2010; Wong *et al.* 2010; Flegel *et al.* 2011); however, its efficacy without adjunct immunosuppression in the treatment of MUE has been evaluated in only a limited number of studies. (Munana & Luttgen 1998; Jung *et al.*2007; Pakozdy *et al.* 2009; Flegel *et al.* 2011) Use of GC drugs, with variable dosing within each study, has been reported in 59 dogs. The doses have ranged from 5–30 mg/kg per day (Pakozdy *et al.* 2009), 0.17–2.5 mg/kg per day (Flegel *et al.* 2011), 1 mg/kg per day (Jung *et al.* 2007), and 0.5–4 mg/kg per day. (Munana & Luttgen 1998) Therefore, the aims of the current study were compare the CSF analysis at diagnosis and after treatment with a standard GC dose in dogs with MUE. The second aim was to determine the survival time in dogs with MUE treated with GC monotherapy. We hypothesized that abnormal CSF findings would normalize in dogs with MUE, and survival time would be longer than in previous studies utilizing variable GC protocols.

MATERIALS AND METHODS

Study population and inclusion criteria

In this prospective study, client-owned dogs were accrued continuously between September 2006 and May 2009. All clients signed informed consent forms prior to enrollment. Complete physical and neurologic examinations were performed by 1 of the authors. Dogs were included in the study if the following inclusion criteria were met: (1) normal minimum database; (2) GC was not administered within 5 days prior to presentation; (3) MRI consistent with meningoencephalitis/myelitis; (4) negative infectious disease titres, including, tick-borne agents (*Borrelia bergdorferi*,*Rickettsia rickettsii*, and *Ehrlichia canis*), protozoa (*Neospora caninum*), fungi (*Histoplasma, Blastomyces, Aspergillus, Coccidioidomyces*, and*Cryptococcus*) and paired serum and CSF distemper virus titers; and (5) abnormal CSF findings without evidence of neoplastic or infectious etiology. A minimum database was defined as a complete blood count, serum biochemical panel, urinalysis, and three-view thoracic radiographs. Large breed dogs with cervical hyperpathia only were excluded from the study.

Diagnostic testing

Magnetic resonance imaging (GE Horizon 1.0 Tesla magnet, Pittsburg, PA, USA) was performed under general anesthesia in all dogs based on lesion localization from the neurologic examination. Dogs were pre-medicated with hydromorphone (Baxter Pharmaceutical, Deerfield, IL, USA) at 0.1 mg/kg IV and diazepam (Valium; Hospira, Lake Forest, IL, USA) at 0.25 mg/kg IV and induced with propofol (PropoFlo; Abbott Animal Health, Abbott Park, IL, USA) at 4 mg/kg IV to effect. Anesthesia was maintained with isoflurane (IsoFlo®; Abbott Animal Health). The standard MRI protocol for this study included T1- and T2- weighted images in sagittal and transverse planes, fluid attenuated inversion recovery images in the transverse planes, and T1-weighted images after administration of Gadolinium (MultiHance; Bracco Diagnostics, Monroe Township, NJ, USA) in transverse and sagittal planes. Magnetic resonance imaging findings were classified as normal, focal or multifocal for this study.

Cerebrospinal fluid (CSF) was collected from the cerebellomedullary or lumbar cisterns during the same anesthetic episode as neuroimaging. Normal CSF analysis was defined as nucleated cell count (TNCC) <5 cells/μL and protein concentration <25 mg/dL for cerebellomedullary cistern puncture and <40 mg/dL for lumbar puncture. (Platt & Olby 2004) After collection, the CSF sample was divided into two aliquots for transportation; in 1 sample, a 1:10 dilution of CSF to autologous serum was made to improve cell stabilization for transportation, and the other sample was CSF only. (Cellio 2001) All samples were transported in additive-free sterile glass tubes. Analysis was performed by an affiliated laboratory (Antech Diagnostic Laboratory, Oakbrook, IL, USA) within 12 h of collection and analysed according to standard procedure. Correction factors were not applied to the data, and all reported values were uncorrected. (Summers *et al.* 1995) Approximately 1 month after initial CSF analysis, a second CSF sample was collected from the same cistern, using the same anesthetic protocol, and analysed as detailed above.

Treatment protocol

Immediately upon recovery from anesthesia all dogs received intravenous methylprednisolone (Solu-Medrol; Pfizer, New York, NY, USA) at 30 mg/kg IV followed by 15 mg/kg IV 3 h after the initial dose and 10 mg/kg IV 3 h after the second dose was administered. Following treatment with methylprednisone, prednisone (West-Ward Pharmaceutical, Eatontown, NJ, USA) or prednisolone (Lloyd, Inc., Shenandoah, IA, USA) at 1 mg/kg PO q12 h, sulfadimathoxine/ormetoprim (Primor® tablets; Pfizer) at 15 mg/kg PO q12 h, doxycycline (Doxycycline tablets; West Ward Pharmaceutical) at 5–10 mg/kg PO q24 h, and famotidine (Famotidine tablets; Wockhardt, Ltd, Morton Grove, IL, USA) at 1 mg/kg PO q24 h were initiated. After obtaining negative results for infectious disease testing, sulfadimathoxine/ormetoprim and doxycycline were discontinued.

If the second CSF results were within reference intervals, the dog was classified as a CSF responder and a gradually decreasing dose of prednisone or prednisolone was administered as follows: 1 mg/kg *per os* q24 h × 30 days, then 1 mg/kg *per os* q48 h × 30 days and then discontinued. If the second CSF results were abnormal, the dog was classified as a CSF non-responder and the same dose of prednisone or prednisolone was continued for an additional 30 days. If dogs did not improve at 60 days or greater following the above treatment, or worsened during treatment, additional immunosuppressive agents were recommended.

Referring veterinarians were contacted by telephone within 48 months after diagnosis of MUE and questioned about the survival of each dog. If the dog had died, the reason for the death was noted. Referring veterinarians were asked if clinical signs had recurred for CSF responders. Relapse was defined as a reoccurrence of clinical signs in CSF responders, after discontinuing GC therapy.

Statistical analysis

Descriptive statistics including medians, minimums and maximums were recorded for continuous data. A Kaplan–Meier survival curve was created for survival data. Overall survival time and survival time of CSF responders and CSF non-responders was evaluated with the Mantel-Cox Log-Rank test comparison.

RESULTS

Sixteen dogs met the inclusion criteria. Breeds included Lhasa apso ($n = 2$), Dachshund ($n = 2$), and 1 each of the following breeds: Golden Retriever, Retriever mix, Pug, Welsh Springer Spaniel, Boston Terrier, Pug-Beagle mix, Beagle, Jack Russell Terrier, Rottweiler, Collie, Maltese terrier and mixed breed. The median age was 4.5 years (2–11 years) and the median weight was 12.0 kg (5.2–38.4 kg). Neuroanatomical lesion localization, based on the neurologic examination, was prosencephalon (5/16 dogs), brainstem (3/16 dogs), T3-L3 myelopathy (2/16 dogs), L6-S2 radiculopathy (1/16 dogs) and peripheral neuropathy (1/16 dogs) involving the vestibulocochlear nerves. Four of 16 dogs were diagnosed with multifocal lesion localization. Magnetic resonance imaging findings were normal in 2 dogs, focal in 3 dogs and multifocal in 11 dogs. Abnormalities on MRI corresponded with the neuroanatomic lesion localization in all dogs. The median prednisone or prednisolone dose was 1 mg/kg (0.8–1.2 mg/kg) PO q12 h. Sulfadimethoxine/ormetoprim and doxycycline were discontinued by day 7 of treatment in all dogs.

Initial CSF analysis

Initial CSF samples were collected from the cerebellomedullary cistern in 13 dogs and the lumbar cistern in 3 dogs. See Table 1 for median CSF TNCC and protein concentration. Results indicated mixed mononuclear or lymphocytic pleocytosis ($n = 15$) and neutrophilic pleocytosis ($n = 1$); in 3 dogs the TNCC was within the reference interval, but the protein concentration was increased.

Table 1: Median CSF TNCC and protein concentration for dogs diagnosed with MUE

	Median CSF TNCC (cell/μL)		**Median CSF protein (mg/dL)**	
	Initial	**1 month**	**Initial**	**1 month**
1. CSF, cerebrospinal fluid; TNCC, total nucleated cell count; MUE, meningoencephalomyelitis of unknown etiology. Responders achieved normal CSF results at 1 month; non-responders did not achieve normal CSF results at 1 month. Combined values refer to CSF responders and CSF non-responders together.				
Responder	8.5 (0–1160)	0 (0–1)	40.5 (25–251)	19 (13–24)

Non-responder	59 (0–1400)	15 (0–120)	68.5 (28–293)	38 (17–175)
Combined	39 (0–1400)	49 (25–293)	1 (0–120)	24 (13–175)

Second evaluation and CSF analysis

In seven of 16 dogs (44%), CSF analytes were within reference intervals and they were therefore considered CSF responders. One dog did not have sufficient sample to perform CSF protein concentration therefore this dog was considered a CSF responder based on the TNCC. Median TNCC and protein concentration for CSF responders and CSF non-responders are listed in Table 1.

The neurologic examination was normal in 10 of 16 dogs (63%) and abnormal in 6 dogs (38%). In 5 of 10 dogs (50%) with normal neurologic examinations, CSF analysis was also normal. In 2 of 6 dogs (33%) with abnormal neurologic examinations, CSF analysis was normal. All abnormalities on neurologic examination indicated persistent changes; no new abnormalities were detected. Three CSF non-responders started adjunct immunosuppression at a median of 68 days (62–75 days) from diagnosis due to a failure to improve on GC treatment. All 3 dogs received cytosine arabinoside (Generic; Hospira Inc, Lake Forrest, IL, USA) at 50 mg/m^2 *subcutaneous* q 12 h. for 48 h, repeated every 3 weeks as needed.

Survival time

Follow-up information was obtained within 48 months (45–1100 days) of initial diagnosis in all dogs. One of seven CSF responders (14%) was reported to have clinical signs consistent with relapse and was euthanized without additional diagnostic testing or treatment. Two CSF non-responders were euthanized because of progressive disease; two CSF non-responders and one CSF responder were euthanized due to unrelated causes; and two CSF responders and one CSF non-responder were euthanized or died acutely of unknown causes. The remaining three CSF responders and four CSF non-responders dogs were alive at the time of writing (Median 485 days). Median survival for all dogs based on Kaplan–Meier survival analysis was 602 days (45–654 days). Median survival for CSF responders was 602 days and the median was not reached in the CSF non-responders. (Fig. 1) There was no significant difference in survival between the CSF responders and CSF non-responders (P = 0.85). Due to the small number of dogs that died due to disease, reporting of survival time between CSF responders and CSF non-responders was not accurate. Additional statistical analysis was not performed due to small sample size.

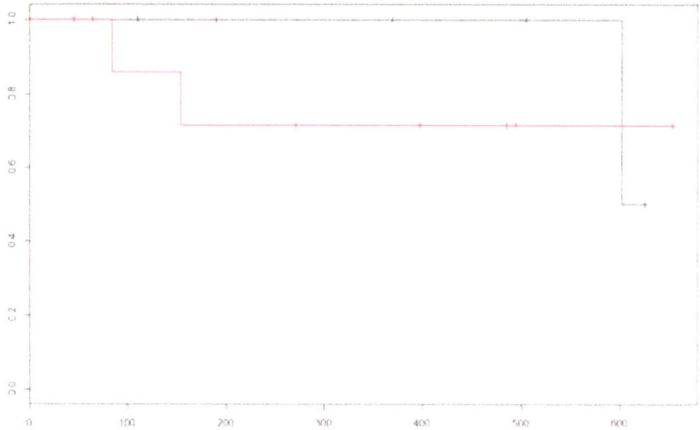

Figure 1: Kaplan-Meier survival curves for 7 responder dogs (black line) and 8 non-responder dogs (red line) with meningoencephalomyelitis of unknown etiology (MUE). Tick marks represent dogs censured for events other than progression of disease.

DISCUSSION

Treatment of dogs with MUE using standardized GC monotherapy resulted in normalization of the CSF analytes in 44% of dogs. None of the previous studies evaluating solo GC therapy has evaluated repeated CSF analysis as a marker for immunosuppression in canine MUE. However, repeated CSF analysis has been evaluated for other immunosuppressant protocols used in treating MUE (Lowrie *et al.* 2013), as well as other inflammatory CNS diseases. (Cizinauskas *et al.* 2000) One study suggested that serial monitoring of CSF TNCC and protein concentrations is a sensitive indicator of successful treatment of inflammatory disease; however, clinical relapse was not evaluated statistically. (Cizinauskas *et al.* 2000) Another study failed to find an association between normal CSF analysis and improved outcome, but did find an association between abnormal CSF analysis and relapse or poor outcome. (Lowrie *et al.* 2013) In the current study, only one CSF responder was reported to have relapsed, suggesting that CSF analysis may be a valid tool for monitoring success or failure of treatment in dogs diagnosed with MUE and treated with GC monotherapy. Larger studies are needed to evaluate this association more fully.

Survival times for dogs in the current study were longer than those in all previous studies of dogs treated with GC monotherapy. Median survival times were reported to be 28 (Pakozdy *et al.* 2009), 91 (Lowrie *et al.* 2013), and 323 (Lowrie *et al.* 2013) days, compared with 602 days in this study. The difference in survival times among studies may reflect different immunosuppression protocols or the prospective nature of the current study. In the current study, we evaluated an immunosuppressive dose of GC that was standardized for all 16 dogs. Methylprednisolone was administered intravenous following the initial diagnosis in all dogs to try to achieve rapid immunosuppression. In studies of treatment protocols using GC in combination with other immunosuppressant agents, median survival times ranged from 26 to 1834 days (Adamo *et al.* 2007; Coates*et al.* 2007; Menaut *et al.* 2008; Pakozdy *et al.* 2009; Talarico & Schatzberg 2010; Wong *et al.* 2010; Flegel *et al.* 2011; Lowrie *et al.* 2013), with a combined median survival time of 375 days. Some of these studies attributed the survival times exclusively to the alternative immunosuppressant. Based on the current study, GC immunosuppression may be a contributing factor to survival times reported for studies, using combination treatments. Furthermore, the long median survival time in this study supports the use of GC monotherapy for dogs diagnosed with MUE.

Lack of a histopathologic diagnosis was a limitation of this study. Although antemortem diagnostic criteria have been established for MUE, inclusion of patients with acute phase infectious disease or neoplasia is an inherent risk in the diagnosis of MUE. (Granger *et al.* 2010) To partially address this possibility, extensive serologic testing was performed at the time of diagnosis for the most common infectious disease in the geographic area as well as paired CSF and serum titres for distemper virus. Serologic testing evaluates immune response to a specific pathogen, therefore it is possible that a dog with acute infectious disease may not yet have mounted an immune response and therefore had negative serology when initially tested. Death or euthanasia due to worsening signs would be expected for dogs with infectious diseases receiving immunosuppressive treatment without concurrent long-term antimicrobial treatment. All dogs included in the study survived for the first 30 days of treatment; therefore it is unlikely that dogs with infectious meningoencephalomyelitis were included. Although neoplastic cells were not identified in CSF, histopathologic examination of the CNS would be expected to be more sensitive than CSF analysis for detection of neoplasia. Brain biopsy was not performed in the dogs in this study due to the risk of complications. Additionally, necropsy was not required and was not obtained in any of the deceased dogs. Requiring diagnosis by either CNS biopsy or necropsy may have resulted in bias towards shorter survival. Therefore, although considered unlikely, occurrence of neoplastic diseases mistakenly diagnosed as meningoencephalomyelitis cannot be excluded. Other limitations of this study included the small size of the study population and limited follow-up time. Larger studies may be able to detect prognostic variables, such normalization differences in CSF protein or TNCC for dogs with MUE that were not evaluated in the current study.

CONCLUSIONS

In dogs with MUE, 44% had normal CSF analysis after 1 month of GC immunosuppression; further studies are needed to determine if a relationship exists between prognosis and results of CSF analysis. Dogs with normal CSF findings at 1 month had longer survival times than dogs with abnormal CSF findings at 1 month. Glucocorticoid therapy in this study, resulted in median survival time longer than previously reported times in studies evaluating combination immunosuppressant protocols; therefore a positive GC effect on survival time in those studies should be considered. Dogs may benefit from the administration of combination immunosuppression protocols if the side effects of GC warrant limited use of GC. In conclusion, this study supports the use of immunosuppression with GC monotherapy in dogs diagnosed with MUE.

REFERENCES

1. Adamo P.F., Rylander H. & Adams W.M. (2007) Ciclosporin use in multi-drug therapy for meningoencephalomyelitis of unknown aetiology in dogs. The Journal of Small Animal Practice 48, 486–496.
2. Cellio B.C. (2001) Collecting, processing, and preparing cerebrospinal fluid in dogs and cats. Compendium Continuing Education for Veterinarians 23, 786–792.
3. Cizinauskas S., Jaggy A. & Tipold A. (2000) Long-term treatment of dogs with steroid-responsive meningitisarteritis: clinical, laboratory and therapeutic results. The Journal of Small Animal Practice 41, 295–301.
4. Coates J.R., Barone G., Dewey C.W., Vitale C.L., Holloway-Azene N.M., Sessions J.K. (2007) Procarbazine as adjunctive therapy for treatment of dogs with presumptive antemortem diagnosis of granulomatous meningoencephalomyelitis: 21 cases (1998–2004). Journal of Veterinary Internal Medicine 2, 100–106.
5. Flegel T., Boettcher I.C., Matiasek K., Oevermann A., Doherr M.G., Oechtering G., Henke D. (2011) Comparison of oral administration of lomustine and prednisolone or prednisolone alone as treatment for granulomatous meningoencephalomyelitis or necrotizing encephalitis in dogs. Journal of the American Veterinary Medical Association 238, 337–345.
6. Granger N., Smith P.M. & Jeffery N.D. (2010) Clinical findings and treatment of non-infectious meningoencephalomyelitis in dogs: a systematic review of 457 published cases from 1962 to 2008. Veterinary Journal 184, 290–297.
7. Jung D.I., Kang B.T., Park C., Yoo J.H., Gu S.H., Jeon H.W., Kim J.W., Heo R.Y., et al. (2007) A comparison of combination therapy (cyclosporine plus prednisolone) with sole prednisolone therapy in 7 dogs with necrotizing meningoencephalitis. Journal of Veterinary Medical Science 69, 1303–1306.
8. Lowrie M., Smith P.M. & Garosi L. (2013) Meningoencephalitis of unknown origin: investigation of prognostic factors and outcome using a standard treatment protocol. The Veterinary Record 172, 527–533.
9. Menaut P., Landart J., Behr S., Lanore D., Trumel C. (2008) Treatment of 11 dogs with meningoencephalomyelitis of unknown origin with a combination of prednisolone and cytosine arabinoside. The Veterinary Record 162, 241–245.
10. Munana K.R. & Luttgen P.J. (1998) Prognostic factors for dogs with granulomatous meningoencephalomyelitis: 42 cases. Journal of the American Veterinary Medical Association 212, 1902–1906
11. Pakozdy A., Leschnik M., Kneissl S., Gumpenberger M., Gruber A., Tichy A., Thalhammer J.G. (2009) Improved survival time in dogs with suspected GME treated with cyclosporin. The Veterinary Record 164, 89–91.
12. Platt S.R. & Olby N.J. (2004) In BSAVA Manual of Canine and Feline Neurology, 35–53. British Small Animal Veterinary Association: Gloucester
13. Summers B.A., Cummings J.F., deLahunta A. (1995) Inflammatory diseases of the central nervous system. In: Veterinary Neuropathology, (This is the only edition of this book), pp. 95–162. Mosby: St. Louis.

14. Talarico L.R. & Schatzberg S.J. (2010) Idiopathic granulomatous and necrotizing inflammatory disorders of the canine central nervous system: a review and future perspectives. The Journal of Small Animal Practice 51, 138–149.
15. Wong M.A., Hopkins A.L., Meeks J.C., Clarke J.D. (2010) Evaluation of treatment with a combination of azathioprine and prednisone in dogs with meningoencephalomyelitis of undetermined etiology: 40 cases (2000–2007). Journal of the American Veterinary Medical Association 237, 929–935.
16. Zarfoss M., Schatzberg S., Venator K., Cutter-Schatzberg K., Cuddon P., Pintar J., et al. (2006) Combined cytosine arabinoside and prednisone therapy for meningoencephalitis of unknown aetiology in 10 dogs. The Journal of Small Animal Practice 47, 588–595.

5
CHAPTER

GRAPIPRANT: AN EP4 PROSTAGLANDIN RECEPTOR ANTAGONIST AND NOVEL THERAPY FOR PAIN AND INFLAMMATION

Kristin Kirkby Shaw, Lesley C. Rausch-Derra and Linda Rhodes

Keywords: Osteoarthritis, EP4, grapiprant, pain, piprant, prostaglandin

INTRODUCTION

Prostanoids are metabolites of arachidonic acid (AA) and have been the target of medicinal therapies for centuries (Appelboom 2002). However, until recently, preparations aimed at inhibiting the action of prostanoids have, with varying degrees of prostanoid specificity, prevented their production and thus impacted both pathologic and homeostatic activity (Curry *et al.* 2005; KuKanich *et al.* 2012). The evolution of pain management has entered a new era – that of selectively blocking the single prostanoid receptor that is primarily responsible for pain and inflammation, thereby preserving the production and activity of homeostatic prostanoids (Nakao *et al.* 2007; Kawabata 2011).

This manuscript reviews the mechanism of action of anti-inflammatory drugs for use in animals and introduce the first-in-class drug for managing pain and inflammation associated with osteoarthritis (OA) in veterinary patients: grapiprant, an EP4 prostaglandin receptor antagonist (PRA).

Citation: Kristin Kirkby Shaw, Lesley C. Rausch-Derra and Linda Rhodes, Grapiprant: an EP4 prostaglandin receptor antagonist and novel therapy for pain and inflammation, DOI: 10.1002/vms3.13.

AA cascade revisited

Arachidonic acid is an omega 6 polyunsaturated lipid that is an integral part of cell membranes and is liberated from the cell membrane by the enzyme phospholipase A_2 (PLA_2) as part of normal cellular metabolism and following cell injury (Curry *et al.* 2005; KuKanich *et al.* 2012). The freed AA molecule is then shuttled into one of three pathways that generate three groups of molecules: prostanoids, leukotrienes and epoxides (Curry *et al.* 2005; KuKanich *et al.* 2012). This manuscript will focus on the prostanoid group.

The enzymes cyclo-oxygenase 1 and 2 (COX-1 and COX-2) convert AA into prostaglandin H_2 (PGH_2), and PGH_2 is subsequently converted, via tissue-specific isomerases and oxidoreductases, to five active prostanoid molecules: thromboxane (TXA), PGD_2, PGI_2 (prostacyclin), PGF_2 and PGE_2 (Simmons *et al.* 2004; Ricciotti & FitzGerald 2011). COX-1 is expressed constitutively in most cells and is the dominant source of prostanoids that are involved in gastric epithelial cytoprotection and homeostasis. COX-2 is constitutively expressed in some tissues, but is also inducible by inflammatory stimuli, and is an important source of prostanoid formation in periods or locations of inflammation. In inflammation, the profile of prostanoid production is determined by the differential expression of these enzymes within cells at the site of inflammation (Ricciotti & FitzGerald 2011). Production of PGE_2 and PGI_2 predominates in sites where COX-2 is activated (Simmons *et al.* 2004).

In the mid-1990s, prostanoid receptors were identified and continue to be characterized (Woodward *et al.* 2011). These receptors have varying distributions throughout the body and mediate the activities of each prostanoid. Each prostanoid interacts with at least one distinct receptor to mediate specific physiological effects, and in some cases this includes specific receptor subtypes for a particular prostanoid.

Inhibiting prostanoid production: the good and the bad

Prostanoids are responsible for a wide range of homeostatic functions in mammals including regulation of renal haemodynamics and ion transport, gastrointestinal cytoprotection and motility, vascular and bronchial smooth muscle activity, immune function and platelet aggregation (Woodward *et al.* 2011; KuKanich *et al.* 2012). Pain and inflammation are also mediated by prostanoids, in particular PGE_2, and thus therapeutic drugs are often used to decrease the production and activity of this molecule (Curry *et al.* 2005; KuKanich *et al.* 2012). Steroids and cyclo-oxygenase inhibiting drugs have until now been the primary options for treating pain and inflammation, and because of their mechanism of action, these approaches have some drawbacks that are discussed below (Stahn *et al.* 2007; KuKanich *et al.* 2012).

Corticosteroids inhibit the enzyme PLA_2, acting up-stream of the COX enzymes in inhibiting the metabolism of AA (Stahn *et al.* 2007). Corticosteroids prevent the synthesis of prostanoids, leukotrienes and epoxides, and thus have broad anti-inflammatory action, but also inhibit the production of many homeostatic AA metabolites. Short-acting corticosteroids can be important therapeutics in the management of acute allergic reactions, and while they may also provide some degree of pain relief, the untoward side effects make them a poor choice for long-term treatment of pain in veterinary patients. Salicylic acid is a natural product derived from plants such as willow bark and meadowsweet, and its medicinal properties of pain relief and fever reduction have been utilized for centuries (Vane 1971). Aspirin, or acetylsalicylic acid, is a synthetic drug made from salicylic acid. Aspirin irreversibly binds to the COX enzymes and inhibits the formation of all prostanoids (Flower 2003; KuKanich *et al.* 2012). While aspirin is effective in reducing fever, pain and inflammation, there are significant adverse effects of treatment with aspirin that are well-recognized in humans and animals, in particular gastrointestinal irritation and ulceration. Furthermore, irreversible inhibition of platelet TXA by aspirin leads to reduced aggregation that lasts up to 7–10 days (the life span of the affected platelets). This anti-thrombotic property can be useful in clinical conditions where reducing blood clotting is called for, but should also be recognized as a potentially significant unwanted side effect of aspirin administration.

Cyclo-oxygenase inhibiting non-steroidal anti-inflammatory drugs (COX inhibiting NSAIDs) decrease inflammation through inhibition of COX enzymes and subsequent inhibition of prostaglanoid production (Curry *et al.* 2005; KuKanich *et al.* 2012). This class includes aspirin, as described above, as well as other non-selective COX inhibitors (i.e. drugs that inhibit both COX 1 and COX 2 enzymes) such as ketoprofen and indomethacin. In addition, drugs have been developed that preferentially inhibit COX-2, such as carprofen, meloxicam, deracoxib, firocoxib and robenacoxib.

The two cyclo-oxygenase isoenzymes, COX-1 and COX-2, were isolated in the 1980s and shortly thereafter it was discovered that COX-2 is induced in response to tissue injury and is associated with inflammation and pain (Vane 1971; KuKanich *et al.* 2012). Drug development then concentrated on molecules that preferentially inhibited this enzyme in the hope of sparing the so-called ‘house-keeping’ prostaglandins produced by COX-1. The coxib class of drugs, or selective COX-2 inhibitors, were first marketed in human medicine in 1999. In humans, COX-2 selective products such as rofecoxib (Vioxx® Merck & Co., Inc. Kenilworth, NJ USA) and celecoxib (Celebrex® Pfizer Inc. New York, NY USA) did show improved GI tolerability; however, in some cases, the FDA reviewed evidence leading the agency to conclude that their use was related to significant cardiovascular side effects and thus, all but one product have been removed from the US market (Harirforoosh *et al.* 2013). The underlying cause for these adverse cardiovascular events may be attributed to inhibition of COX-2 synthesis of PGI_2 (prostacyclin). PGI_2 is a potent vasodilator and has anti-thrombotic properties (an endogenous antagonist of TXA), thus decreased production of PGI_2 by coxib-inhibiting NSAIDs may lead to increased thrombosis and vasoconstriction, two methods of potentiating cardiovascular disease (Harirforoosh *et al.* 2013). The cardiovascular adverse events associated with COX-2 selective NSAIDs in humans have not been observed in dogs taking COX-2 selective NSAIDs. However, severe gastrointestinal, renal and hepatic adverse events have been reported in dogs taking these products (Lascelles *et al.* 2005; KuKanich *et al.* 2012; Monteiro-Steagall *et al.* 2013).

Both COX-1 and COX-2 activity are important in maintaining gastrointestinal integrity and renal haemodynamics in dogs, primarily through the actions of PGE_2 and PGI_2 (Wilson *et al.* 2004; KuKanich *et al.* 2012). COX-2 is expressed in the canine kidney and involved in regulation of vessel tone and salt and water balance via synthesis of PGE_2 and PGI_2. In the stomach and intestinal tract, COX-1 is the primary mediator of gastro-protective prostanoid (PGE_2 and PGI_2) production in the healthy animal. COX-2 is up-regulated in areas of gastrointestinal irritation and it is important in promoting the healing of gastrointestinal ulcerations (KuKanich *et al.* 2012). This suggests that administration of a selective COX-2 inhibitor drug in the face of gastrointestinal ulceration, such as due to stress or administration of corticosteroids or a non-selective cyclo-oxygenase-inhibiting NSAID such as aspirin, may reduce healing and potentiate ulceration and perforation (Lascelles *et al.* 2005). Another potential mechanism for gastrointestinal injury secondary to cyclo-oxygenase inhibiting NSAID administration is the increased production of inflammatory leukotrienes (Curry *et al.* 2005). Inhibition of the COX pathways may result in increased AA that must be metabolized by the lipo-oxygenase enzyme (LOX) pathway.

The four FDA approved COX inhibitor NSAIDs for use in dogs, unless contra-indicated, are considered to be effective treatments for the pain associated with OA. However, these COX-inhibiting NSAIDs, as a class, carry the potential for adverse effects including gastrointestinal ulceration and perforation and renal insufficiency (Lascelles *et al.* 2005; Monteiro-Steagall *et al.* 2013). While COX-2 selective and preferential NSAIDs are associated with fewer side effects compared to aspirin and older, non-selective COX inhibitor NSAIDs, many dogs do not tolerate these drugs, and alternative pharmacologic pain relief is indicated. Currently, no other class of pharmaceuticals is approved by the FDA for the treatment of pain and inflammation associated with OA in dogs. Thus, it is evident that an FDA approved product that demonstrates targeted pain relief with improved tolerability is needed.

THE PIPRANT CLASS: PRA

After the identification of prostanoid receptors in the 1990s, significant research ensued into methods of targeting each receptor with synthetic agonists and antagonists (Woodward *et al.* 2011). In October 2013, the World Health Organization defined a newly recognized class of drugs that act as PRAs as the piprant class (World Health Organization, 2013).

EP4 PRAs and anti-inflammatory effects: experimental models

Prostaglandin E_2 (PGE_2) is a key mediator of swelling, redness and pain, the classic signs of inflammation, with pain resulting from PGE_2-mediated sensitization of sensory neurons and swelling and redness resulting from PGE_2-mediated vasodilation and increased vascular permeability (Ricciotti & FitzGerald 2011). PGE_2 exerts its effects via four receptors, EP1, EP2, EP3 and EP4 (Woodward *et al.* 2011). The EP4 receptor is the primary mediator of the PGE_2-elicited sensitization of sensory neurons and PGE_2-elicited inflammation (Southall & Vasko 2001; McCoy *et al.* 2002; Lin *et al.* 2006; Nakao *et al.* 2007; Clark *et al.* 2008; Chen *et al.* 2010; Boyd *et al.* 2011). Grapiprant (AT-001) is a new analgesic and anti-inflammatory drug in the piprant class that functions as a selective EP4 PRA (Nakao *et al.* 2007). The following is a review of the literature and studies that demonstrate the anti-inflammatory effects of EP4 PRAs and of grapiprant in particular. The use of receptor knockout mice has been helpful in understanding the roles of the specific EP receptors in inflammation. Collagen antibody-induced arthritis (CAIA) in mice is a model for the human inflammatory disorder rheumatoid arthritis (RA). The individual PGE_2 receptors were evaluated by inducing CAIA in mice which were genetically modified to knock out the EP1, -2, -3, or -4 receptors and measuring the clinical, histopathological and cellular markers of disease (McCoy *et al.* 2002). When mice with one of these four receptors knocked out were evaluated for signs of pain and inflammation, the EP4 receptor knock-out mice, but not the EP1, EP2 or EP3 receptor knock-out mice, had decreased incidence and severity of disease, decreased histopathological deterioration associated with arthritis and decreased levels of inflammatory markers, implicating EP4 as a key mediator of inflammation. In a mouse model of acute inflammation, EP1, 2, 3 or 4 receptor knock-out mice were subjected to UV irradiation of the skin. EP4 and EP2 knock-out mice, but not EP1 or EP3 knock-out mice, had significantly decreased ear swelling compared to control mice. The reduction in swelling was also seen when the wild-type mice were treated with an EP4 PRA (Kabashima*et al.* 2007).

The anti-inflammatory effects of EP4 receptor antagonism have also been investigated in animal models of inflammation. In a study by Clark *et al.* (2008), joint inflammation (as measured by paw swelling) was created using an adjuvant-induced arthritis (AIA) model in rats. Rats treated with an EP4 PRA (MF498), but not an EP1 or an EP3 PRA, demonstrated reduced paw swelling. The reduction in swelling was similar to that seen in mice treated with a cyclo-oxygenase-2 (COX-2) inhibitor. In a study by Murase *et al.* (2008), the selective EP4 PRA, CJ-042,794, caused decreased paw swelling in a complete Freund's adjuvant model of chronic inflammatory pain in rats. The reductions in paw swelling in the CJ-042,794 treated rats were again similar to those seen with rofecoxib (a COX-2 inhibitor) treated rats. Using a complete Freund's adjuvant administration as a rodent model for pain and inflammation, treatment with an EP4 PRA, identified as 1a, also demonstrated reduced swelling of the paw (Boyd *et al.* 2011). In a series of experiments reported by Chen *et al.* (2010), an EP4 PRA, ER-819762, suppressed inflammatory cytokine production, suppressed disease and slowed disease progression in collagen and GPI-induced arthritis in mice. These data support the anti-inflammatory role of EP4 receptor antagonism in rodents. Indeed, these results demonstrated that EP4 PRAs can reduce inflammation as effectively as COX-2 inhibitors.

Several studies have been conducted examining the anti-inflammatory and analgesic effects of grapiprant (AT-001, referred to as CJ-023,423 in the publications) in rats (Nakao *et al.* 2007). Studies using rat models have demonstrated grapiprant's ability to reduce acute and chronic pain and inflammation (Nakao *et al.* 2007; RaQualia 2007a,b). The anti-inflammatory effect of grapiprant on paw swelling, inflammatory biomarkers in the serum and synovial inflammation was examined in the tarsal joint in AIA in rats (RaQualia 2007b). Grapiprant exhibited dose-dependent and significant anti-inflammatory effects on all parameters tested. The efficacy of grapiprant on paw swelling was comparable to those of rofecoxib and piroxicam (COX-inhibiting drugs). In another study, the anti-inflammatory activity of grapiprant on rat carrageenan-induced foot swelling was investigated (RaQualia 2007a). Grapiprant inhibited foot swelling in a dose-dependent manner compared to rats treated with placebo control. Nakao *et al.* (2007) investigated three different models of pain in rats: mechanical hyperalgesia, thermal hyperalgesia and weight bearing deficit. Oral administration of CJ-023,423 significantly reduced hyperalgesia in rodents in all three models, including significantly reversing complete Freund's adjuvant-induced chronic inflammatory pain.

Not only is the EP4 receptor prominently involved in inflammation and pain, but importantly this receptor may mediate central sensitization and play a role in chronic pain. Lin *et al.* (2006) reported that in rodents, the EP4 receptor is expressed by sensory neurons, and the level of EP4 receptors increased following peripheral inflammation. Administration of an EP4 PRA decreased pain and hypersensitivity in rodents.

EP4 PRA in veterinary medicine: targeted pain management

The EP4 receptor in mice, humans and dogs has been cloned and characterized. The canine EP4 receptor has approximately 90% homology to the human receptor (Castleberry *et al.* 2001). Grapiprant is a PRA that selectively blocks the EP4 receptor in rodents, humans, and dogs (RaQualia 2007c). Grapiprant has undergone experimental and pilot studies in laboratory and client-owned dogs. A multi-site, masked, placebo-controlled, randomized field trial for the control of pain and inflammation associated with OA in dogs was recently completed and was submitted to and accepted by the FDA in support of regulatory approval (www.aratana.com). The results of these studies in client-owned dogs demonstrate that this drug provides control of the pain associated with OA. Studies are currently underway investigating the use of grapiprant in cats, and at this time data are not yet available.

As part of development of grapiprant for FDA approval for dogs with OA, a safety study in healthy Beagles investigated the effects of daily orally administered doses up to 50 mg kg^{-1} day^{-1} oral suspension (equivalent to approximately 30.5 mg kg^{-1} day^{-1} of the tablet formulation) for nine consecutive months (Rausch-Derra *et al.* 2015a,b). There were no drug-related effects on liver enzyme values, BUN/creatinine, or platelet function. Mild and reversible dose- and time-dependent decreases in total protein, albumin and calcium were seen. Clinical signs were also dose dependent and restricted to mild gastrointestinal signs including soft stool, occasional stool with mucus or blood, and sporadic vomiting. There were no histopathological changes to any tissues, including the stomach, kidneys or liver except in one dog in the 50 mg kg^{-1} group had mild mucosal regeneration of the ileum seen on histopathology.

The relative lack of toxic effects with grapiprant compared to those that have been reported in dogs treated with COX-inhibiting NSAIDs is not surprising. Grapiprant is a targeted approach to pain management – it selectively blocks the EP4 receptor, does not interfere with the production of prostanoids, and therefore does not affect the other PG receptor pathways that are affected in animals treated with COX inhibitor NSAIDs.

CONCLUSION

PGE_2 is a key mediator of pain and inflammation and has its effect through binding to the EP4 receptor. Grapiprant directly and specifically blocks the EP4 receptor, and therefore blocks PGE_2-elicited pain and inflammation. An EP4 PRA, such as grapiprant, which has been demonstrated to provide relief from arthritic pain in canine clinical patients, acts without affecting the synthesis and widespread activity of PGE_2 and other prostanoids.

Safety studies in laboratory dogs have demonstrated an excellent safety profile, and a wide safety margin, and this has been confirmed in two large field effectiveness studies in dogs with OA (Rausch-Derra *et al.* 2015a,b). The relative lack of toxic effects with grapiprant compared to those that have been reported in dogs treated with COX-inhibiting NSAIDs is consistent with grapiprant's unique mechanism of action, although until FDA review and approval, claims of safety and effectiveness cannot be made. Grapiprant may offer a more targeted, and potentially better tolerated, method of pain management in dogs with OA.

ACKNOWLEDGEMENT

We would like to acknowledge the scientists at RaQualia who pioneered basic research and development of EP4 PRAs.

CONFLICTS OF INTEREST

At the time of writing, all authors were employees of Aratana Therapeutics, Inc., Kansas City, KS, USA At the time of publication, KK Shaw will be a full time employee of Animal Surgical Clinic of Seattle; Seattle, WA, USA and a paid consultant for Aratana Therapeutics, Inc.

REFERENCES

1. Appelboom T. (2002) Arthropathy in art and the history of pain management – through centuries to cyclooxygenase-2 inhibitors. Rheumatology 41, 28–34.
2. Boyd M.J., Berthelette C., Chiasson J.F., Clark P., Colucci J., Denis D. et al. (2011) A novel series of potent and selective EP4 receptor ligands: facile modulation of agonism and antagonism. Bioorganic & Medicinal Chemistry Letters 21, 484–487
3. Castleberry T.A., Lu B., Smock S.L. & Owen T.A. (2001) Molecular cloning and functional characterization of the canine prostaglandin E2 receptor EP4 subtype. Prostaglandins & Other Lipid Mediators 65, 167–187
4. Chen Q., Muramoto K., Masaaki N., Ding Y., Yang H., Mackey M. et al. (2010) A novel antagonist of the prostaglandin E(2) EP(4) receptor inhibits Th1 differentiation and Th17 expansion and is orally active in arthritis models. British Journal of Pharmacology 160, 292–310.
5. Clark P., Rowland S. E., Denis D., Mathieu M. C., Stocco R., Poirier H. et al. (2008) MF498 [N-{[4-(5,9-Diethoxy- 6-oxo-6,8-dihydro-7H-pyrrolo[3,4-g] quinolin-7-yl)-3-m ethylbenzyl]sulfonyl}-2-(2-methoxyphenyl)acetamide], a selective E prostanoid receptor 4 antagonist, relieves joint inflammation and pain in rodent models of rheumatoid and osteoarthritis. The Journal of Pharmacology and Experimental Therapeutics 325, 425–434

6. Curry S.L., Cogar S.M. & Cook J.L. (2005) Nonsteroidal anti-inflammatory drugs: a review. Journal of the American Animal Hospital Association 41, 298–309.
7. Flower R. (2003) What are all the things that aspirin does? BMJ 327, 572–573.
8. Harirforoosh S., Asghar W. & Jamali F. (2013) Adverse effects of nonsteroidal anti-inflammatory drug: an update of gastrointestinal, cardiovascular and renal complications. Journal of Pharmacy and Pharmaceutical Sciences 16, 821–847.
9. Kabashima K., Nagamachi M., Honda T., Nishigori C., Miyachi Y., Tokura Y., Narumiya S. (2007) Prostaglandin E2 is required for ultraviolet B-induced skin inflammation via EP2 and EP4 receptors. Laboratory Investigation 87, 49–55.
10. Kawabata A. (2011) Prostaglandin E2 and pain–an update. Biological and Pharmaceutical Bulletin 34, 1170–1173.
11. KuKanich B., Bidgood T. & Knesl O. (2012) Clinical pharmacology of nonsteroidal ant-inflammatory drugs in dogs. Veterinary Anaesthesia and Analgesia 39, 69–90.
12. Lascelles B.D.X., Blikslager A.T., Fox S.M. & Reece D. (2005) Gastrointestinal tract perforation in dogs treated with a selective cyclooxygenase-2 inhibitor: 29 cases (2002–2003). Journal of the American Veterinary Medical Association 227, 1112–1117.
13. Lin C. R., Amaya F., Barrett L., Wang H., Takada J., Samad T. A., Woolf C. J. (2006) Prostaglandin E2 receptor EP4 contributes to inflammatory pain hypersensitivity. Journal of Pharmacology and Experimental Therapeutics 319, 1096–1103.
14. McCoy J.M., Wicks J.R. & Audoly L.P. (2002) The role of prostaglandin E2 receptors in the pathogenesis of rheumatoid arthritis. The Journal of Clinical Investigation 110, 651–658.
15. Monteiro-Steagall B.P., Steagall P.V.M. & Lascelles B.D.X. (2013) Systematic review of nonsteroidal antiinflammatory drug-induced adverse effects in dogs. Journal of Veterinary Internal Medicine 27, 1011–1019.
16. Murase A., Okumura T., Sakakibara A., Tonai-Kachi H., Nakao K., Takada J. (2008) Effect of prostanoid EP4 receptor antagonist, CJ-042,794, in rat models of pain and inflammation. European Journal of Pharmacology 580, 116–121
17. Nakao K., Murase A., Ohshiro H., Okumura T., Taniguchi K., Murata Y. et al. (2007) CJ-023,423, a novel, potent and selective prostaglandin EP4 receptor antagonist with antihyperalgesic properties. Journal of Pharmacology and Experimental Therapeutics 322, 686–694
18. RaQualia (2007a) Determination of the Dose Response Relationship of CJ-023423 in the Rat CarrageeninInduced Foot Edema Model. SR_DB1_CJ-023423_RAT_CFE_1_2007.
19. RaQualia (2007b) Investigation of the Inhibitory Effects of CJ-023423 on Inflammation and Bone Destruction in Adjuvant-Induced Arthritis Rats. SR_DB1_CJ- 023423_AIA_1_2007
20. RaQualia (2007c) Determination of the Binding Affinity of CJ-023423 for the

Cloned Dog EP4 Receptor. SR_PPL_CJ-02423_dog_EP4BD_2007

21. Rausch-Derra L., Rhodes L., Freshwater L. (2015a) Pharmacokinetic Comparison of Oral Tablet and Suspension Formulations of Grapiprant, a Novel Therapeutic for the Pain and Inflammation of Osteoarthritis in Dogs. Presented at AAVPT Biennial Symposium, Fort Collins, CO.

22. Rausch-Derra L., Huebner M. & Rhodes L. (2015b) Evaluation of the safety of long-term, daily oral administration of grapiprant, a novel drug for treatment of osteoarthritic pain and inflammation, in health dogs. American Journal of Veterinary Research 76, 853–859.

23. Ricciotti E. & FitzGerald G.A. (2011) Prostaglandins and inflammation. Arteriosclerosis, Thrombosis, and Vascular Biology 31, 986–1000

24. Simmons D.L., Botting R.M. & Hla T. (2004) Cyclooxygenase isozymes: the biology of prostaglandin synthesis and inhibition. Pharmacological Reviews 56, 387–437.

25. Southall M.D. & Vasko M.R. (2001) Prostaglandin receptor subtypes, EP3C and EP4, mediate the prostaglandin E2-induced cAMP production and sensitization of sensory neurons. The Journal of Biological Chemistry 276, 16083–16091.

26. Stahn C., Lowenberg M., Hommes D.W. & Buttgereit F. (2007) Molecular mechanisms of glucocorticoid action and selective glucocorticoid receptor agonists. Molecular and Cellular Endocrinology 275, 71–78.

27. Vane J.R. (1971) Inhibition of prostaglandin synthesis as a mechanism of action for aspirin-like drugs. Nature: New Biology 231, 232–235.

28. Wilson J.E., Chandrasekharan N.V., Westover K.D. et al. (2004) Determination of expression of cyclooxygenase-1 and -2 isozymes in canine tissues and their differential sensitivity to nonsteroidal anti-inflammatory drugs. American Journal of Veterinary Research 65, 810–818

29. Woodward D.F., Jones R.L. & Narumiya S. (2011) International Union of basic and clinical pharmacology. LXXXIII: classification of prostanoid receptors, updating 15 years of progress. Pharmacological Reviews 63, 471–538.

30. World Health Organization (2013) Pre-stems: Suffixes Used in the Selection of INN.

6
CHAPTER

COMPARATIVE ASPECTS OF CANINE MELANOMA

Adriana Tomoko Nishiya, Cristina Oliveira Massoco, Claudia Ronca Felizzola, Eduardo Perlmann, Karen Batschinski, Marcello Vannucci Tedardi, Jéssica Soares Garcia, Priscila Pedra Mendonça, Tarso Felipe Teixeira and Maria Lucia Zaidan Dagli

Keywords: Melanoma, canine, cancer, histopathology, therapy

INTRODUCTION

Melanoma is a malignant neoplasm originating from melanocytes. Melanocytic neoplasms have been described in men and in most domesticated animal species, including dogs, cats, horses, and also in wild terrestrial and marine animals [1].

Since dogs live in close proximity to humans, they are influenced by similar environmental factors that may lead to chronic diseases and cancer. In fact, the domestic dog (*Canis familiaris*) reportedly presents more naturally inherited chronic diseases than any other animal species. Hence, those aspects have to be considered in the selection of an animal model for a multifactorial human disease, and the dog appears to be the one with the best characteristics [2,3,4]. Dogs are considered recommended models due to their relatively high susceptibility to cancers, including melanomas, and many behavioral similarities [5].

While many genetic alterations of melanomas have recently been discovered and studied, control of this disease is still challenging in both humans and animals, particularly in dogs and cats. The aim of this review is to report a comparative approach

Citation: Adriana Tomoko Nishiya, Cristina Oliveira Massoco, Claudia Ronca Felizzola, Eduardo Perlmann, Karen Batschinski, Marcello Vannucci Tedardi, Jéssica Soares Garcia, Priscila Pedra Mendonça, Tarso Felipe Teixeira and Maria Lucia Zaidan Dagli, Comparative Aspects of Canine Melanoma, doi:10.3390/vetsci3010007.

of the etiological, epidemiological, pathological, and molecular aspects of melanomas in dogs.

CANINE MELANOMA EPIDEMIOLOGY

Melanoma is one of the most devastating types of cancer, killing around 50,000 people worldwide every year [6,7]. In 2015, according to the American Cancer Society, it is estimated that about 73,870 new melanoma cases will be diagnosed (about 42,670 in men and 31,200 in women), and 9940 people are expected to die of melanoma (about 6640 men and 3300 women).

Human malignant mucosal melanoma of the head and neck is increasing rapidly in incidence in the United States. It is an uncommon and fatal malignancy that does not appear to have the same etiologic basis as cutaneous melanoma. In 452 observed cases, the majority of patients had sino-nasal location (72.6%) and white women ages 70 or older were most affected [8]. This kind of human malignant melanoma is uncommon and has aggressive behavior with increasing rates of recurrence and regional and distant metastasis [9]. Regional lymphatic metastasis occurred in 57.9% to 21% of patients and recurrence rates were 57.9% to 26.3% for patients treated with surgery alone and for those treated with surgery and radiotherapy, respectively. Distant metastases occurred in 52.6% receiving surgery alone and in 47.3% receiving both therapies [10].

Canine oral malignant melanomas in dogs accounted for 0.99% of all (338/33826) canine pathology cases received from 1992 through 1999 at the University of Missouri—Veterinary. The most common sites are the gingiva and labial mucosa [11].

In a retrospective study of neoplasms in domestic animals (data collected between 1993 and 2002 at the School of Veterinary Medicine and Animal Science of the University of São Paulo, Brazil), of 1813 cases of neoplasms in dogs, 58 were melanocytic neoplasms, accounting for 3% of the total in this species [12]. In another retrospective study, 2154 neoplasms were diagnosed at the University of São Paulo between 2000 and 2006. A total of 193 cases (8.9%) were melanocytic neoplasms, of which 186 cases occurred in dogs (96.4%), and only seven in cats (3.6%). Male mixed-breed dogs with black hair coats, with ages varying from 8 to 11 years, were the most commonly affected animals [13].

Canine malignant melanomas are located at different anatomical sites, such as the mouth (Figure 1A,B), lips, skin (Figure 1C), eyes, and digits (Table 1). Studies are controversial about the most common location for this disease in dogs; however, most studies point to the oral cavity and skin as the most common sites [14,15,16,17]. In a survey of 384 melanocytic canine tumors, oral, cutaneous, lips/feet, and eye sites comprised 19%, 59%, 19%, and 3%, respectively [18]. In another study considering malignant melanomas, oral cavity and cutaneous localization were the most common in 40%–62% and 27%–31%, respectively [13,19].

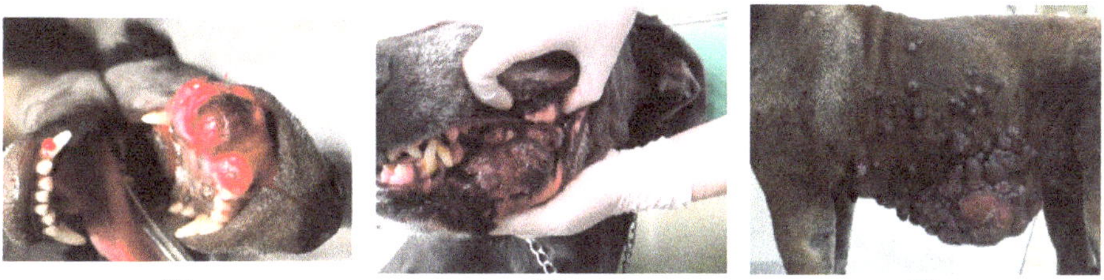

(A) (B) (C)

Figure 1: Clinical aspect of malignant oral melanomas (A) in maxilla; (B) in mandible. Clinical aspect of malignant cutaneous melanoma (C) in thoracic and abdominal wall (*Adriana Nihiya*).

Table 1: Common sites of malignant melanomas in dogs

Sites/Total Number of Cases	*n* = 1652	*n* = 143	*n* = 209
Oral	1026	57	67
Cutaneous	448	44	88
Scrotum	-	4	-
Digit	94	21	-
Ungual	60	-	-
Ocular	24	17	-
Lips/Feet	-	-	54
Reference	Gillard *et al.*, 2014 [19]	Teixeira *et al.*, 2010 [13]	Spangler and Kass, 2006 [18]

Data obtained from historical studies indicated that the following breeds of dogs are considered at risk to develop melanocytic tumors: Airedale Terrier, Boston Terrier, Boxer, Chihuahua, Chow Chow, Cocker Spaniel, Doberman Pinscher, English Springer Spaniel, Golden Retriever, Irish Setter [20], Miniature Schnauzer, Scottish Terrier [19,20], Poodles, Beauce Shepherds, Rottweilers, and Labrador Retrievers [19]. Some breeds of dogs, specifically the Schnauzer family (miniature and standard), Scottish Terriers, and Irish Setters are at risk for developing digital malignant melanomas [21,22].

Malignant melanomas typically occur in middle-aged to older dogs, as Miller *et al.* [23] found an average age of nine years, and with no gender predilections.

Teixeira *et al.* [24] studied 25 canine oral melanomas, including 16 melanotic and nine amelanotic specimens. In this study, 25% of the melanotic melanoma-bearing dogs were eight-year old animals, and 22.2% of amelanotic melanoma-bearing group were younger, with ages varying from four to eight years.

Most information on animal cancer epidemiology in the literature comes from laboratories or hospitals, usually from a unique center and using non-standard coding protocols. This may lead to epidemiological bias, and the data rarely generate reliable information useful to establish comparisons. Cancer registries are the most important source of epidemiological data for neoplasms [25]. There are some animal cancer registries around the world, situated mostly in Europe and the USA. In 2013, the São

Paulo Animal Cancer Registry was created at the University of São Paulo, Brazil, serving as the first animal cancer registry in Latin America [25,26]. This system will allow for better and more accurate epidemiologic studies in domestic animals in this region.

CANINE MALIGNANT MELANOMA ETIOLOGY

In humans, malignant melanoma is the most aggressive, therapy-resistant, and deadly form of skin cancer [27]. The major risk factors for human melanoma include family history, skin and mucosal pigmentation characteristics, sun exposure, particularly to UVB light, and skin reactions to sun exposure. Another type of melanoma, oral malignant melanoma, is a rare aggressive neoplasm usually seen in middle-aged adults.

Several etiological factors are supposed to be involved in canine malignant melanomas, including consanguinity, trauma, chemical exposure, hormones, and genetic susceptibility [28]. However, there is no consensus regarding the etiology of malignant melanomas in dogs [29]. Sunlight may be involved in the development of this disease in the sun-exposed skin areas of the body, such as the face and pinnae; however, sunlight probably is not involved in mucosal melanomas, like the ones found in the canine buccal cavity. Other factors, like the presence of pigmented cells, trauma, chemical agents, or even the buccal microbiota, and inflammation may be associated with the etiology of these tumors [30].

Although melanomas can arise in any dog, the prevalence of this disease is higher in purebred dogs, especially Standard and Miniature Schnauzers, Doberman Pinschers, Scottish Terriers, Irish and Gordon Setters, and Golden Retrievers. This fact supports the theory that melanomas in dogs could have a genetic basis [28]. Genetic and epigenetic modifications in melanocytes that lead to alterations in expression or function of genes and proteins involved in cell cycle control and apoptosis are certainly involved in the development of melanomas.

CANINE MELANOMA PATHOLOGICAL ASPECTS AND PROGNOSIS

Melanocytic neoplasms can be classified as benign or malignant tumors [31]. Malignant melanomas are considered malignant neoplasms arising from melanocytes, while melanocytomas are the benign counterparts [31].

Melanocytes, which are dendritic cells derived from the neuroectoderm and melanoblasts of the neural crest, migrate during embryogenesis to the dermis and epidermis, mucous membranes, and eyes [29,32]. These dendritic cells in melanoma development have demonstrated altered expression of cell–cell adhesion molecules, such as decreased expression of E-cadherin and V-CAM 1 and increased expression of N-cadherin, Mel-CAM 1, ICAM 1, and $\alpha \beta$ integrins [33]. The development of malignant melanoma is generally characterized by a series of transitions that are outlined in [34], and arises from melanocytes that normally reside within the basal layer of epidermis [35].

According to Head *et al.* [36], a melanocytoma is a benign tumor composed of melanocytes in the basal region of the epithelium and extending into the submucosa (junctional melanocytoma) or in the sub-epithelial connective tissue under normal epithelium (dermal melanocytoma). Malignant melanoma can be subdivided into three patterns on the basis of cell shape [36]:

- -epithelioid—round and polygonal cells (Figure 2)

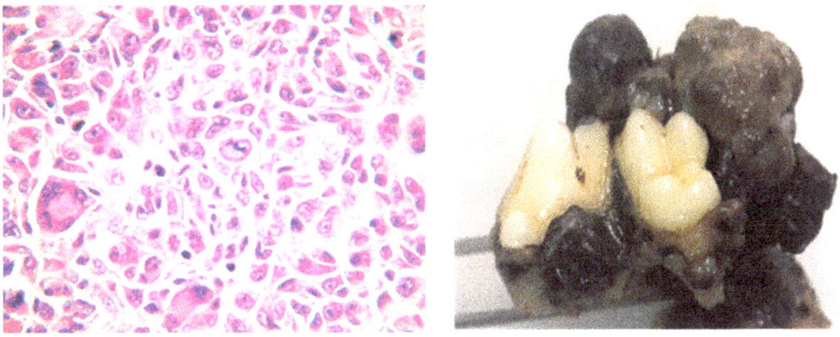

(A) (B)

Figure 2: Photomicrograph of the most common histopathology type of malignant melanoma (epithelioid), showing formation of cell nests, with the presence of multinucleated giant cells and atypical mitotic figures, HE, Objective 40 × (A). Canine oral malignant melanoma, pigmented, exophytic mass protruding from the gingiva (B). Formalin-fixed tissue. Photographs are courtesy of Professor Dr. José Guilherme Xavier.

- -spindle cell—tumor resembles fibroblasts
- -mixed tumors—show both cell types

Malignant melanoma histologically can be the highly melanotic type or the highly anaplastic amelanotic type. Anaplastic melanocytes can be large with abundant cytoplasm with one or more oval or elongated nuclei, with obvious nucleoli. These are frequently characterized to form nests in the submucosa by a mixed structure of epithelial-like cells and fusiform cells and junctional infiltration between basal cells and in the submucosa [36] (Figure 3).

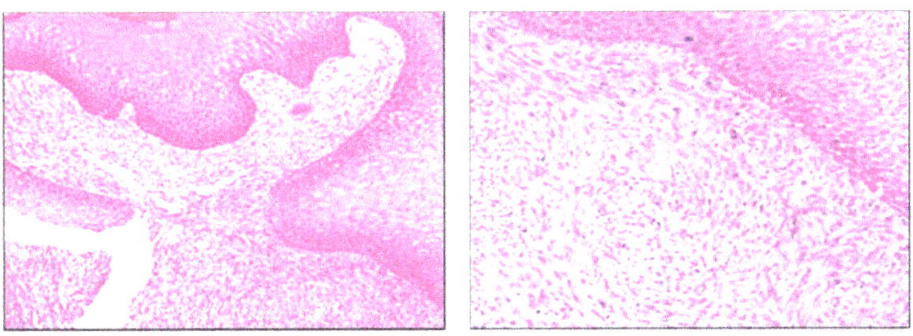

(A) (B)

Figure 3: Photomicrograph of oral amelanotic melanoma ((A), Objective 10 ×; (B), Objective 20 ×). Hematoxylin and eosin.

The most prominent biological property of melanoma cells is the ability to produce melanin [37]. The disruption of homeostasis of close association between melanocytes and basal keratinocytes may trigger a continuous proliferation of the melanocytes, which may lead to the development of a malignant melanoma [7]. Once malignant melanoma cells have escaped from the keratinocyte control, they become able to invade the tissue by the degradation of extracellular matrix through the action of metalloproteinases [38].

The histopathological diagnosis of melanoma may be difficult if the tumor does not contain melanin. Amelanotic malignant melanomas may represent one third of all melanoma cases in dogs.

Their histopathological aspect may resemble carcinomas, sarcomas, lymphomas, and osteogenic tumors. For this reason, the diagnosis of malignant melanoma should be made with the use of immunohistochemistry [11,39,40]. Teixeira *et al.* [13] used two different antibodies to confirm the diagnosis of malignant melanoma in amelanotic cases: HMB 45 (Mouse monoclonal anti-human HMB45, from Dako) and Melan A (Monoclonal mouse anti-human Melan-A, from Dako), and both were considered suitable to immunostain canine melanocytes. Ramos-Vara *et al.* [11] considered Melan A as a specific and sensitive marker for malignant melanomas. Smedley *et al.* [41] evaluated 49 amelanotic melanomas and created a cost-effective and efficient immunodiagnostic cocktail panel containing antibodies against PNL2, Melan-A, TRP-1, and TRP-2 that had 100% specificity and 93.9% sensitivity in identifying canine oral amelanotic melanocytic neoplasms. In addition, malignant melanomas are positive for vimentin and variably positive for S-100 protein and neuron-specific enolase (NSE) [42].

In order to use immunohistochemical techniques to study melanoma cell characteristics, it is frequently necessary to remove melanin from the histopathological specimen. There are several methods to do bleaching in melanoma cells, but the one described by Silva *et al.* [43] is one of the most effective, in which slides were immersed only in 10% hydrogen peroxide in pH 7.4 0.2 mol/L Tris-HCl buffer solution for 24 h in the dark at room temperature.

CANINE MELANOMA: MOLECULAR ASPECTS

Melanomas in humans seem to arise from normal melanocytes that suffer a number of molecular events that lead to their transformation. The progression from normal melanocytes to melanoma sometimes involves its transformation to melanocytic nevus. The genetic alterations involved in this progression are still under study. Several genes/genetic pathways were identified in human melanomas, and these are important for the diagnosis, establishment of prognosis, and drug targeting [44]. Some of these genes are described below:

- CDKN2A Locus—about 70% of melanomas harbor mutations or deletions in this locus on chromosome 9p21.
- Genes that are altered when normal melanocytes generate a nevus: BRAF, NRAS, and INK4a/ARF.

- Genes that are mutated or deregulated when a nevus is transformed to a melanoma: BRAF, NRAS, INK4a/ARF, PTEN, c-kit, NEDD9, and MITF.

Genetic alterations in canine malignant melanomas from mucosal or acral sites have not been fully described. Activating mutations in BRAF exon 15 have not been found [6,45]. Activating mutations of NRAS and c-kit appear to be absent in canine mucosal melanoma, in contrast to human mucosal melanoma, where these genes are mutated in 15% of tumors [44,46,47]. Further studies are necessary to understand the molecular basis of canine malignant melanomas.

Genetic alterations in canine malignant melanomas from human mucosal melanomas have not been fully studied (Table 2). Mutations in exon 15 of BRAF are not found [6], similar to human mucosal malignant melanoma [48]. Activating mutations of NRAS are presented in three of 77 cases [19] and c-kit appears absent in canine mucosal melanomas [49], in contrast to human mucosal melanoma, where these genes are mutated in 4% and 14% of tumors, respectively [50].

Table 2: Genes altered by mutations in canine and human mucosal malignant melanomas

	Human	Dog
BRAF	4% [50], 2% [48], 6% [14]	0% [6,19]
C-KIT	12.5% [16], 4% [50]	0% [49]
NRAS	22% [15], 14% [50], 10% [14]	6% [19]
PTEN	48.1% [15]	4% [19]
GNAQ	0% [16]	0% [19]
CDK4	0% [17]	0% [19]

In 2014, Gillard *et al.* [19] compared the histopathology and genetic alterations of canine and human melanomas. They observed that dog malignant melanomas present cytological characteristics similar to human melanoma simulating "nevus" and "animal type," suggesting a new melanoma classification. They also studied six genes in canine melanomas that are recurrent mutations in human melanomas, BRAF, NRAS, PTEN, KIT, GNAQ, and CDK4. In total, out of the 95 cases (77 oral and 18 cutaneous melanomas), no mutations were found in BRAF, KIT, GNAQ, and CDK4 genes; only three had a positive NRAS mutation and two had a PTEN gene mutation, of which one case had both changes [19]. BRAF mutations were seen in 57% of human cutaneous melanomas and NRAS was mutated in 17% of samples. Both changes were seen in 15.4% [51].

The low frequency of BRAF mutations associated with UV-independent carcinogenesis and oral anatomical distribution of canine melanomas supports the dog as a spontaneous model for investigation of non-UV-associated human melanomas [52].

Human and canine melanoma share differential gene expression patterns of MAPK, but similar sensitivity in cell culture to therapeutic inhibitors of MAPK (AZD6244) and PI3K/AKT (rapamycin) [6]. Dog malignant melanomas share numerous immunohistochemistry similarities (KIT, PTEN, and phosphorylated forms of AKT and ERK1/2) with human melanoma subtypes; particularly with mucosal, digital and ungual localizations that usually show high growth and aggressive behavior [5].

CANINE ORAL MELANOMAS

Melanoma is considered the most common oral malignancy in dogs [53], accounting for 14.4% to 45.5% of all oral tumors [54,55,56,57,58,59]. Some studies describe melanomas as the second most frequent oral cancer in dogs [54,56]. Oral malignant melanoma may also occur in cats and humans, but it is infrequent [60,61].

Malignant melanoma can be located in any portion of the oral cavity, but the gingival mucosa is the most common site [54,62]. The mandibular labial mucosa was the most common area, affected in 53% of cases, as described by Ramos-Vara *et al.* [11]. Although malignant melanoma rarely affects the tongue, it is considered the most common tumor type of this anatomic site as described by Dennis *et al.* [63], and large-breed dogs, particularly Chow Chow and Shar Pei, are at increased risk for malignant lingual melanoma [62,63].

Small-breed dogs and dogs with pigmented oral mucosa appear to be at increased risk for the development of oral malignant melanoma [61,62]. Cocker Spaniel, Poodle, Pekinese, Gordon Setter, Chow Chow, Golden Retriever, mixed-breed dogs, and Dachshund are the most commonly affected breeds [11,61]. Boxers and German Shepherds appear to be less affected by the disease, as described by Ramos-Vara *et al.* [11].

Dogs with oral malignant melanoma are usually 10.5 to 12 years old, with an average age of 11.4 years [11,54,61]. Males are supposed to be more predisposed to oral malignant melanomas, as verified by Todoroff *et al.* [54] and Vos *et al.* [55]; however, Ramos-Vara *et al.* [11], in a study of 328 dogs diagnosed with oral melanoma, and Teixeira *et al.* [13] found no such predisposition.

Oral malignant melanoma is a highly locally aggressive disease, with local invasion into bones occurring in 57% of lesions, with metastasis to regional lymph nodes (Figure 4) in 30.3% to 74% of cases, and to the lungs and other distant organs in 14% to 92% of affected dogs [11,61,64].

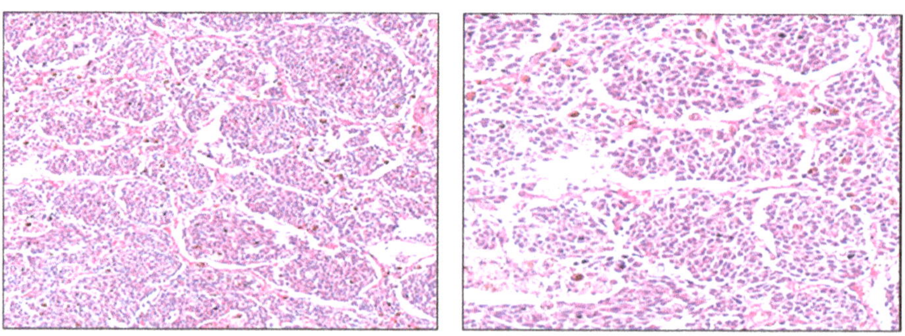

(A) (B)

Figure 4: Photomicrograph of lymph node metastasis from oral melanocytic neoplasm ((A), Objective 10x; (B), Objective 20x). Hematoxylin and eosin.

Melanoma is one of the few neoplasms in animals for which location is an important prognostic indicator [65]. The statement that all oral melanocytic neoplasms should be considered malignant is commonly found throughout the literature and has become dogma [41].

The prognosis for oral melanoma varies from favorable to unfavorable, with an overall median survival time (MST) of less than 36 months, depending on the intrinsic characteristics of the tumor, and the stage of the disease [61,66,67,68,69].

Historically, many studies confirm that oral and lip melanomas have a poorer prognosis when compared to skin melanomas. The differences concerning the results of different studies of lip melanomas are directly related to the real site of the tumor, that is, either in the skin or in the mucocutaneous junction. In one study, oral melanomas had an MST of 147 days, while the MST of melanoma of the lips and digits were 676 days and 725 days, respectively [18]. Large and poorly or non-pigmented tumors, necrosis, ulceration, high rate of cell proliferation (PCNA expression), and p53 expression are considered poor prognostic factors [29]. Amelanotic melanomas showed a significantly higher amount of mitotic cells when compared to melanotic melanomas [24]. The PCNA (proliferating cell nuclear antigen) in pigmented and non-pigmented melanomas was also assessed. It was demonstrated that cells of all samples stained positive for PCNA, confirming the proliferative activity of this tumor.

The World Health Organization (WHO) staging scheme for dogs with oral melanoma is based on the size of the tumor and the presence of regional and distant metastasis (Table 3) [70]. These staging systems are old and size is not considered a prognostic factor for malignant melanoma [18,28,36], but they are still cited in veterinary practice.

Dogs with stage I melanomas have tumors smaller than 2 cm in diameter, while dogs with stage II and III have tumors measuring between 2 to 4 cm, and more than 4 cm, respectively. Dogs with lymph node metastasis are also classified as stage III disease, and dogs with distant metastasis are classified as stage IV disease. Median survival times for dogs with oral melanoma treated with surgery are approximately 17–18 months, 5–6 months, and 3 months for stage I, II, and III disease, respectively [67].

In a study of 70 dogs with oral melanoma, Tuohy *et al.* [71] observed that 11.4% of dogs had mandibular lymph node metastasis and 1.4% of dogs had lung metastasis at the time of diagnosis. After 821 days (mean time of follow-up), 8.6% of mandibular lymph node metastasis, 17.1% of lung metastasis, 5.7% of metastasis to both sites, and 4.2% of metastasis to lung and other locations were observed. Williams *et al.* [64] reported that 70% of canines with melanomas had metastasis when lymphadenomegaly was present, and that 40% had metastasis in the absence of lymphadenomegaly. Harvey *et al.* [72] observed that dogs with untreated oral melanomas have a median survival time of 65 days.

Gillard *et al.* [19] performed clinical and histopathological analyses of 153 malignant canine melanomas with a four-year follow-up. These samples were histopathological characterization by human classification and showed that most canine tumors are intradermal and homologous to human nevocytoid (72%) type, animal type (16.5%), composite type (6.5%), pleomorphic type (4.5%), and superficial spreading melanoma type (0.5%) [19]. Figure 5 shows a representative histology of canine oral malignant melanoma on which local invasion, sparsely pigmented cells, and pleomorphism with variation in shape and cell or nuclear size can be seen.

Table 3: TNM classification of tumors in domestic animals, WHO, Geneva, 1980.

Clinical Staging System for Oral Tumor			
Primary Tumor (T)			
Tis	Tumor *in situ*		
T1	Tumor <2 cm in diameter at greatest dimension		
T1a	Without evidence of bone invasion		
T1b	With evidence of bone invasion		
T2	Tumor 2–4 cm in diameter at greatest dimension		
T2a	Without evidence of bone invasion		
T2b	With evidence of bone invasion		
T3	Tumor >4 cm in diameter at greatest dimension		
T3a	Without evidence of bone invasion		
T3b	With evidence of bone invasion		
Regional Lymph Nodes (N)			
N0	No regional lymph node metastasis		
N1	Movable ipsilateral lymph nodes		
N1a	No evidence of lymph mode metastasis		
N1b	Evidence of lymph mode metastasis		
N2	Movable contralateral lymph nodes		
N2a	No evidence of lymph mode metastasis		
N2b	Evidence of lymph mode metastasis		
N3	Fixed lymph nodes		
Metastasis (M)			
M0	No distance metastasis		
M1	Distance metastasis		
Stage Group	**Tumor (T)**	**Nodes (N)**	**Metastasis (M)**
I	T1	N0, N1a, N2a	M0
II	T2	N0, N1a, N2a	M0
III	T3	N0, N1a, N2a	M0
	Any T	N1b	M0
IV	Any T	N2b, N3	M0
	Any T	Any N	M0

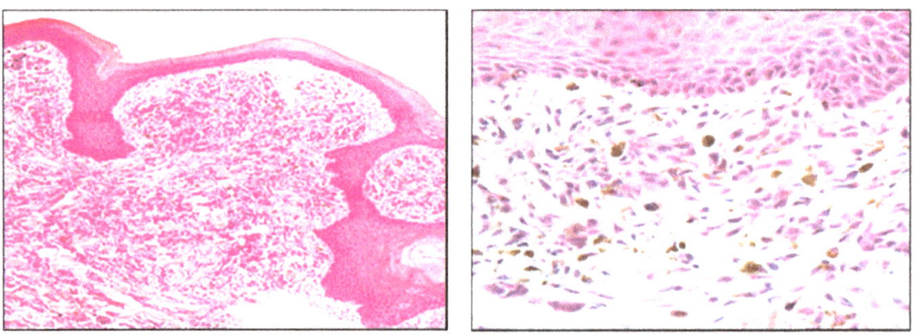

(A) (B)

Figure 5: Photomicrograph of oral melanocytic neoplasm ((A), Objective 4 ×; (B), Objective 40 ×); Hematoxylin and Eosin.

A recent study of over 382 canine oral melanomas did not find statistically significant differences in survival among different sites or mitotic indices [11].

CANINE OCULAR MELANOMAS

Ocular melanocytic tumors, benign or malignant, may occur in humans and domestic animals. These tumors may affect the eyelids, conjunctiva, orbit, limbo, and uvea [73,74]. Melanomas have different biological behaviors depending on the location in the eye [75]. In general, canine ocular melanomas are less aggressive than oral melanomas. Within the ocular melanoma group, the uveal melanoma is characterized by being more aggressive than the epibulbar melanoma [75].

Eyelid tumors in dogs are usually benign, such as sebaceous adenomas and sebaceous epitheliomas. Among all eyelid tumors, the melanocytic neoplasms account for 20%, and only 8% of these are melanomas [73]. Most, if not all, eyelid skin melanomas are benign [75]. Eyelid melanomas in dogs are usually pedunculated with nodular internal infiltration [73]. They are generally non-aggressive tumors, but occasionally some pigmented melanomas act aggressively and become locally invasive with the development of metastasis [73]. When compared to dogs, melanomas of the eyelid in humans carry a worse prognosis, especially when the tumor is located on the lid margin [76].

Conjunctival melanomas generally affect the nictitating membrane and the bulbar and/or eyelid conjunctiva [77]. Rottweilers and Cockers Spaniels are predisposed [74]. Lesions appear as dark, raised solid masses. Metastasis is rarely seen, but when it occurs it is typically associated with melanomas of the conjunctival eyelid. Complete surgical removal is warranted in early-diagnosed cases [77]. Due to the high risk of local recurrence, enucleation should be considered for invasive tumors [74]. Although conjunctival melanomas in humans are unusual, they have the potential to cause vision impairment and reduce life expectancy, with a mortality rate varying from 18% to 44% [74,78].

Canine and feline limbal melanomas have a benign biological behavior. They appear as raised, well-circumscribed heavily pigmented masses that arise from scleral and subconjunctival connective tissue melanocytes. Most of them develop slowly and are located closely to the superior aspect of the limbus. Labrador Retrievers are genetically predisposed [79].

Among the intraocular melanocytic tumors in the dog, melanocytomas are the most common tumors encountered, representing approximately 80% of the neoplasms. Melanomas account for only 20% of tumors [74]. It is difficult and unreliable to clinically differentiate between melanocytomas and melanomas, since melanocytomas can be locally aggressive and even invade the drainage angle and adjacent tissues [73,80]. Therefore, histopathological analysis is indispensable for a definitive diagnosis [81]. Despite the fact that melanocytomas are benign, when located in the iris, they can spontaneously cause necrosis and pigment dispersion, which may lead to obstruction of drainage and cause glaucoma in dogs and humans [82] (Figure 6).

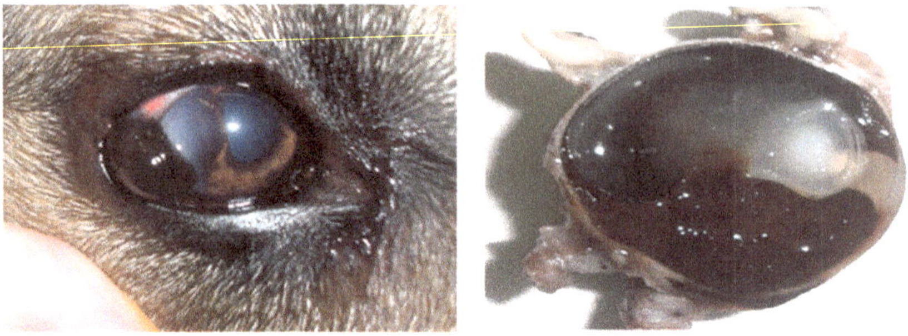

(A) (B)

Figure 6: Photographs showing: blackened mass in the iris with extraocular extension (A) and sagittal section of the eyeball revealing melanocytic neoplasia of iris, ciliary body, and choroid (B) (*Eduardo Perlmann*).

Melanocytomas most commonly affect the anterior uvea in dogs, but rarely affect the choroid [29]. When located in the uvea, they may cause several changes, such as intraocular hemorrhage, uveitis, and secondary glaucoma. Despite the fact that human intraocular melanocytomas are commonly located at the level of the optical disk or adjacent tissues, this location was never described in dogs [74]. An early diagnosis and rapid surgical treatment increase the chances of a favorable prognosis [83]. Wilcock *et al.* [75] studied 91 canine uveal melanocytic neoplasms, and only three developed metastatic disease. These data emphasize the low metastatic rate of uveal melanoma in dogs. Giuliano *et al.* [84], however, showed that animals affected by uveal melanomas had a lower life expectancy when compared with patients diagnosed with uveal melanocytomas. Tumors located in the uvea most frequently are consistent with primary neoplasia; however, animals presenting with intraocular-pigmented tumors should have a complete diagnostic work-up and physical exam to rule out metastasis [85].

In general, when tumors are only confined to the intraocular space, the recommended treatment is enucleation. Exenteration is indicated when the tumor extends to the extraocular space [83]. Other treatment options include iridectomy or diode laser photocoagulation in small-pigmented tumors of the iris [86]. There is no evidence that chemotherapy is effective in the treatment of ocular melanomas [87], but long-term follow-up evaluation would be needed. Ocular malignant melanoma had significantly shorter survival time than benign melanocytomas [84].

CANINE DIGITAL MELANOMAS

Melanoma is considered the second most common type of cancer of the digits in dogs [22,29,88]. Local invasion is a common feature of digital melanomas and 5%–58% of dogs with this disease have evidence of bone lysis [22,88,89,90]. Tumors of the footpad and interdigital region are less likely to invade into the bone [22,90]. Besides possible local invasion, regional and distant metastasis via lymphatics is frequently noted. It is estimated that 30%–40% of dogs have metastasis at the time of presentation and that even after appropriate local treatment with surgery, subsequent metastasis is frequently seen [22,88].

Due to its aggressive behavior, canine digital melanomas often require digital amputation. The median survival time for dogs without metastasis at the time of diagnosis treated with digital amputation is approximately 12 months, with 42%–57% of dogs surviving one year, and 11%–13% surviving two years [22,88,90,91].

Canine Cutaneous Melanomas

In contrast to digital melanomas, cutaneous melanomas typically have benign behavior in dogs, with the exception of melanomas that develop on the mucocutaneous junctions [18,92]. They account for 0.8%–2% of all canine cutaneous tumors [64] and are more commonly seen in dogs with heavily pigmented skin. Predisposed breeds include Scottish Terrier, Poodle, Golden Retriever, Dachshund, Cocker Spaniel, Miniature Poodle, Chow Chow, and Gordon Setter [93]. Benign skin melanomas are usually solitary, small, pigmented, firm, and freely moveable over deeper structures. Malignant melanomas tend to be fast-growing tumors, and often are ulcerated, and pigmented (grey, brown, or black) [21].

The most common sites for benign cutaneous melanomas are the face (near the eyelids), trunk, and extremities. Malignant melanoma is found most frequently on the head, ventral abdomen, and scrotum. When metastases occur, lymph nodes, followed by lungs, are the main organs involved [29].

Brockley *et al.* [94] studied 63 dogs diagnosed with melanomas at different locations. Surgery was performed in 24 cutaneous melanomas, with 88% of dogs alive a year after treatment.

Most dogs are cured with complete surgical excision, although some characteristics of the tumor, such as a mitotic index of ≥3/10 HPF, the presence of ≥20% of nuclear atypia, a Ki67 index ≥15%, ulceration, lymphatic invasion, and tumors extending beyond dermis, may have a negative influence on prognosis [18,41,92].

TREATMENT MODALITIES FOR CANINE MELANOMAS

Surgery

Surgery is the most common and main treatment option for local management of all melanomas, including oral [69], ocular [74], cutaneous, and digital melanomas [90,92]. Due to its high metastatic potential, systemic therapy should also be considered [61,62].

Tuohy *et al.* [71] studied 70 cases of canine oral malignant melanomas treated with curative intent surgery. Surgical resections were done with wide margins, including 2 to 3 cm of bone margins, and 1 cm of soft tissue margins. Histopathological analysis showed that 72.9% of tumors were completely excised, with 10% of these patients developing local tumor recurrence. In this study, dogs that had surgery as their sole treatment option had a progression-free interval (PFI) longer than 567 days, and an MST of 874 days. In a survey performed by Boston *et al.* [69], among wide-margin surgeries performed, 79.3% (73/92) were completely excised based on histologic evaluation, and the recurrence rate was 8.3% (6/73) in this group. The MST of these dogs was 354 days. Esplin [65] studied 61 dogs diagnosed with well-differentiated oral melanomas that were surgically excised, and reported an MST of 34 months with 3.2% of local recurrence.

Regional lymph node resection has been studied in maxillofacial tumors. The analysis of sentinel lymph nodes provides essential information regarding the clinical stage of disease, and also helps determine the appropriate treatment plan [95,96]. As previously shown, in a survey of 100 dogs with oral malignant melanoma, 53% had cytological or histopathological evidence of mandibular lymph node metastasis, even in normal sized nodes [64]. Therefore, regional lymph node removal is warranted, especially in dogs with oral melanomas.

Radiation Therapy

Radiation therapy is effective for malignant melanomas in dogs and may be useful for the control of local disease and involved regional lymph nodes [97]. Response rates are generally best for smaller tumors rather than for salvage therapy against large tumor burdens late in their clinical progression [98]. Another prognostic factor that appears to affect therapy outcome includes the presence of bone lysis. Proulx *et al.* [97] found that dogs without evidence of radiologic bone destruction experienced longer disease-free intervals and overall survival when compared to dogs with bone invasion.

Although melanoma has traditionally been viewed as a "radio-insensitive" disease, many studies suggest a significant role for radiation therapy in the treatment of melanoma [99]. Optimal fractionation schedules have not yet been established for canine malignant melanoma; however, hypofractionated protocols have been utilized with some success [93]. Overall response rates range from 82% to 94.4%, with the complete and partial resolution of tumors in 51% to 69% and 25% to 31% of cases, respectively [91,92,93,94,95,96,97,98,99,100,101,102]. The reported median time to progression ranges from 3.6 to 7.9 months with a median survival time varying from 5.3 to 11.9 months [97,98,100,101,102,103].

Chemotherapy alone has generally offered little benefit in terms of clinical outcome for the control of local canine melanomas; however, a few published studies have shown that the association of radiation with chemotherapy may potentially slow local progression and/or improve overall survival. Cancedda *et al.* [102] compared the efficacy of radiation therapy (5 × 6 Gy) alone and radiation therapy with post-radiation temozolamide (60 mg/m^2 PO for five consecutive days every 28 days) in dogs with measurable malignant melanoma. Dogs treated with temozolamide had a significantly longer median time to progression (6.8 months) than dogs treated only with radiation (3.6 months). Freeman *et al.* [103] retrospectively looked at dogs with incompletely resected oral melanoma treated with either cisplatin (10–30 mg/m^2 IV) or carboplatin (90 mg/m^2 IV) given once weekly 1 h before receiving radiation therapy (6 × 6 Gy). The reported median survival time was 11.9 months, representing the longest survival time when compared to the survival time previously reported for dogs with incompletely resected oral malignant melanoma [103]. Other studies combining radiation with chemotherapy agents, such as carboplatin, cisplatin, or melphalan, did not have a significant impact on either time to progression or overall survival [97,101,104].

Chemotherapy

Despite treating dogs with appropriate local therapies, such as surgery and/or radiation therapy, the ultimate cause of death, especially in oral melanomas, is metastasis. Therefore, the use of systemic therapies is typically recommended. Many chemotherapy protocols have been published in the veterinary literature with minimal improvement in survival times when compared to local treatment alone.

Many chemotherapy protocols using platinum agents have been studied. Rassnick *et al.* [104] reported an overall response rate of 28% using carboplatin as a single agent (300 to 350mg/m²/IV/ every 21 days) prior to surgery in dogs with oral (25/27) and cutaneous melanomas (2/27). Boria *et al.* [105] reported an overall response rate of 18% and a MST of 119 days using cisplatin (50 to 55 mg/m²/IV/ every three weeks) in combination with piroxicam (0.3 mg/kg/PO/24 hs) in oral melanomas.

Brockley *et al.* 2013 [94] evaluated the effect of carboplatin on the survival of 63 canine patients diagnosed with oral, cutaneous, or digital malignant melanomas. In this survey, carboplatin was administered at 300 mg/m² IV every 21 days for a total of 4–6 cycles. The addition of carboplatin after local therapy did not lead to a significant increase in survival times, and the anatomic site was significantly associated with survival. The overall median survival time for patients with oral, digital, and cutaneous melanomas were 389 days, 1350 days, with a median follow-up of 776 days, respectively.

In another survey, Dank *et al.* [106] compared the outcome of 17 dogs treated with surgery, adjuvant carboplatin (150 to 300 mg/m²/IV every three weeks), with or without radiation therapy. The MST was 387 days for the group treated with radiotherapy and 440 days for the group without the addition of radiotherapy.

In a comparative study reported by Tuohy *et al.* [71], surgery with or without any adjuvant therapy (carboplatin, cyclophosphamide as a metronomic therapy, radiotherapy, or xenogeneic canine melanoma vaccine) did not improve overall survival time in dogs with oral melanoma. The MST reported was 874 and 396 days for dogs that had surgery or surgery plus adjuvant therapy, respectively. Boston *et al.* [69] treated 151 dogs with oral melanoma and also concluded that there were no benefits in survival times among dogs that had surgery alone (MST of 335 days for 98 dogs) *versus* dogs that had surgery followed by systemic adjuvant therapy (MST of 352 for 53 dogs). Carboplatin, lomustine, dacarbazine, doxorubicin, metronomic chemotherapy, or commercial melanoma vaccine were the adjuvant therapies used in this study. Postoperative radiation therapy was associated with a longer survival time (MST of 1747 days), but was not significant in the multivariate analysis of this study.

Immunotherapy

Many researchers are currently using and developing therapies to activate the immune system of dogs. The immune responses by therapeutic vaccine represent a potential and powerful strategy for the treatment of melanomas [107]. There is wide evidence that the immune system could modulate the progression and metastasis of melanoma.

Many biological agents have the capacity to demonstrate antitumor activation, such as BCG, IFN-alpha, IL-2, and immunization activators, using an anticancer vaccine [108].

Bacillus Calmette–Guérin (BCG) is used intralesionally in melanomas to activate an immune response and induce tumor regression; however, there may be some complications, such as granulomas and hypersensitivity reactions [109].

Corynebacterium parvum is a bacterial substance that has antitumor activity in humans and canines with melanoma. MacEwen *et al.* [67] used *C. parvum* in dogs with stage II and III oral melanomas and compared the outcomes between surgical excision alone and surgery plus *C. parvum* immunotherapy. Animals who received *C. parvum* and surgery had a better prognosis than those with surgery only.

In rodents, dogs, and men, a liposome-encapsulad muramyl tripeptide phosphatidyl ethanolamine (L-MTP-PE), when used *in vivo*, actives monocytes and macrophages, resulting in antitumor activity, which can lead to melanoma metastasis tumor regression or at least stable disease. According to MacEwen *et al.* [108], when L-MTP-PE was used alone or in combination with GM-CSF the antitumor response was minimal, and only prolonged the survival time in dogs with stage I melanoma.

Bianco *et al.* [110], demonstrated that peripheral blood mononuclear cells with apoptotic melanoma cells significantly increased the antitumor immune response, leading to a reduction of the melanoma in three out of five dogs treated intralesionally with FasL-DNA.

Alexander *et al.* [111] used an allogeneic melanoma vaccine in combination with human a glycoprotein 100 (hgp 100), which is a xenogeneic melanoma protein. The vaccine was well tolerated in dogs, and the tumor response rate was 35% for six weeks (including complete response and stable disease).

Hogge *et al.* [112] used an autologous vaccine made of lysate cells transfected with GM-CSF in dogs with soft tissue sarcoma or melanoma. There was a large concentration of inflammatory cells at the site of vaccine administration, different from the ones that received a vaccine placebo only.

A xenogeneic human DNA-encoding tyrosinase protein vaccine (Oncept®) has been developed and used in dogs with stage II and III oral malignant melanoma [113]. This vaccine was generally well tolerated in a study of 111 dogs. No systemic reactions occurred, only local hematomas and pain at the injection site [114]. In another retrospective study, medical records from 45 dogs were reviewed, including 30 dogs with stage II and III disease, treated with the Oncept® vaccine after appropriate achievement of loco-regional cancer control. The review found that dogs that received the vaccine did not achieve a greater progression-free survival, disease-free interval, or median survival time than dogs that did not receive the vaccine [115].

The role of dendritic cells (DCs) as a biological adjuvant against malignant melanoma through the induction of an active immune response in the oncologic patient has been explored. Dendritic cells, as professional antigen-presenting cells with an ability to initiate the immune response, could therefore qualify for vaccination strategies to treat human or canine cancers. Compared with the human clinical trials using DC-based vaccines, reports of testing in dogs are scarce.

For humans, at least 13 clinical trials conducted in the United States have been registered using *ex vivo* autologous DCs [116] and, for dogs, only a few reports have been published to strengthen the rational use of DC vaccination for canine malignant melanoma [117,118]. Both protocols used bone marrow-derived DC of dogs with or without malignant melanoma. Gyorffy *et al.* [117] conducted a study using a few canine melanoma bearers and employed DC transduced with an adenovirus vector encoding a xenoantigen, human melanoma antigen gp100, as a coadjuvant of radiation therapy. One dog had an antigen-specific cytotoxic T lymphocyte (CTL) activity in peripheral blood lymphocytes, with no clinical signs, either locally or systemically, with melanoma recurrence 48 months after initial DC injection. However, another dog, which had a negative CTL activity, relapsed 22 months after vaccination. Tamura *et al.* [118], using an autologous DC pulsed with canine melanoma CMM2 cell lysate, efficiently elicited T cell-mediated immunity against CMM-2 cells *in vivo*, reinforcing the rationale to use DC as a therapeutic vaccine.

Although the immunotherapeutic approach using a DC vaccine to drive tumor-specific immune responses appears to be a promising strategy to control malignant melanoma, there are limitations, such as the cost of vaccine production for veterinary use as well as the very fragmentary designed strategies available.

Outcomes after Treatment

Table 4 describes the reported outcomes for canine oral malignant melanoma treated with different protocols.

Table 4: Outcomes for canine oral malignant melanoma after different therapeutic protocols

Summary of Treatment Outcome for Canine Oral Malignant Melanoma
Radiation Therapy (RT)
- Response Rate = 82%–94.4% - Local Recurrence = 11%–27% MST (Median Survival Time) = 5.3–11.9 months
References: Theon *et al.*, 1997 (98); Bateman *et al.*, 1994 (100); Murphy *et al.*, 2005 (101); Cancedda *et al.*, 2014 (102); Proulx *et al.*, 2003 (97); Freeman *et al.*, 2003 (103).
Surgery (SX) with Wide Margins
- Local Recurrence = 3.2%–10% - MST = 11.8–34 months
References: Tuohy *et al.*, 2014 (71); Boston *et al.*, 2014 (69); Esplin *et al.*, 2008 (65).
Chemotherapy (CT) for Macroscopic Disease
Carboplatin response rate = 28% - Cisplatin + piroxicam response rate = 18%
References: Rassnick *et al.*, 2001 (104); Boria *et al.*, 2004 (105).
Adequate Local Treatment + Systemic Therapy
- SX ± RT + adjuvant carboplatin: MST = 14.6 months - SX ± RT + adjuvant carboplatin, metronomic therapy, or melanoma vaccine: MST = 13.2 months (adjuvant therapy did not improve overall MST) - SX + adjuvant carboplatin, lomustine, dacarbazine, doxorubicin, or melanoma vaccine: MST = 11.7 months (adjuvant therapy did not improve overall MST) - RT + post-RT temozolamide: CT did not improve MST, but was associated with a longer median time to progression when compared to dogs treated with RT alone (6.8 months *versus* 2.6 months) - SX + RT + cisplatin or carboplatin once weekly 1 h before RT: MST = 11.9 months
References: Dank *et al.*, 2012 (106); Tuohy *et al.*, 2014 (71); Boston *et al.*, 2014 (69); Cancedda *et al.*, 2014 (102); Freeman *et al.*, 2003 (103).

Abbreviations: RT = radiotherapy, SX = surgery, CT = chemotherapy, MST = median survival time.

New Perspectives for the Treatment of Canine Melanomas

The aggressive nature of melanomas in canines and humans, with short survival times and minimal clinical outcome benefits after surgery and adjuvant therapy, emphasizes the importance of new studies to find an effective therapy for treatment and prevention of melanomas metastasis.

A canine therapeutic vaccine has been commercially available since 2007. The Merial melanoma vaccine for dogs (Oncept®) consists of DNA encoding the gene for the human melanocyte protein tyrosinase but apparently seems not to cure all melanoma cases. Published studies evaluating the survival times in dogs with melanoma in the mouth undergoing surgery and treatment with the Merial melanoma vaccine report average survival times of 599 days (20 months) or longer [113,114]. These results, though not from randomized studies, are promising and have prompted many veterinary oncologists to recommend the vaccine for patients with stage II and III melanoma despite the lack of FDA-standard clinical trials. The vaccine is well tolerated and has not been reported to be associated with side effects requiring medical intervention. In patients with very large and aggressive melanoma, there may not be sufficient time for an immune response to be mounted against the tyrosinase protein to prevent progression of the melanoma. In fact, 15% of patients treated with the vaccine reportedly die within three months of initiation of treatment, presumably due to the aggressive nature of the melanoma and insufficient time for the vaccine to be effective [119].

Lupeol [120] is among the new therapies under study. Lupeol is a triterpene extracted from various fruits and vegetables that reportedly inhibits melanoma cell proliferation *in vitro* and *in vivo*. A total of 11 dogs bearing buccal melanomas (three, five, and three dogs diagnosed with clinical stage I, II, and III melanoma, respectively) were evaluated. Subcutaneous lupeol (10 mg/kg) was administered postoperatively at various time points. Of the 11 subjects, seven exhibited no local recurrence 180 days postoperatively and no severe adverse effects were observed in any of these cases. Furthermore, no metastases have been detected during the period of the trial.

The current and promising immunotherapy to further augment the options for treatment in malignant melanomas, at least in humans, has been based on checkpoint–blocking antibodies, which can restore anticancer immune responses. Immune checkpoint molecules regulate the immune response avoiding autoimmunity and deleterious effects of an inflammatory response, but when expressed on tumors cells they work as a mechanism of immune evasion. Good examples of immune checkpoint molecules include PD-1 immune checkpoint inhibitor antibody (Pembrolizumab-humanized IgG4; Nivolumab- human IgG4), which was the first drug to gain FDA approval to a phase I trial in patients with BRAF inhibitor-resistant advanced melanoma and BRAFV600 mutation-positive melanoma [121]; and a checkpoint inhibitor (ipilimumab) directed against the cytotoxic T lymphocyte Antigen (CTLA-4). Data from clinical trials has demonstrated the important role this therapeutic approach can play—even with the development of immune-related side effects—since it has been proved a meaningful clinical improvement and an impressive increase in overall survival in melanoma patients [122] when compared to conventional chemotherapy. In the veterinary medicine field, the perspective of this therapy was described by Maekawa*et* *al.* [123], who demonstrated that an antibovine PD-L1 monoclonal antibody effectively blocked the binding of recombinant PD-1 with PD-L1-expressing tumor cells in a dose-dependent manner, including canine melanoma cells.

Other therapy as future treatment strategy for canine malignant melanoma can be based on oncolytic virotherapy. Basically, the virus infects and kills tumor cells when replication, lysis, and release of viruses occur. Tumor oncolysis by reovirus infection that was related in Ras-transformed cells was studied in six canine malignant melanoma cell lines CMeC1, CMeC2, KMeC, LMeC, CMGD2, and CMGD5. All of them were susceptible to reovirus infection, although Ras activation was not related in these cells, and only one of them (CMGD2) demonstrated more than 50% of cell death [124].

All efforts are geared toward better characterization of malignant melanomas in dogs, for the benefit of these companion animals, and also in an attempt to benefit the treatment of melanoma in humans.

CONCLUSIONS

Melanomas are very aggressive tumors and dogs are considered good models to study this disease. All efforts are geared toward better characterization and control of malignant melanomas in dogs, for the benefit of these companion animals, and also in an attempt to benefit the treatment of human melanomas.

ACKNOWLEDGMENTS

Karen Batschinski is the recipient of a fellowship from Fundação de Amparo a Pesquisa do Estado de São Paulo, FAPESP, Proc. Number 2013/16423-8. The authors are grateful to Jose Guilherme Xavier for supplying photos of canine melanomas.

AUTHOR CONTRIBUTIONS

Adriana Tomoko Nishiya, Claudia Ronca Felizzola, Eduardo Perlmann, Claudia Ronca Felizzola, Priscila Pedra Mendonça, Jéssica Soares Garcia, Tarso Felipe Teixeira, Maria Lucia Zaidan Dagli and Maria Lucia drafted the manuscript, Karen Batschinski, Marcello Vannucci Tedardi and the others revised the manuscript. All authors read and approved the final manuscript.

REFERENCES

1. Sweet, M.; Kirkham, N.; Bendall, M.; Currey, L.; Bythell, J.; Heupel, M. *PLoS ONE* 2012.
2. Starkey, M.P.; Scase, T.J.; Mellersh, C.S.; Murphy, S. Dogs really are man's best friend—Canine genomics has applications in veterinary and human medicine! *Brief. Funct. Genomic. Proteomic.* 2005, *4*, 112–128.
3. Paoloni, M.; Khanna, C. Translation of new cancer treatments from pet dogs to humans. *Nat. Rev. Cancer* 2008, *8*, 147–156. [Google Scholar]
4. Nowend, K.L.; Starr-Moss, A.N.; Murphy, K.E. The function of dog models in

developing gene therapy strategies for human health. *Mamm. Genome* 2011, *22*, 476–485.

5. Khanna, C.; Lindblad-Toh, K.; Vail, D.; London, C.; Bergman, P.; Barber, L.; Breen, M.; Kitchell, B.; McNeil, E.; Modiano, J.F.; *et al.* The dog as a cancer model. *Nat. Biotechnol.* 2006, *24*, 1065–1066.
6. Fowles, J.S.; Denton, C.L.; Gustafson, D.L. Comparative analysis of MAPK and PI3K/AKT pathway activation and inhibition in human and canine melanoma. *Vet. Comp. Oncol.* 2015, *13*, 288–304.
7. Haass, N.K.; Smalley, K.S.; Herlyn, M. The role of altered cell–cell communication in melanoma progression. *J. Mol. Histol.* 2004, *35*, 309–318.
8. Marcus, D.M.; Marcus, P.M.; Prabhu, R.S.; Owonikoko, T.K.; Lawson, D.H.; Switchenko, J.; Beither, J. Rising incidence of mucosal melanoma of the head and neck in the United States. *J. Skin Cancer* 2012, 231693.
9. Gavriel, H.; McArthur, G.; Sizeland, A.; Henderson, M. Review: Mucosal melanoma of the head and neck. *Melanoma Res.* 2011, *21*, 257–266.
10. Meleti, M.; Leemans, C.R.; De Bree, R.; Vescovi, P.; Sesenna, E.; van der Waal, I. Head and neck mucosal melanoma: Experience with 42 patients, with emphasis on the role of postoperative radiotherapy. *Head Neck* 2008, *30*, 1543–1551.
11. Ramos-Vara, J.A.; Beissenherz, M.E.; Miller, M.A.; Johnson, G.C.; Pace, L.W.; Fard, A.; Kottler, S.J. Retrospective study of 338 canine oral melanomas with clinical, histologic, and immunohistochemical review of 129 cases. *Vet. Pathol.*2000, *37*, 597–608.
12. Kimura, K.C.; Garate, A.P.; Dagli, M.L.Z. Retrospective study of neoplasms in domestic animals: A survey between 1993 and 2002 of the service of animal pathology, department of pathology, school of veterinary medicine and animal science, University of Sao Paulo, Southeast Brazil. *Braz. J. Vet. Pathol.* 2012, *5*, 60–69.
13. Teixeira, T.F.; Silva, T.C.; Cogliati, B.; Nagamine, N.K.; Dagli, M.L.Z. Retrospective study of melanocytic neoplasms in dogs and cats. *Braz. J. Vet. Pathol.* 2010, *3*, 100–104.
14. Omholt, K.; Grafström, E.; Kanter-Lewensohn, L.; Hansson, J.; Ragnarsson-Olding, B.K. KIT pathway alterations in mucosal melanomas of the vulva and other sites. *Clin. Cancer Res.* 2011, *17*, 3933–3942.
15. Zanoni, M.T.; Medicina, D.; Lombardi, D.; Ungari, M.; Balzarini, P.; Rossini, C.; Pellegrini, W.; Battaglia, P.; Capella, C.; Castelnuovo, P.; *et al.* Sinonasal mucosal melanoma: Molecular profile and therapeutic implications from a series of 32 cases. *Head Neck* 2013, *35*, 1066–1077.
16. Lyu, J.; Wu, Y.; Li, C.; Wang, R.; Song, H.; Ren, G.; Guo, W. Mutation scanning of BRAF, NRAS, KIT, and GNAQ/GNA11 in oral mucosal melanoma: A study of 57 cases. *J. Oral Pathol. Med.* 2015.
17. Curtin, J.A.; Fridlyand, J.; Kageshita, T.; Patel, H.N.; Busam, K.J.; Kutzner, H.; Cho, K.H.; Aiba, S.; Bröcker, E.B.; LeBoit, P.E.; *et al.* Distinct sets of genetic

alterations in melanoma. *N. Engl. J. Med.* 2005, *353*, 2135–2147.

18. Spangler, W.L.; Kass, P.H. The histologic and epidemiologic bases for prognostic consideration in canine melanocytic neoplasia. *Vet. Pathol.* 2006, *43*, 136–149.
19. Gillard, M.; Cadieu, E.; De Brito, C.; Abadie, J.; Vergier, B.; Devauchelle, P.; Degorce, F.; Dreano, S.; Primot, A.; Dorso, L.; *et al.* Naturally occurring melanomas in dogs as models for non-UV pathways of human melanomas. *Pigment Cell Melanoma Res.* 2014, *27*, 90–102.
20. Priester, W.A. Skin tumors in domesticated animals. Data from 12 United States and Canadian Colleges of Veterinary Medicine. *J. Natl. Cancer Insit.* 1973, *50*, 457–466.
21. Goldschmidt, M.H. Pigmented lesions of the skin. *Clin. Dermatol.* 1994, *12*, 507–514.
22. Marino, D.J.; Matthiesen, D.T.; Stefanacci, J.D.; Moroff, S.D. Evaluation of dogs with digit masses: 117 cases (1981–1991). *J. Am. Vet. Med. Assoc.* 1995, *207*, 726–728. [PubMed]
23. Miller, W.H.; Griffin, I.; Campbell, K.L. *Muller and Kirk's Small Animal Dermatology*, 7th ed.; Elsevier Mosby: St. Louis, MO, USA, 2013; pp. 774–843.
24. Teixeira, T.F.; Gentile, L.B.; Silva, T.C.; Mennecier, G.; Chaible, L.M.; Cogliati, B.; Roman, M.A.; Gioso, M.A.; Dagli, M.L.Z. Cell proliferation and expression of connexins differ in melanotic and amelanotic canine oral melanomas. *Vet. Res. Commun.* 2014, *38*, 29–38.
25. Tedardi, M.V.; Biondi, L.R.; Kimura, K.C.; Pedra Mendonça, P.; Grandi, F.; Latorre, A.M.; Dagli, M.L.Z. Comparative oncology in Sao Paulo, Brazil—What to learn from cancer registry. *Source J. Vet. Sci.* 2014, *1*, 1–8.
26. Tedardi, M.V.; Veneziano, D.B.; Kimura, K.C.; Pedra Mendonça, P.; Biondi, L.R.; Grandi, F.; Latorre, A.M.; Dagli, M.L.Z. Sao Paulo animal cancer registry, the first in Latin America. *Vet. Comp. Oncol.* 2015, *13*, 154–155.
27. Haass, N.K.; Ripperger, D.; Wladykowski, E.; Dawson, P.; Gimotty, P.A.; Blome, C.; Fischer, F.; Schmage, P.; Moll, I.; Brandner, J.M. Melanoma progression exhibits a significant impact on connexin expression patterns in the epidermal tumor microenvironment. *Histochem. Cell Biol.* 2010, *133*, 113–124.
28. Modiano, J.F.; Ritt, M.G.; Wojcieszyn, J. The molecular basis of canine melanoma: Pathogenesis and trends in diagnosis and therapy. *J. Vet. Intern. Med.* 1999, *13*, 163–174.
29. Smith, H.; Goldschmidt, H.; Mcmanus, P.M. A Comparative review of melanocytic neoplasms. *Vet. Pathol.* 2002, *39*, 651–678.
30. Dzutsev, A.; Goldszmid, R.S.; Viaud, S.; Zivtogel, L.; Trinchieri, G. The role of the microbiota in inflammation, carcinogenesis, and cancer therapy. *Eur. J. Immunol.* 2015, *45*, 17–31.
31. Goldschmidt, M.H.; Hendrick, M.J. Tumors of the skin and soft tissues. In *Tumors in Domestic Animals*, 4th ed.; Meuten, D.J., Ed.; Iowa State Press: Ames, IA, USA, 2002; pp. 78–82.

32. Scott, D.W.; Miller, W.H., Jr.; Griffin, C.E. *Muller & Kirk's Small Animal Dermatology*, 6th ed.; Elsevier Saunders: Philadelphia, PA, USA, 2001; pp. 1–70.

33. Li, G.; Herlyn, M. Dynamics of intercellular communication during melanoma development. *Mol. Med. Today* 2000, *6*, 163–169.

34. Chin, L. The genetics of malignant melanoma: Lessons from mouse and man. *Nat. Rev. Cancer* 2003, *3*, 559–570.

35. Gaggioli, C.; Sahai, E. Melanoma invasion—Current knowledge and future directions. *Pigment Cell Res.* 2007, *20*, 161–172.

36. Head, K.W.; Else, R.W.; Dubielzig, R.R. Tumors of the Alimentary Tract. In *Tumors in Domestic Animals*, 4th ed.; Meuten, D.J., Ed.; Iowa State Press: Ames, IA, USA, 2002; pp. 426–430.

37. Tajima, S.; Ura-Ishiko, A.; Hayashi, A. Melanogenesis, biosynthetic phenotype of fibronectin and collagen, and migrating activity in cloned B16 mouse melanoma cells. *J. Dermatol. Sci.* 1996, *12*, 24–30.

38. Simonetti, O.; Lucarini, G.; Brancorsini, D.; Nita, P.; Bernardini, M.L.; Biagini, G.; Offidani, A. Immunohistochemical expression of vascular endothelial growth factor, matrix metalloproteinase 2 and matrix metalloproteinase 9 in cutaneous melanocytic lesions. *Cancer* 2002, *95*, 602–624.

39. Nakhleh, R.E.; Wick, M.R.; Rocamora, A.; Swanson, P.E.; Dehner, L.P. Morphologic diversity in malignant melanomas. *Am. J. Clin. Pathol.* 1990, *93*, 731–740.

40. Chénier, S.; Doré, M. Oral Malignant Melanoma with Osteoid Formation in a Dog. *Vet. Pathol.* 1999, *36*, 74–76.

41. Smedley, R.C.; Spangler, W.L.; Esplin, D.G.; Kitchell, B.E.; Bergman, P.J.; Ho, H.Y.; Bergin, I.L.; Kiupel, M. Prognostic markers for canine melanocytic neoplasms: A comparative review of the literature and goals for future investigation. *Vet. Pathol.* 2011, *48*, 54–72.

42. Sandusky, G.E.; Carlton, W.W.; Wightman, K.A. Diagnostic immunohistochemistry of canine round cell tumors. *Vet. Pathol.* 1987, *24*, 495–499.

43. Silva, A.P.; Silva, R.G.; Cogliati, B.; Dias, A.S.M.; Le Bas, A.E.; Hernandez-Blazquez, F.J. Bleaching of melanin in the epidermis of South American fur seal and its application on enzyme immunohistochemistry. *Pesqui. Vet. Bras.* 2011, *31*, 267–270.

44. Fisher, D.E.; Kwong, L.N.; Chin, L. Melanoma. In *DeVita VT, Hellman and Rosenberg's Cancer Principles & Practice of Oncology*, 8th ed.; De Vita, V.T., Jr., Lawrence, T.S., Rosenberg, S.A., Eds.; Lippincott Williams & Wilkins: Philadelphia, PA, USA, 2008; pp. 1889–1951.

45. Shelly, S.; Chien, M.B.; Yip, B.; Kent, M.S.; Theon, A.P.; McCallan, J.L.; London, C.A. Exon 15 BRAF mutations are uncommon in canine oral malignant melanomas. *Mamm. Genome* 2004, *16*, 211–217.

46. Chu, P.Y.; Pan, S.L.; Liu, C.H.; Lee, J.; Yeh, L.S.; Liao, A.T. KIT gene exon 11 mutations in canine malignant melanoma. *Vet. J.* 2013, *196*, 226–230.

47. Curtin, J.A.; Busam, K.; Pinkel, D.; Bastian, B.C. Somatic activation of KIT in distinct subtypes of melanoma. *J. Clin. Oncol.* 2006, *24*, 4340–4346.

48. Maldonado, J.L.; Fridlyand, J.; Patel, H.; Jain, A.N.; Busam, K.; Kageshita, T.; Ono, T.; Albertson, D.G.; Pinkel, D.; Bastian, B.C. Determinants of BRAF mutations in primary melanomas. *J. Natl. Cancer Inst.* 2003, *95*, 1878–1890.

49. Murakami, A.; Mori, T.; Sakai, H.; Murakami, M.; Yanai, T.; Hoshino, Y.; Maruo, K. Analysis of KIT expression and KIT exon 11 mutations in canine oral malignant melanomas. *Vet. Comp. Oncol.* 2011, *9*, 219–224.

50. Zebary, A.; Jangard, M.; Omholt, K.; Ragnarsson-Olding, B.; Hansson, J. KIT, NRAS and BRAF mutations in sinonasal melanoma. *Br. J. Cancer* 2013, *109*, 559–564.

51. Goel, V.K.; Lazar, A.J.; Warneke, C.L.; Redston, M.S.; Haluska, F.G. Examination of mutations in BRAF, NRAS, and PTEN in primary cutaneous melanoma. *J. Investig. Dermatol.* 2006, *126*, 154–160.

52. Mochizuki, H.; Kennedy, K.; Shapiro, S.G.; Breen, M. BRAF Mutations in Canine Cancers. *PLoS ONE* 2015.

53. Bergman, P.J. Canine Oral Melanoma. *Clin. Tech. Small Anim. Pract.* 2007, *22*, 55–60.

54. Todoroff, R.J.; Brodey, R.S. Oral and pharyngeal neoplasia in the dog: A retrospective survey of 361 cases. *J. Am. Vet. Med. Assoc.* 1979, *175*, 567–571.

55. Vos, J.H.; Gaag, I.V.D. Canine and feline oral-pharyngeal tumours. *J. Vet. Med.* 1987, *34*, 420–427.

56. Guerra, J.L.; Dagli, M.L.; Godoy, L.F.; Birman, E.G. A retrospective study of oral neoplasms in dogs: A survey from 1941 to 1986. *Rev. Fac. Med. Vet. Zootec. Univ. S. Paulo* 1989, *26*, 207–212.

57. Stopiglia, A.J.; Felizzola, C.R.; Dagli, M.L.Z.; Xavier, J.G.; Guerra, J.L.; Birman, E. Estudo clínico e anátomo-patológico das formações neoplásicas e não neoplásicas da cavidade bucal de cães. *Comun. Cient. Fac. Med. Vet. Zootec. USP* 1992,*16*, 33–39

58. Ghirelli, C.D.O. In Biblioteca Digital USP. Available online: http://www.teses.usp.br/teses/disponiveis/10/10137/tde-22072008-090727/pt-br.php (assecced on 15 November 2015).

59. Requicha, J.F.M.F. Repositório Universidade de Trás-os-Montes e Alto Douro. Available online: https://repositorio.utad.pt/bitstream/10348/711/1/MsC_jfmfrequicha.pdf (accessed on 15 November 2015).

60. Bronden, L.B.; Eriksen, T.; Kristensen, A.T. Oral malignant melanomas and other head and neck neoplasms in Danish dogs-data from the Danish Veterinary Cancer Registry. *Acta Vet. Scand.* 2009, *51*, 1–6.

61. Liptak, J.M.; Withrow, S.J. Cancer of gastrointestinal tract. In *Small Animal Clinical Oncology*, 5th ed.; Withrow, S.J., Vail, D.M., Page, R.L., Eds.; Elsevier Saunders: St. Louis, MO, USA, 2013; pp. 381–395.

62. McEntee, M.C. Clinical behavior of nonodontogenic tumors. In *Oral and*

Maxillofacial Surgery in Dogs and Cats; Verstraete, F.J.M., Lommer, M.J., Eds.; Elsevier Saunders: Pennsylvania, PA, USA, 2012; pp. 387–402.

63. Dennis, M.; Ehrhart, N.; Duncan, C.; Barnes, A.; Ehrhart, E. Frequency of and risk factors associated with lingual lesions in dogs: 1196 cases (1995–2004). *J. Am. Vet. Med. Assoc.* 2006, *228*, 1533–1537.
64. Williams, L.E.; Packer, R.A. Association between lymph node size and metastasis in dogs with oral malignant melanoma: 100 cases (1987–2001). *J. Am. Vet. Med. Assoc.* 2003, *222*, 1234–1236.
65. Esplin, D.G. Survival of dogs following surgical excision of histologically well-differentiated melanocytic neoplasms of the mucous membranes of the lips and oral cavity. *Vet. Pathol.* 2008, *45*, 889–896.
66. White, R.A.S.; Jefferies, A.R.; Freedman, L.S. Clinical staging for oropharyngeal malignancies in the dog. *J. Small Anim. Pract.* 1985, *26*, 581–594.
67. MacEwen, E.G.; Patnaik, A.K.; Harvey, H.J.; Hayes, A.A.; Matus, R. Canine oral melanoma: Comparison of surgery*versus* surgery plus Corynebacterium parvum. *Cancer Investig.* 1986, *4*, 397–402.
68. Hahn, K.A.; Denicola, D.B.; Richardson, R.C.; Hahn, E.A. Canine oral malignant melanoma: Prognostic utility of an alternative staging system. *J. Small Anim. Pract.* 1994, *35*, 251–256.
69. Boston, S.E.; Lu, X.; Culp, W.T.N.; Montinaro, V.; Romanelli, G.; Dudley, R.M.; Liptak, J.M.; Mestrinho, L.A.; Buracco, P. Efficacy of systemic adjuvant therapies administered to dogs after excision of oral malignant melanomas: 151 cases (2001–2012). *J. Am. Vet. Med. Assoc.* 2014, *245*, 401–407.
70. Owen, L.N. *TNM Classification of Tumours in Domestic Animals*; World Health Organization: Geneve, Switzerland, 1980.
71. Tuohy, J.L.; Selmic, L.E.; Worley, D.R.; Ehrhart, N.P.; Withrow, S.J. Outcome following curative-intent surgery for oral melanoma in dogs: 70 cases (1998–2011). *J. Am. Vet. Med. Assoc.* 2014, *245*, 1266–1273.
72. Harvey, H.J.; MacEwen, E.G.; Braun, D.; Patnaik, A.K.; Withrow, S.J.; Jongeward, S. Prognostic criteria for dogs with oral melanoma. *J. Am. Vet. Med. Assoc.* 1981, *178*, 580–582.
73. Mould, J.R.B.; Petersen-Jones, S.M.; Peruccio, C.; Ratto, A.; Sassani, J.W.; Harbour, J.W. Uveal melanocytic tumors. In*Ocular Tumors in Animals and Humans*; Peiffer, R.L., Jr., Simons, K.B., Eds.; Iowa State Press: Ames, IA, USA, 2002; pp. 225–282.
74. Dubielzig, R.R.; Ketring, K.L.; Mclellan, G.J.; Albert, D.M. *Veterinary Ocular Pathology: A Comparative Review*; W.B. Saunders: Philadelphia, PA, USA, 2010; p. 472.
75. Wilcock, B.P.; Peiffer, J.R. Morphology and behavior of primary ocular melanomas in 91 dogs. *Vet. Pathol.* 1986, *23*, 418–424.
76. Garner, A.; Koornneef, L.; Levene, A.; Collin, J.R. Malignant melanoma of the eyelid skin: Histopathology and behaviour. *Br. J. Ophthalmol.* 1985, *69*, 180–186.

77. Conceição, L.F.; Ribeiro, A.P.; Piso, D.Y.T.; Laus, J.L. Considerations about ocular neoplasia of dogs and cats. *Cienc. Rural* 2010, *40*, 2235–2242.

78. Lim, L.A.; Madigan, M.C.; Conway, R.M. Conjunctival melanoma: A review of conceptual and treatment advances.*Clin. Ophthalmol.* 2013, *7*, 521–531.

79. Donaldson, D.; Sansom, J.; Scase, T.; Adams, V.; Mellersh, C. Canine Limbal melanoma: 30 cases (1992–2004). Part 1. Signalment, clinical and histological features and pedigree analysis. *Vet. Ophthalmol.* 2006, *9*, 115–119.

80. Perlmann, E.; Barros, P.S.M.; Fernandez, L.; Di Cesare, S.; Bakalian, S.; Burnier, M.N., Jr. Histopathological evaluation of pigmented intraocular tumors in dogs. *Investig. Ophthalmol. Vis. Sci.* 2010, *5*, 5159.

81. Esson, D.; Fahrer, C.; Zarfoss, M.K.; Dubielzig, R.R. Suspected uveal metastasis of a nail bed melanoma in a dog. *Vet. Ophthalmol.* 2007, *10*, 262–266.

82. Fineman,M.S.;Eagle,R.C.;Shields,J.A.;Shields,C.L.;Potter,P.Melanocytomalytic glaucoma in eyes with necrotic iris melanocytoma. *Ophthalmology* 1998, *105*, 492–496.

83. Ryan, A.M.; Diters, R.W. Clinical and pathologic features of canine ocular melanomas. *J. Am. Med. Assoc.* 1984, *184*, 60–67.

84. Giuliano, E.A.; Chappell, R.; Fischer, B.; Dubielzig, R.R. A matched observational study of canine survival with primary intraocular melanocytic neoplasia. *Vet. Ophthalmol.* 1999, *2*, 185–190.

85. Konrade, K.A.; Hoffman, A.; Schubert, C.S.; Dubielzig, R.R. A histologic series of secondary uveal melanomas in eleven dogs. In Proceedings of the 40th Annual Meeting of the American College of Veterinary Ophthalmologist, Chicago, IL, USA, 4–7 November 2009.

86. Willis, A.M.; Wilkie, D.A. Ocular oncology. *Clin. Tech. Small Anim. Pract.* 2001, *16*, 77–85.

87. Cazalot, G., Raymond-Letron, I.; Regnier, A. Choroidal melanoma presented as glaucoma in a dog: Case report and review of the literature. *Rev. Med. Vet.* 2008, *159*, 74–78.

88. Henry, C.J.; Brewer, W.G.; Whitley, E.M.; Tyler, J.W.; Ogilvie, G.K.; Norris, A.; Fox, L.E.; Morrison, W.B.; Hammer, A.; Vail, D.M.; *et al.* Canine digital tumors: Veterinary cooperative oncology group retrospective study of 64 dogs. *J. Vet. Intern. Med.* 2005, *19*, 720–724.

89. Aronsohn, M.G.; Carpenter, J.L. Distal extremity melanocytic nevi an malignant melanomas in dogs. *J. Am. Anim. Hosp. Assoc.* 1990, *26*, 605–612.

90. Wobeser, B.K.; Kidney, B.A.; Powers, B.E.; Withrow, S.J.; Mayer, M.N.; Spinato, M.T.; Allen, A.L. Diagnosis and clinical outcomes associated with surgically amputated canine digit submitted to multiple veterinary diagnostic laboratories. *Vet. Pathol.* 2007, *44*, 355–361.

91. Manley, C.A.M.; Leibman, N.F.; Wolchok, J.D.; Riviere, I.C.M.; Bartido, S.; Craft, D.M.; Bergman, P.J. Xenogeneic Murine Tyrosinase DNA Vaccine for Malignant Melanoma of the Digit of Dogs. *J. Vet. Intern. Med.* 2011, *25*, 94–99.

92. Bostock, D.E. Prognosis after surgical excision of canine melanoma. *Vet. Pathol.* 1979, *16*, 32–40.

93. Bergman, P.J.; Kent, M.S.; Farese, J.P. Melanoma. In *Small Animal Clinical Oncology*, 5th ed.; Withrow, S.J., Vail, D.M., Page, R.L., Eds.; Elsevier Saunders: St. Louis, MO, USA, 2013; pp. 321–334.

94. Brockley, L.K.; Cooper, M.A.; Bennett, P.F. Malignant melanoma in 63 dogs (2001–2011): The effect of carboplatin chemotherapy on survival chemotherapy on survival. *N. Z. Vet. J.* 2013, *61*, 25–31.

95. Smith, M.M. Surgical approach for lymph node staging of oral and maxillofacial neoplasms in dogs. *J. Am. Anim. Hosp. Assoc.* 1995, *31*, 514–518.

96. Herring, E.S.; Smith, M.M.; Robertson, J.L. Lymph node staging of oral and maxillofacial neoplasms in 31 dogs and cats. *J. Vet. Dent.* 2002, *19*, 122–126.

97. Proulx, D.R.; Ruslander, D.M.; Dodge, R.K.; Hauck, M.L.; Williams, L.E.; Horn, B.; Price, G.S.; Thrall, D.E. A retrospective analysis of 140 dogs with oral melanoma treated with external beam radiation. *Vet. Radiol. Ultrasound.*2003, *44*, 352–359.

98. Théon, A.P.; Rodriguez, C.; Madewell, B.R. Analysis of prognostic factors and patterns of failure in dogs with malignant oral tumors treated with megavoltage irradiation. *J. Am. Vet. Med. Assoc.* 1997, *210*, 778–784.

99. Khan, N.; Mohammad, K.K.; Almasan, A.; Singh, A.D.; Macklis, R. The evolving role of radiation therapy in the management of malignant melanoma. *Int. J. Radiat. Oncol. Biol. Phys.* 2011, *80*, 645–654.

100. Bateman, K.E.; Catton, P.A.; Pennock, P.W.; Kruth, S.A. 0-7-21 radiation therapy for the treatment of canine oral melanoma. *J. Vet. Intern. Med.* 1994, *8*, 267–272.

101. Murphy, S.; Hayes, A.M.; Blackwood, L.; Maglennon, G.; Pattinson, H.; Sparkes, A.H. Oral malignant melanoma: The effect of coarse fractionation alone or with adjuvant carboplatin therapy. *Vet. Comp. Oncol.* 2005, *3*, 222–229.

102. Cancedda, S.; Bley, C.R.; Aresu, L.; Dacasto, M.; Leone, V.F.; Pizzoni, S.; Gracis, M.; Marconato, L. Efficacy and side effects of radiation therapy in comparison with radiation therapy and temozolomide in the treatment of measurable canine malignant melanoma. *Vet. Comp. Oncol.* 2014.

103. Freeman, K.P.; Hahn, K.A.; Harris, F.D.; King, G.K. Treatment of dogs with oral melanoma by hypofractionated radiation therapy and platinum-based chemotherapy (1987–1997). *J. Vet. Intern. Med.* 2003, *17*, 96–101.

104. Rassnick, K.M.; Ruslender, D.M.; Cotter, S.M.; Al-Sarraf, R.; Bruyette, D.S.; Gamblin, R.M.; Meleo, K.A.; Moore, A.S. Use of carboplatin for treatment of dogs with malignant melanoma: 27 cases (1989–2000). *J. Am. Vet. Med. Assoc.* 2001,*218*, 1444–1448.

105. Boria, P.A.; Murry, D.J.; Bennett, P.F.; Glickman, N.W.; Snyder, P.W.; Merkel, B.L.; Schlittler, D.L.; Mutsaers, A.J.; Thomas, R.M.; Knapp, D.W. Evaluation of cisplatin combined with piroxicam for the treatment of oral malignant melanoma and oral squamous cell carcinoma in dogs. *J. Am. Vet. Med. Assoc.* 2004, *224*,

388–394.

106. Dank, G.; Rassnick, K.M.; Sokolovsky, Y.; Garrett, L.D.; Post, G.S.; Kitchell, B.E.; Sellon, R.K.; Kleiter, M.; Northrup, N.; Segev, G. Use of adjuvant carboplatin for treatment of dogs with oral malignant melanoma following surgical excision. *Vet. Comp. Oncol.* 2014, *12*, 78–84.

107. Bergman, P.J.; Mcknight, J.; Novosad, A.; Charney, S.; Farrelly, J.; Craft, D.; Wulderk, M.; Jeffers, Y.; Sadelain, M.; Hohenhaus, A.E.; *et al.* Long-term survival of dogs with advanced malignant melanoma after DNA vaccination with xenogeneic human tyrosinase: A phase I trial. *Clin. Cancer Res.* 2003, *9*, 1284–1290.

108. MacEwen, E.G.; Kurzman, I.D.; Vail, D.M.; Dubielzig, R.R.; Everlith, K.; Madewell, B.R.; Rodriguez, C.O., Jr.; Phillips, B.; Zwahlen, C.H.; Obradovich, J.; *et al.* Adjuvant therapy for melanoma in dogs: Results of randomized clinical trials using surgery, liposome-encapsulated muramyl triptide, and granulocyte macrophage colony-stimulang factor. *Clin. Cancer Res.* 1999, *5*, 4249–4258.

109. Moff, S.L.; Corey, G.R.; Gottfredsson, M. Distant cutaneous granulomas after bacille Calmette-Guérin immunotherapy for malignant melanoma: Case for direct infection. *Clin. Infect. Dis.* 1999, *29*, 1569–1570.

110. Bianco, S.R.; Sun, J.; Fosmire, S.P.; Hance, K.; Padilla, M.L.; Ritt, M.G.; Getzy, D.M.; Duke, R.C.; Withrow, S.J.; Lana, S.;*et al.* Enhancing anti melanoma immune responses through apoptosis. *Cancer Gene Ther.* 2003, *10*, 726–736.

111. Alexander, A.N.; Huelsmeyr, M.K.; Mitzey, A.; Dubielzig, R.R.; Kurzman, I.D.; MacEwen, E.G.; Vail, D.M. Development of an allogenic whole-cell tumor vaccine expressing xenogenic gp100 and implementation in phase II clinical trial in canine patients with malignant melanoma. *Cancer Immunol. Immunother.* 2006, *55*, 433–442.

112. Hogge, G.S.; Burkholder, J.K.; Culp, J.; Albertini, M.R.; Dubielzig, R.R.; Keller, E.T.; Yang, N.S.; MacEwen, E.G. Development of human granulocyte-macrophage colony-stimulating factor- transfected tumor cell vaccines for treatment of spontaneous canine cancer. *Hum. Gene Ther.* 1998, *9*, 1851–1861.

113. Bergman, P.J.; Wolchok, J.D. Of mice and men (and dogs): Development of a xenogeneic DNA vaccine for canine oral malignant melanoma. *Cancer Ther.* 2008, *6*, 817–826.

114. Grosenbaugh, D.A.; Leard, A.T.; Bergman, P.J.; Klein, M.K.; Meleo, K.; Susaneck, S.; Hess, P.R.; Jankowski, M.K.; Jones, P.D.; Leibman, N.; *et al.* Safety and efficacy of a xenogeneic DNA vaccine encoding for human tyrosinase as adjunctive treatment for oral malignant melanoma in dogs following surgical excision of the primary tumor. *Am. J. Vet. Res.* 2011, *72*, 1631–1638.

115. Ottnod, J.M.; Smedley, R.C.; Walshaw, R.; Hauptman, J.G.; Kiupel, M.; Obradovich, J.E. A retrospective analysis of the efficacy of Oncept vaccine for the adjunct treatment of canine oral malignant melanoma. *Vet. Comp. Oncol.* 2013, *11*, 219–229.

116. Rotte, A.; Bhandaru, M.; Zhou, Y.; Mcelwee, K.J. Immunotherapy of melanoma:

Present options and future promises. *Cancer Metastasis Rev.* 2015, *34*, 115–128.

117. Gyorffy, S.; Rodriguez-Lecompte, J.C.; Woods, J.P.; Foley, R.; Kruth, S.; Liaw, P.C.; Gauldie, J. Bone marrow-derived dendritic cell vaccination of dogs with naturally occurring melanoma by using human gp100 antigen. *J. Vet. Intern. Med.* 2005, *19*, 56–63.
118. Tamura, K.; Yamada, M.; Isotani, M.; Arai, H.; Yagihara, H.; Ono, K.; Washizu, T.; Bonkobara, M. Induction of dendritic cell-mediated immune responses against canine malignant melanoma cells. *Vet. J.* 2008, *175*, 126–129.
119. Elmslie, R. VRCC Veterinary Speciality & Emergency Hospital. Available online: http://www.vetcancerspecialists.com/blog/2013/1/31/the-controversy-surrounding-the-melanoma-vaccine-for-dogs/ (accesse on 15 November 2015).
120. Yokoe, I.; Azuma, K.; Hata, K.; Mukaiyama, T.; Goto, T.; Tsuka, T.; Imagawa, T.; Itoh, N.; Murahata, Y.; Osaki, T.; *et al.* Clinical systemic lupeol administration for canine oral malignant melanoma. *Mol. Clin. Oncol.* 2015, *3*, 89–92.
121. Robert, C.; Ribas, A.; Wolchok, J.D.; Hodi, F.S.; Hamid, O.; Kefford, R.; Weber, J.S.; Joshua, A.M.; Hwu, W.J.; Gangadhar, T.C.; *et al.* Anti-programmed-death-receptor-1 treatment with pembrolizumab in ipilimumab-refractory advanced melanoma: A randomised dose-comparison cohort of a phase 1 trial. *Lancet* 2014, *384*, 1109–1117.
122. Schadendorf, D.; Hodi, F.S.; Robert, C.; Weber, J.S.; Margolin, K.; Hamid, O.; Patt, D.; Chen, T.T.; Berman, D.M.; Wolchok, J.D. Pooled analysis of long-term survival data from phase II and phase III trials of ipilimumab in unresectable or metastatic melanoma. *J. Clin. Oncol.* 2015, *33*, 1889–1894.
123. Maekawa, N.; Konnai, S.; Ikebuchi, R.; Okagawa, T.; Adachi, M.; Takagi, S.; Kagawa, Y.; Nakajima, C.; Suzuki, Y.; Murata, S.; *et al.* Expression of PD-L1 on canine tumor cells and enhancement of IFN-c production from tumor infiltrating cells by PD-L1 blockade. *PLoS ONE* 2014.
124. Igase, M.; Hwang, C.C.; Coffey, M.; Okuda, M.; Noguchi, S.; Mizuno, T. The oncolytic effects of reovirus in canine solid tumor cell lines. *J. Vet. Med. Sci.* 2015, *77*, 541–548.

7
CHAPTER

UNDERSTANDING THE OSTEOSARCOMA PATHOBIOLOGY: A COMPARATIVE ONCOLOGY APPROACH

Jyotika Varshney, Milcah C. Scott , David A. Largaespada and Subbaya Subramanian

Keywords: Osteosarcoma, comparative oncology, microRNAs, prognosis, canine osteosarcoma

INTRODUCTION

Osteosarcoma is an aggressive primary bone tumor most prevalent in human patients. It mostly occurs during adolescence, with a second peak at middle age (older than 40) [1,2]. The tumor is characterized by increased production of osteoid (abnormal bone matrix) and by exceptionally complex karyotypes [3,4]. While the target cell for malignant transformation in the formation of osteosarcoma is not known with certainty, it is thought to be a mesenchymal stem cell (MSC) or a cell committed to the osteoblast lineage [5]. Evidence from mouse models indicates that any of several cell stages could serve as target cells for osteosarcoma development [6]. There are three common histologic types of osteosarcoma: osteoblastic, where tumor cells produce large amounts of tumor osteoid; chondroblastic, where tumor cells produce chondroid (cartilage) in addition to some amount of tumor osteoid; and fibroblastic, where tumor cells are predominantly fibroblasts and can produce both collagen and tumor osteoid [7]. The disease is highly metastatic, with distant spread mostly to lungs and other sites

---

Citation: Jyotika Varshney, Milcah C. Scott, David A. Largaespada and Subbaya Subramanian, Understanding the Osteosarcoma Pathobiology: A Comparative Oncology Approach, doi:10.3390/vetsci3010003.

in bone, but osteosarcoma can also metastasize to lymph nodes and intra-abdominal organs [8,9]. The metastatic pattern (lungs, bones, lymph nodes) is similar for dogs and humans [10]. Osteosarcoma may present with macroscopic metastatic disease or metastatic disease can occur after therapy. In either case, prognosis is significantly worse once metastasis has been detected [11,12].

In canine patients, osteosarcoma is a disease primarily of adult dogs; the median age at diagnosis is approximately eight years, with a small peak of incidence in young animals (younger than 3 years) [10,13]. This differs from the situation in human patients where the peak age of incidence is in adolescence. Nevertheless, the natural history of the disease is similar in canine and human osteosarcoma patients [14]. Moreover, we have observed that genome wide expression profiles of canine osteosarcoma are indistinguishable from human pediatric osteosarcoma and more like human osteosarcoma than any other human cancer [14,15]. In dogs, there is generally a strong breed preference in the risk for cancer, such as osteosarcoma [16,17]. Many large breed dogs have an increased risk for osteosarcoma compared to other breeds [4,18,19]. The genetic determinants of osteosarcoma susceptibility in dogs are not fully elucidated, and it is possible that these factors will also be important in human osteosarcoma susceptibility. The development of treatment strategies in dogs and people has proven mutually beneficial for both species [20]. In fact, current treatment options are similar in both species.

Osteosarcoma is treated using surgery, radiation and chemotherapy. Surgical techniques have greatly improved with time, and in many cases limb salvage is feasible with low rates of local recurrence in humans [21]. Combination chemotherapies are vital for effective treatment of osteosarcoma [22]. However, despite decades of effort, nothing better than the most often used combination of three chemotherapeutic agents (*i.e.*, methotrexate, doxorubicin and cisplatin) has been found [22].The adjuvant chemotherapy is generally administered prior to surgery and, according to many studies, the extent of necrosis observed in the primary tumor after surgical removal is correlated with the outcome. [21]. The goal of the adjuvant chemotherapy is to eliminate the micrometastases that are thought to be present in >80% of all patients at the time of diagnosis, thus preventing relapse [1]. New research is underway to define specific molecular targets that could be utilized to treat this disease, but their elucidation has been proven difficult. It is possible that osteosarcoma may also be treated using recently developed immunotherapies, such as immune checkpoint blockade or chimeric antigen receptor-engineered T cells [21].

Osteosarcoma is characterized by aneuploidy and extensive genetic instability [23]. Due to this extreme genetic instability, common causes of osteosarcoma development have largely been limited to implicating loss of *RB* and *TP53* regulated cellular activities and upregulation of *MYC* transcriptional activity reviewed by Morrow *et al.* [24]. Beyond these, few alterations are common or well accepted as osteosarcoma drivers. Gene amplification and protein overexpression of the*RUNX2* transcription factor, which is a regulator of bone renewal, has been proposed to drive osteosarcoma [25]. Conflicting data on activation of beta-catenin dependent transcription in osteosarcoma has been reported [26]. In addition, TGF-β signaling has been proposed to promote the acquisition of metastatic disease [27]. Notable, expression of Ezrin at high levels has been found in metastatic human and canine osteosarcoma and functionally validated in model systems as a driver of osteosarcoma metastasis [28]. Recently, a large scale *Sleeping Beauty* (SB) transposon-based forward genetic screen was carried out for osteosarcoma in mice [29]. From this screen, a large number of new candidate osteosarcoma proto-oncogene and tumor suppressors were reported. These included the candidate oncogenes *SEMA4D* and *SEMA6D*, which were partially functionally validated as well as tumor suppressors like *NF1*, *NF2* and *PTEN* [29]. Beyond protein encoding genes, several micro RNAs (miRNAs) and miRNA clusters have been suggested as drivers or suppressors of osteosarcoma development and progression [30]. What remains unclear is which common oncogenic drivers for osteosarcoma should be targeted and how they would be targeted. Unlike the case for other malignancies, osteosarcoma is genetically heterogeneous and common molecular targets may not be present.

Osteosarcoma is much more common in dogs than in people (greater than 15 times) and can be experimentally induced in mice via transgenesis. Perceivably, the opportunity to study osteosarcoma in three different species may make it possible to identify core genes and pathways, whose alterations are central to the osteosarcoma phenotype and that would make good targets for therapy. In the past, the main challenges were the development of improved surgical techniques for limb salvage, prevention of local recurrence and the identification of effective combination chemotherapies. Currently, a major pressing need is the development of new therapies to prevent the outgrowth of metastatic disease and to treat it once it has occurred. It is possible that germline or somatic mutations or tumor gene expression signatures identified through multi-species approaches could help predict which patients will respond well to current treatment regimes and which need to be referred for more intensive therapy or follow-up screening. However, much remains to be learned about what allows microscopic osteosarcoma lesions to resist chemotherapy and to suddenly break tumor dormancy and form a macroscopic mass. Until these questions are answered, we are not fully capable to help many human and canine osteosarcoma patients.

This review is an attempt to address many of the unanswered questions pertaining to osteosarcoma by focusing on recently acquired knowledge from a multi-species approach.

HUMAN OSTEOSARCOMA

Osteosarcoma in human patients is a rare tumor with a peak incidence in the second decade of life. The incidence is roughly 25 cases per 10 million per year in the United States [31]. A second wave of osteosarcoma is diagnosed in individuals between 70 and 80 years of age, often in association with Paget's disease. Paget's disease is an abnormality of bone homeostasis in which excessive bone reabsorption and reformation occur. Genetic and viral origins of Paget's disease have been suggested. While osteosarcoma is a rare manifestation of the disease, risk for osteosarcoma is increased. Osteosarcoma can occur in nearly any part of the skeleton, but commonly affects one of the long bones. As it occurs during a period of intense bone growth, there may be an association between this growth and sensitivity to osteoblast transformation [31]. Indeed, children with osteosarcoma are on average tall for their age [32]. Genetic studies also have suggested an association between the inheritance of certain forms of growth control genes and risk for osteosarcoma [33]. Other risk factors for human osteosarcoma include prior radiation therapy, male gender, and possibly African ancestry [34,35]. A genome-wide association study (GWAS) revealed possible risk alleles in the glutamate receptor, metaotropic 4 (*GRM4*) gene and a gene desert at chromosome 2p25.2 [36]. A recent GWAS also identified a potential high-risk allele for osteosarcoma metastasis at presentation within the transcriptional activator *NFIB* [37], a gene that was also identified as a potential tumor/metastasis suppressor in a transposon-based genetic screen in mice [29].

Some rare inherited cancer predisposition syndromes increase the risk for osteosarcoma. These rare cancers include Li-Fraumeni syndrome, hereditary retinoblastoma and Rothman-Thompson syndrome caused by germline mutations in *TP53, RB1*, and *RECQL4*, respectively [38]. Certain other cancer predisposition syndromes also seem to increase the risk of osteosarcoma development including Neurofibromatosis Type 1 syndrome, Werner's syndrome and Diamond-Blackfan anemia [24]. Patients with hereditary multiple osteochondromas, due to inheritance of mutations in the *EXT1* or *EXT2*genes, are predisposed to development of osteosarcoma also [24].

Human osteosarcoma is typically diagnosed due to swelling and pain often in the limbs. This can cause a limp if the involved limb is a leg or immobility of a joint. Pain may be constant or associated with exertion. In rare cases osteosarcoma will trigger a bone fracture. Diagnosis is made following a complete medical exam and imaging studies. Often an X-ray is done, followed by positron emission tomography or a bone scan. As osteosarcoma can often metastasize to the lungs, lung X-rays are utilized. A definitive diagnosis requires a biopsy. Staging of osteosarcoma is controversial. Most believe that all osteosarcoma should be considered high grade and treated as such although low grade osteosarcoma seems to be a distinct entity [38]. The only commonly accepted staging is localized *versus* metastatic disease.

Human osteosarcoma is commonly treated using surgery and chemotherapy [38]. Chemotherapy for roughly ten weeks that precedes surgery and the extent of necrosis in the surgically removed primary tumor has been suggested to be associated with long term risk for disease recurrence [38]. Chemotherapy is also given after surgery for a period of up to a year. Usually two or three chemotherapeutic agents are given for osteosarcoma treatment. Common combinations include high-dose methotrexate, doxorubicin and cisplatin (sometimes with ifosfamide); doxorubicin and cisplatin; ifosfamide and etoposide; ifosfamide, cisplatin (or carboplatin) and epirubicin [38]. Radiation therapy is used in some cases for non-resectable tumors [38].

The prognosis of human osteosarcoma is affected largely by the presence or absence of metastases. The 5-year survival rate for localized osteosarcoma is estimated to be between 50% and 60%. For metastatic disease the 5-year survival rate is 15% to 30% [39]. There is a better prognosis if metastatic osteosarcoma is present only in the lungs and is all metastatic lesions can be removed surgically [39]. That said, there is a dire need to develop therapies that can be used to treat patients who present with extensive metastatic disease or who recur with metastatic disease. At present, palliative care is often used in such cases or referral for clinical trials [38].

CANINE OSTEOSARCOMA

Canine osteosarcoma accounts for 80%–90% of canine primary bone tumors [40]. Dogs often present with a history of lameness or in some cases with a pathologic fracture of the affected bone. Diagnosis is based on clinical signs, imaging and biopsy. The metaphyseal region of long bones is the most common primary site with front limbs affected twice as often as rear limbs and the distal radius and proximal humerus being the two most common locations [41,42].

It is believed that external factors such as chemical carcinogens, ionization radiation, metallic implants to fix fractures and precedent skeletal disorders such as osteomyelitis and microscopic fractures can lead to canine osteosarcoma [10]. There are implications of genetic factors such as *TP53* and RB1 aberrations, as well as certain viruses and growth factor alterations [43]. Osteosarcoma can affect any breed of dog, but it is more commonly found in the larger breeds. Some breeds, such as the Scottish Deerhound, Great Dane, St. Bernard and Greyhound, are at high risk for developing primary bone tumors suggesting a genetic predilection [40]. In fact, the CDKN2A locus has been recently linked to osteosarcoma risk in dogs, and the risk allele is fixed in certain breeds like Rottweilers and Irish Wolfhounds [4].

Without treatment, the estimated survival for a dog with osteosarcoma is less than 3 months. On the other hand, survival times of approximately 1 year (or about 10% of a dog's lifetime) are achievable for 20%–50% of dogs with osteosarcoma treated using the current standard of care, and a small percentage of dogs can survive up to 5–6 years after diagnosis [44]. Standard of care for dogs is surgery (amputation of limb sparing surgery) with adjuvant chemotherapy [45]. The choice of chemotherapy drugs does not seem to influence survival, thus, toxicity, quality of life and cost tend to be the factors that guide treatment decisions [44]. Chemotherapy is only recommended when the primary tumor is removed and as of current, the drug of choice is carboplatin.

Many well-controlled studies show that a clinical response for osteosarcoma is only achievable with accepted standard of care. In very rare cases, dogs with osteosarcoma that receive palliative care may have prolonged (>1 year) survival, even in face of metastatic disease. Anecdotal benefits reported from herbal or "alternative" treatments, have not been reproducible, and no alternative therapies have been shown to have efficacy or provide consistent clinical benefit in controlled trials.

Metastatic bone cancer is the common cause of death or euthanasia, in 90% of dogs by 1 year [46]. Reducing the primary tumor's ability to metastasize and enhancing the antitumor activity of chemotherapy drugs and yet having minimal negative side effects is still a challenge for veterinary practitioners [10]. Treatment options for canine patients with metastases include pulmonary metastasectomy, but treatment for metastatic disease is only recommended if the primary tumor remains in complete remission [47]. The median survival after pulmonary metastasectomy can be up to 6 months; but without standard surgical procedure, survival outcome is usually less than 2 months [46].

MOUSE MODELS OF OSTEOSARCOMA

The number of genetically engineered or other mouse models of osteosarcoma are fairly restricted. However, these have been useful for studies on the cell of origin for osteosarcoma development and gaining insight into new genes and pathways that influence osteosarcoma initiation, progression and the process of metastasis. Most of the reported models utilize Cre/LoxP mediated deletion of *Trp53* and/or *Rb1* (reviewed in [48]). A few other models have been created by transgenic overexpression of various oncogenes including *Fos* and SV40 large T antigen [49], or co-deletion of one copy of *Twist* and mutation of *Apc* [50]. Osteosarcoma can be induced with high efficiency in mice by osteoblast lineage specific deletion of the*Trp53* gene, although the latency and penetrance is greatly enhanced by co-deletion of both copies of the *Rb1* gene [51].These data are consistent with the centrality of *TP53* and *RB1* loss of function alterations in human osteosarcoma [23]. Mouse osteosarcoma induced by deletion of *Trp53* is genomically unstable, as is seen in human osteosarcoma [52].

Others have created mouse cell lines from spontaneously occurring osteosarcoma. In cases in which these osteosarcoma were induced on a uniform strain background, the osteosarcoma cells can be grown in syngeneic hosts by intravenous, subcutaneous, or orthotopic injections into the tibia (reviewed in [53]). Examples include the K12 and K7M2 derivative that is highly metastatic, and the Dunn along with its metastatic derivative LM8. These cell lines have been useful for testing the role of various components of the immune system on primary osteosarcoma tumor growth and osteosarcoma metastasis [54]. Such cell lines have also been used to create matched pairs of poorly and highly metastatic cell lines for study [53]. These have been useful for developing candidate genes and pathways that may regulate the process of metastasis, such as high-level expression of ezrin [28].

Quist *et al.* reported that osteosarcoma could be induced in mice via homozygous Cre/LoxP-mediated deletion of *Trp53*and *Rb1* in undifferentiated mesenchyme, pre-osteoblasts or infrequently cycling mature osteoblasts [6]. These data suggest that a variety of cell types could be targets for osteosarcoma development. This plasticity may also be the basis for the ready acquisition of new osteosarcoma phenotypes in patients, including chemo/radiotherapy resistance and the ability to readily colonize the lung.

From osteosarcoma mouse models, we have learned that osteosarcoma cells have a predilection to metastatic colonization of the lung, but, interestedly, have observed a metastatic potential spectrum across various cell lines. Intriguingly, in mouse models of Li-Fraumeni, the rate of lung metastasis is influenced by the nature of the p53 mutant allele used and when in the lifetime of the mouse Cre is used to induce mutation of the p53 gene [51]. The rate of spontaneous development of osteosarcoma and the frequency of lung metastasis is higher in mice heterozygous for the $Trp53^{R272H}$ allele than in mice heterozygous for the carry $Trp53^{R270H}$ allele [55]. Recently, a new mouse model of osteosarcoma was developed which utilizes the *Sleeping Beauty* (SB) transposon mutagenesis system [29]. In this project, a SB transposon vector designed to activate proto-oncogenes or inactivate tumor suppressor genes by insertional mutagenesis, was mobilized specifically in *Osx1+* cells using a tissue-specific mutagenesis approach. Mutagenesis by SB was able to induce osteosarcoma in otherwise wild type mice or accelerate osteosarcoma in mice with tissue-specific induction of the $Trp53^{R270H}$ allele. Transposon insertion mutations in specific regions of the genome are found recurrently in SB induced tumors and these regions are called "common insertion sites" or CIS [29]. CIS result from selection for insertions that occur within or near a cancer gene in the right position and the right orientation so as to give the cell a selective advantage and drive the development of a tumor. Thus, the identification of genes at or near CIS defines new candidate drivers of cancer development.

CONSERVED DRIVERS OF OSTEOSARCOMA

Genomic Alterations

It has been reported that genomic alterations are necessary for development of osteosarcoma in mouse models (*TP53*) and are accepted as being commonly shared in humans and dogs [13,29,56].

Highly chaotic karyotypes encompass a key feature that characterizes some mouse models used for osteosarcoma studies, and naturally occurring osteosarcoma in dogs, as well as in human patients. The average human osteosarcoma harbors roughly 30 coding alterations [23,57] while in dog osteosarcoma and mouse models, this figure is not known with certainty. Many of the candidate genes implicated in the pathogenesis and progression of osteosarcoma in people have also been characterized in the canine disease. Notable examples of these genes are *PTEN* (phosphatase and tensin homolog), *RB1*(retinoblastoma), and *TP53* (tumor protein 53), and *MET* (mesenchymal-epithelial transition factor).

Genetic alterations of the retinoblastoma susceptibility (*RB1*) gene have been implicated in the development and progression of osteosarcoma. In people, almost 70% of osteosarcomas have at least one *RB1* gene alteration and the percentage is similar in dog osteosarcomas [13]. We recently reported that an aberrant RB-E2F1 regulatory pathway is predictive of biological behavior [58]. Since our work, another group has reported that RB1 alterations may serve as a prognostic marker for the management of osteosarcoma patients [59].

Approximately 50% of human osteosarcomas have been reported to have somatic *TP53* deletions or point mutations detected using exon sequencing strategies [23]. However, a recent study that used whole genome sequencing of human osteosarcomas suggests that nearly all osteosarcoma tumors have p53 pathways lesions, which in many cases are translocations that break in the first intron of *TP53* gene [57]. Thus, it would appear that p53 pathway loss might be a requirement for osteosarcoma development in people. Clearly, germline *TP53* mutations, which cause Li-Fraumeni syndrome, predispose to osteosarcoma. However, it is unclear whether *TP53* mutations act as initiating mutations or progression mutations in sporadic osteosarcoma. In any case, p53 pathway alterations are common in genetically engineered mouse models as well as spontaneous canine and human osteosarcoma. Therefore, mouse models could be used to develop therapies that exploit p53 pathway alterations in patient osteosarcoma.

In humans and dogs, several oncogenes have been identified as possibly playing a role in osteosarcoma including *MET,FOS*, *IGF1R* (Insulin-Like Growth Factor 1 Receptor), *PVT1/MYC*, *RUNX2*, and *HER2*. Some of these changes involve copy number alterations. Consistent genome and chromosome copy number changes have been reported in canine and human osteosarcoma [17]. For instance, a high copy number gain of the *RUNX2* locus has been reported in both human and dog osteosarcoma [56].

Some of these genes, or the pathways they regulate, including the *PVT1/ MYC* locus, *MET* signaling, and *IGF1R* have been implicated in genetically engineered mouse models of osteosarcoma [29,52].

Recurrent point mutations have been observed in osteosarcoma, but there are few beyond *RB1* and *TP53* that reach statistical significance. This is in part because too few samples have been sequenced. However, point mutations or deletions of several tumor suppressor genes, likely to be drivers of osteosarcomagenesis, were observed in a recent report of human osteosarcoma including *NF1*, *NF2* and *PTEN*, all of which were also recovered in a transposon-based screen for osteosarcoma in mice [29]. Overlap exists between other reported candidate human osteosarcoma genes after genome-wide copy number and whole exome sequencing were done [23], and also after transposon based screening in a mouse model including activation of *PI3KCA*, and *AKT1*, and inactivation of *ARID1A* [29].

Deregulation of Micrornas in Canine and Human Osteosarcoma

microRNAs (miRNAs) are small non coding RNAs that regulate more than 60% of the genome post transcriptionally. Several studies have identified deregulated miRNAs in osteosarcoma [60,61,62,63,64,65,66]. One of the earliest studies reported four differentially expressed miRNAs in a handful of osteosarcoma samples compared to controls [67]. Since these initial studies, additional research has shown that miRNA deregulation is potentially central to osteosarcoma development and progression [68]. Indeed, our group generated a Sarcoma MicroRNA Expression Database (S-MED) that represents 22 different sarcoma types, including osteosarcoma [69]. Through S-MED we found that osteosarcoma clustered separately from all other sarcoma types indicating the presence of potentially biologically important miRNAs. One of the unique miRNA signatures we found revealed the significant downregulation of around 50 miRNAs in the human 14q32 locus compared to the controls [65]. Most importantly, we have also shown a comparable decrease in expression of orthologous 14q32 miRNAs in canine osteosarcoma samples [65]. Interestingly we did not observe any copy number changes at the 14q32 locus, suggesting epigenetic changes at the locus. We confirmed that subset of these 50 miRNAs (miR-382, miR-369-5p, miR-544 and miR-134) could target the 3′ UTR of cMYC transcript. Additionally, overexpression of these miRNAs in osteosarcoma cells decreased the cMYC levels and induced apoptosis [65,70]. Also cMYC has been shown to transactivate a commonly known miRNA cluster, miR-17-92 [71]. We showed that restoration of the 14q32 miRNAs not only did decrease the cMYC levels but also significantly reduced the levels of mir-17-92 [70].

It was observed in other studies that miR-135b, -150, -370, -542-5p, -652, and -654 were highly expressed compared to osteoblasts [72,73,74]. Many of them play crucial roles in bone differentiation and key signaling pathways (miR-206 and -286) [75]. Additionally, miRNAs target *TP53*, which is an important tumor suppressor gene, was mutated in more than 60% osteosarcoma tumors [76]. One of the key miRNAs in the *TP53* pathway is miR-34, which is significantly downregulated in many osteosarcoma tumors that affects the cell cycle and proliferation [77,78,79].

The role of miRNAs in canine osteosarcoma remains to be fully elucidated. Since the discovery of miRNAs, there have been few studies that show a correlation between deregulation of miRNAs and canine osteosarcoma. A recent study investigated the role of miR-196a and its target Annexin V in human (143B, MG63) and canine (DAN) osteosarcoma cell lines to identify potential targets for new therapeutic agents in both the species [80]. They observed that miR-196a is downregulated in many of the canine osteosarcoma tumors compared to the normal bone, which is in contradiction with some earlier studies [66,81]. Further studies need to be performed on a larger cohort to establish that miR-196a is a potential therapeutic target and can impact multiple downstream targets in canine osteosarcoma.

A study led by Fenger *et al.*, sought to characterize miRNA expression in canine primary tumors among the major large breeds (greyhounds, rottweilers, golden retrievers and some mixed breeds) [43,82]. Using Nanominer software, they determined 189 miRNAs that were differentially expressed. Of these, miR-494 was highly expressed in all the breeds compared to normal canine osteoblasts.

As mentioned earlier, our group was among the first groups to observe a significant downregulation of around 50 miRNAs in the human 14q32 chromosomal region, which was highly conserved in the dog genome. Out of the 50 miRNAs, 2 miRNAs, miR-134 and mir-544, shared 100% conservation with the canine genome and mapped to the predicted synteny in canine osteosarcoma [14]. We have comprised a table of key miRNAs that play an important role in survival outcome and chemoresponse that can potentially lead to osteosarcoma diagnosis, subtyping and therapeutics in human and canine osteosarcoma (Table 1).

Table 1: miRNAs as potential markers for survival outcome and/ or chemosensitivity

miRNAs Deregulated in OS	Expression Levels Compared to the Controls	Overall Function	References
miR-382	Down-regulated	Poor survival outcome and metastasis marker	[70,83]
miR-154	Down-regulated	Poor survival outcome	[70]
miR-33a	Up-regulated	Chemoresistance	[84]
miR-34c	Down-regulated	Chemoresistance	[85]

Epigenetic Changes in Osteosarcoma

Most forms of human cancer have changes in the epigenome compared to the normal cellular counterparts from which they are derived. Indeed, changes to the epigenome seem to be a ubiquitous feature of cancer. Epigenetic changes are revealed in alterations to the pattern of DNA methylation, histone modifications and nucleosome remodeling (reviewed in [24]). Osteosarcoma, like other forms of human cancer, seems to have many such epigenome changes compared to normal osteoblasts, the presumptive target cell for transformation. Several studies have analyzed the epigenome in a genome-wide manner, albeit with low numbers of cases [86,87]. These studies confirm that specific methylation events are heterogeneous among different cases of human osteosarcoma and that these differences may help explain differences in the clinical behavior of different osteosarcomas. These genome wide studies in human osteosarcoma have been restricted to the study of DNA methylation. Work on other chromatin modification remains to be done. The study of genome wide epigenetic changes has not been undertaken on a large scale in genetically engineered mouse models or canine osteosarcoma samples.

Many studies in osteosarcoma have focused on methylation of specific genes or gene regions. These studies suggest that certain genes and genetic pathways are subject to control by DNA methylation and attendant modifications to the histone code. Among these are alterations to the RB and p53 pathways. While these specific genes are not frequent targets of methylation based gene silencing, genes in these pathways have been reported as targets for pathogenic methylation. Specifically the *CDKN2A* locus, encoding the cyclin dependent kinase inhibitor $p16^{INK4a}$ and the Mdm2 inhibitor $p14^{Arf}$, has been reported [88,89]. Several genes that are targets of p53, or modulate p53 activity, have been shown to be methylated and silenced in osteosarcoma cell lines or xenograft tumors including *CDKN1A*, *HIC1* and *GADD45* [90,91,92]. Many other tumor suppressor genes are silenced by promoter hypermethylation in osteosarcoma cell lines including *RASSF1A*, *TIMP3*, DAPK1 and others (review in Morrow and Khanna, Critical Reviews in Oncogenesis, 2015). Methylation and silencing of tumor suppressive miRNA genes has also been observed as specific events in human osteosarcoma cell lines and primary tumors. Promoter hypomethyation, and probable overexpression, of oncogenes is less well studied in osteosarcoma, but several reports have been made suggesting such a mechanism, notably for the metastasis promoting gene *IRX1* and the growth factor gene *IGF2* [93,94]. Several candidate osteosarcoma oncogenes found in a transposon-based forward genetic screen in mice are also hypomethylated and overexpressed in human osteosarcoma compared to normal osteoblasts, including *SEMA4D*, *RAF1* and *PAK1* [29]. Some of these epigenetic changes, including aberrant repression and activation, are associated with loss of imprinting control at specific loci in osteosarcoma cells [95,96,97].

Genome wide studies of epigenetic alterations in human osteosarcoma need to incorporate many more samples before we learn to what extent they may explain molecular subtypes and clinical behavior of different cases. No such studies have been reported for canine osteosarcomas or mouse models either. When they are, they will allow cross-species comparisons that could help reveal the most meaningful alterations. Despite these limitations, it is apparent that osteosarcoma development is accompanied by changes to the epigenome that drive progression and confer specific cancer phenotypes. Published data does suggest that epigenome targeted therapies, including histone deacetylase inhibitors and DNA demethylating agents, can alter gene expression and inhibit osteosarcoma growth and/or metastasis [93,98]. Indeed, one study suggests that osteosarcoma cell lines can be reprogrammed using induced pluripotency genes and that the accompanying epigenetic changes reduce tumorigenic potential [99]. Taken together, these data suggest that modification of osteosarcoma epigenomes will be a useful therapeutic approach.

ADVANTAGES OF A MULTI-SPECIES, COMPARATIVE OSTEOSARCOMA STUDY APPROACH

Using comparative genetic studies in multiple organisms, it is possible to understand more about the inherited and somatically acquired genetic alterations that are informative of osteosarcoma risk and clinical behavior, especially metastasis. It is reasonable that genetic alterations that are present in human, dog, and mouse osteosarcomas represent the most likely true drivers of osteosarcoma progression, based on the concept of convergent evolution. Singly, mouse models offer opportunities to discover new genes and pathways important in disease initiation and progression. Dogs bring many other advantages to the table. Notably, since they show remarkable intra-breed homogeneity, which, together with noticeable interbreed heterogeneity, the dog offers distinctive opportunities to understand the genetics underlying osteosarcoma. Taken all together, an interspecies approach offers a possibly broader view and understanding of osteosarcoma since, for example, what is found to be altered at the genetic level in one species may be epigenetically silenced altered in another, but would be hard to pick out based on changes to gene expression alone.

Findings from mouse models and naturally occurring osteosarcoma in dogs need to be translated into therapeutic approaches in a clinically relevant model. Advantages of clinical trials in dogs are numerous and include that there are many more cases of canine osteosarcoma than human osteosarcoma [100,101]. In addition, disease progression in dogs, even with standard of care, is rapid so that assessments of improvement can be made in comparatively short periods of time [102].

It has been shown that histological response is not a good predictor (St. Jude, CTOS 20th Annual Meeting) in human osteosarcoma patients, and so there is an urgent need for informative biomarkers. The 14q32 locus is a new and promising marker, which was discovered by our group through a comparative species approach [65].

CONCLUSIONS

In more than 70% of osteosarcoma patients, current standard-of-care therapies ultimately fail to prevent relapse and metastasis. This dismal outcome has not improved over the past three decades, indicating a desperate need for novel drugs and treatment strategies. As osteosarcoma is genetically heterogeneous, successful therapies will need to target conserved pathobiology. In this review, we discussed the presence of multiple conserved signaling mechanisms as well as some of the approaches for understanding osteosarcoma pathobiology. Recent studies highlight the role of microRNAs in regulation of these conserved signaling pathways. In addition, we have just begun to understand the roles of the regulatory small RNAs and long-noncoding RNAs (lncRNAs). Further, intricacy in gene regulations does not end with identification of regulatory RNAs and its interacting partners. Molecular intricacy is also heavily dependent on our understanding of the implications of other layers of gene regulation such as role for competing endogenous RNAs along with pseudogenes, circular RNAs and lncRNAs. Acquiring such breadth and depth of knowledge is critical for developing therapies that will prevent bypass mechanisms of resistance to therapies. Moreover, cell non-autonomous functions of secreted factors such as exosomes are currently being investigated. In addition, emerging concepts of immune regulation by cancer and recent advancements in immunotherapy hold promise for treating and better outcomes in osteosarcoma.

ACKNOWLEDGMENTS

We thank Jaime Modiano and Aaron Sarver for helpful discussions and Anne Sarver for assisting in manuscript preparation. Due to the space restrictions we could not cite many other significant contributions made by numerous researchers and laboratories in this potentially important and rapidly progressing field. Subbaya Subramanian and David A. Largaespada are supported by research grants funded by American Cancer Society Grant (RSG 13-381-01-RMC), the Sobiech osteosarcoma fund, Children's cancer research funds, the Wyckoff Rein in Sarcoma Foundation.

AUTHOR CONTRIBUTIONS

Jyotika Varshney and Subbaya Subramanian developed the concept for the review. Milcah C. Scott and David A. Largaespada provided input in the canine osteosarcoma and epigenetics of osteosarcoma.

REFERENCES

1. Moore, D.D.; Luu, H.H. Osteosarcoma. *Cancer Treat Res.* 2014, *162*, 65–92.
2. Ottaviani, G.; Jaffe, N. The epidemiology of osteosarcoma. *Cancer Treat Res.* 2009, *152*, 3–13.
3. Letson, G.D.; Muro-Cacho, C.A. Genetic and molecular abnormalities in tumors of the bone and soft tissues. *Cancer Control* 2001, *8*, 239–251.
4. Karlsson, E.K.; Sigurdsson, S.; Ivansson, E.; Thomas, R.; Elvers, I.; Wright, J.; Howald, C.; Tonomura, N.; Perloski, M.; Swofford, R.; *et al.* Genome-wide analyses implicate 33 loci in heritable dog osteosarcoma, including regulatory variants near CDKN2A/B. *Genome Biol.* 2013, *14*, R132.
5. Mutsaers, A.J.; Walkley, C.R. Cells of origin in osteosarcoma: Mesenchymal stem cells or osteoblast committed cells?*Bone* 2014, *62*, 56–63.
6. Quist, T.; Jin, H.; Zhu, J.F.; Smith-Fry, K.; Capecchi, M.R.; Jones, K.B. The impact of osteoblastic differentiation on osteosarcomagenesis in the mouse. *Oncogene* 2015, *34*, 4278–4284.
7. Yoshida, H.; Adachi, H.; Hamada, Y.; Aki, T.; Yumoto, T.; Morimoto, K.; Orido, T. Osteosarcoma. Ultrastructural and immunohistochemical studies on alkaline phosphatase-positive tumor cells constituting a variety of histologic types.*Acta Pathol. Jpn.* 1988, *38*, 325–338.

8. Dirik, Y.; Cinar, A.; Yumrukcal, F.; Eralp, L. Popliteal lymph node metastasis of tibial osteoblastic osteosarcoma. *Int. J. Surg. Case Rep.* 2014, *5*, 840–844.

9. Jeffree, G.M.; Price, C.H.; Sissons, H.A. The metastatic patterns of osteosarcoma. *Brit. J. Cancer* 1975, *32*, 87–107.

10. Morello, E.; Martano, M.; Buracco, P. Biology, diagnosis and treatment of canine appendicular osteosarcoma: Similarities and differences with human osteosarcoma. *Vet. J.* 2011, *189*, 268–277.

11. Gill, J.; Ahluwalia, M.K.; Geller, D.; Gorlick, R. New targets and approaches in osteosarcoma. *Pharmacol. Ther.* 2013,*137*, 89–99.

12. Jaffe, N. Osteosarcoma: Review of the past, impact on the future. The American experience. *Cancer Treat Res.* 2009,*152*, 239–262.

13. Modiano, J.F.; Breen, M.; Lana, S.E.; Ehrhart, N.; Fosmire, S.P.; Thomas, R.; Jubala, C.M.; Lamerato-Kozicki, A.R.; Ehrhart, E.J.; Schaack, J.; *et al.* Naturally occurring translational models for development of cancer therapy. *Gene Ther. Mol. Biol.* 2006, *10*, 31–40. [Google Scholar]

14. Scott, M.C.; Sarver, A.L.; Gavin, K.J.; Thayanithy, V.; Getzy, D.M.; Newman, R.A.; Cutter, G.R.; Lindblad-Toh, K.; Kisseberth, W.C.; Hunter, L.E.; *et al.* Molecular subtypes of osteosarcoma identified by reducing tumor heterogeneity through an interspecies comparative approach. *Bone* 2011, *49*, 356–367.

15. Paoloni, M.; Davis, S.; Lana, S.; Withrow, S.; Sangiorgi, L.; Picci, P.; Hewitt, S.; Triche, T.; Meltzer, P.; Khanna, C. Canine tumor cross-species genomics uncovers targets linked to osteosarcoma progression. *BMC Genom.* 2009, *10*, 625.

16. Schiffman, J.D.; Breen, M. Comparative oncology: What dogs and other species can teach us about humans with cancer. *Philos. Trans. R. Soc. Lond. B Biol. Sci.* 2015, *370*.

17. Thomas, R.; Wang, H.J.; Tsai, P.C.; Langford, C.F.; Fosmire, S.P.; Jubala, C.M.; Getzy, D.M.; Cutter, G.R.; Modiano, J.F.; Breen, M. Influence of genetic background on tumor karyotypes: Evidence for breed-associated cytogenetic aberrations in canine appendicular osteosarcoma. *Chromosome Res.* 2009, *17*, 365–377.

18. McNeill, C.J.; Overley, B.; Shofer, F.S.; Kent, M.S.; Clifford, C.A.; Samluk, M.; Haney, S.; van Winkle, T.J.; Sorenmo, K.U. Characterization of the biological behaviour of appendicular osteosarcoma in Rottweilers and a comparison with other breeds: A review of 258 dogs. *Vet. Comp. Oncol.* 2007, *5*, 90–98.

19. Dobson, J.M. Breed-predispositions to cancer in pedigree dogs. *ISRN Vet. Sci.* 2013, *2013*, 941275.

20. Paoloni, M.; Khanna, C. Translation of new cancer treatments from pet dogs to humans. *Nat. Rev. Cancer* 2008, *8*, 147–156.

21. Isakoff, M.S.; Bielack, S.S.; Meltzer, P.; Gorlick, R. Osteosarcoma: Current treatment and a collaborative pathway to success. *J. Clin. Oncol.* 2015, *33*, 3029–3035.

22. Ferrari, S.; Serra, M. An update on chemotherapy for osteosarcoma. *Expert Opin.*

Pharmacother. 2015, *16*, 2727–2736.

23. Perry, J.A.; Kiezun, A.; Tonzi, P.; van Allen, E.M.; Carter, S.L.; Baca, S.C.; Cowley, G.S.; Bhatt, A.S.; Rheinbay, E.; Pedamallu, C.S.; *et al.* Complementary genomic approaches highlight the PI3K/mTOR pathway as a common vulnerability in osteosarcoma. *Proc. Natl. Acad. Sci. USA* 2014, *111*, 5564–5573.
24. Morrow, J.J.; Khanna, C. Osteosarcoma genetics and epigenetics: Emerging biology and candidate therapies. *Crit. Rev. Oncog.* 2015, *20*, 173–197.
25. Li, N.; Luo, D.; Hu, X.; Luo, W.; Lei, G.; Wang, Q.; Zhu, T.; Gu, J.; Lu, Y.; Zheng, Q. RUNX2 and osteosarcoma.*Anticancer Agents Med. Chem.* 2015, *15*, 881–887.
26. Tian, J.; He, H.; Lei, G. Wnt/beta-catenin pathway in bone cancers. *Tumour Biol.* 2014, *35*, 9439–9445.
27. Lamora, A.; Talbot, J.; Bougras, G.; Amiaud, J.; Leduc, M.; Chesneau, J.; Taurelle, J.; Stresing, V.; Le Deley, M.C.; Heymann, M.F.; *et al.* Overexpression of smad7 blocks primary tumor growth and lung metastasis development in osteosarcoma. *Clin. Cancer Res.* 2014, *20*, 5097–5112.
28. Khanna, C.; Wan, X.; Bose, S.; Cassaday, R.; Olomu, O.; Mendoza, A.; Yeung, C.; Gorlick, R.; Hewitt, S.M.; Helman, L.J. The membrane-cytoskeleton linker ezrin is necessary for osteosarcoma metastasis. *Nat. Med.* 2004, *10*, 182–186.
29. Moriarity, B.S.; Otto, G.M.; Rahrmann, E.P.; Rathe, S.K.; Wolf, N.K.; Weg, M.T.; Manlove, L.A.; LaRue, R.S.; Temiz, N.A. A Sleeping Beauty forward genetic screen identifies new genes and pathways driving osteosarcoma development and metastasis. 2015, *47*, 615–624.
30. Chang, L.; Shrestha, S.; LaChaud, G.; Scott, M.A.; James, A.W. Review of microRNA in osteosarcoma and chondrosarcoma. *Med. Oncol.* 2015, *32*, 613.
31. Geller, D.S.; Gorlick, R. Osteosarcoma: A review of diagnosis, management, and treatment strategies. *Clin. Adv. Hematol. Oncol.* 2010, *8*, 705–718.
32. Mirabello, L.; Pfeiffer, R.; Murphy, G.; Daw, N.C.; Patino-Garcia, A.; Troisi, R.J.; Hoover, R.N.; Douglass, C.; Schuz, J.; Craft, A.W.; *et al.* Height at diagnosis and birth-weight as risk factors for osteosarcoma. *Cancer Causes Control* 2011, *22*, 899–908.
33. Savage, S.A.; Woodson, K.; Walk, E.; Modi, W.; Liao, J.; Douglass, C.; Hoover, R.N.; Chanock, S.J. Analysis of genes critical for growth regulation identifies Insulin-like Growth Factor 2 Receptor variations with possible functional significance as risk factors for osteosarcoma. *Cancer Epidemiol. Biomark. Prev.* 2007, *16*, 1667–1674.
34. Miller, R.W. Contrasting epidemiology of childhood osteosarcoma, Ewing's tumor, and rhabdomyosarcoma. *Natl. Cancer Inst. Monogr.* 1981, *56*, 9–15.
35. Jawad, M.U.; Cheung, M.C.; Min, E.S.; Schneiderbauer, M.M.; Koniaris, L.G.; Scully, S.P. Ewing sarcoma demonstrates racial disparities in incidence-related and sex-related differences in outcome: An analysis of 1631 cases from the SEER database, 1973–2005. *Cancer* 2009, *115*, 3526–3536.
36. Savage, S.A.; Mirabello, L.; Wang, Z.; Gastier-Foster, J.M.; Gorlick, R.; Khanna,

C.; Flanagan, A.M.; Tirabosco, R.; Andrulis, I.L.; Wunder, J.S.; *et al.* Genome-wide association study identifies two susceptibility loci for osteosarcoma.*Nat. Genet.* 2013, *45*, 799–803.

37. Mirabello, L.; Koster, R.; Moriarity, B.S.; Spector, L.G.; Meltzer, P.S.; Gary, J.; Machiela, M.J.; Pankratz, N.; Panagiotou, O.A.; Largaespada, D.; *et al.* A Genome-wide scan identifies variants in NFIB associated with metastasis in patients with osteosarcoma. *Cancer Discov.* 2015, *5*, 920–931.
38. Gorlick, R.; Khanna, C. Osteosarcoma. *J. Bone Miner. Res.* 2010, *25*, 683–691.
39. Hameed, M.; Dorfman, H. Primary malignant bone tumors—Recent developments. *Semin. Diagn. Pathol.* 2011, *28*, 86–101.
40. Anfinsen, K.P.; Grotmol, T.; Bruland, O.S.; Jonasdottir, T.J. Breed-specific incidence rates of canine primary bone tumors—A population based survey of dogs in Norway. *Can. J. Vet. Res.* 2011, *75*, 209–215.
41. Liptak, J.M.; Dernell, W.S.; Straw, R.C.; Rizzo, S.A.; Lafferty, M.H.; Withrow, S.J. Proximal radial and distal humeral osteosarcoma in 12 dogs. *J. Am. Anim. Hosp. Assoc.* 2004, *40*, 461–467.
42. Boerman, I.; Selvarajah, G.T.; Nielen, M.; Kirpensteijn, J. Prognostic factors in canine appendicular osteosarcoma—A meta-analysis. *BMC Vet. Res.* 2012, *8*, 56–56.
43. Fenger, J.M.; London, C.A.; Kisseberth, W.C. Canine osteosarcoma: A naturally occurring disease to inform pediatric oncology. *ILAR J.* 2014, *55*, 69–85.
44. Szewczyk, M.; Lechowski, R.; Zabielska, K. What do we know about canine osteosarcoma treatment? Review. *Vet. Res. Commun.* 2015, *39*, 61–67.
45. Berg, J. Canine osteosarcoma: Amputation and chemotherapy. *Vet. Clin. N. Am. Small Anim. Pract.* 1996, *26*, 111–121.
46. Straw, R.C.; Withrow, S.J.; Powers, B.E. Management of canine appendicular osteosarcoma. *Vet. Clin. North Am. Small Anim. Pract.* 1990, *20*, 1141–1161.
47. Gilson, S.D. Principles of surgery for cancer palliation and treatment of metastases. *Clin. Tech. Small Anim. Pract.* 1998, *13*, 65–69.
48. Guijarro, M.V.; Ghivizzani, S.C.; Gibbs, C.P. Animal models in osteosarcoma. *Front. Oncol.* 2014, *4*, 189.
49. Ruther, U.; Komitowski, D.; Schubert, F.R.; Wagner, E.F. c-fos expression induces bone tumors in transgenic mice.*Oncogene* 1989, *4*, 861–865.
50. Entz-Werle, N.; Choquet, P.; Neuville, A.; Kuchler-Bopp, S.; Clauss, F.; Danse, J.M.; Simo-Noumbissie, P.; Guerin, E.; Gaub, M.P.; Freund, J.N.; *et al.* Targeted apc;twist double-mutant mice: A new model of spontaneous osteosarcoma that mimics the human disease. *Transl. Oncol.* 2010, *3*, 344–353.
51. Walkley, C.R.; Qudsi, R.; Sankaran, V.G.; Perry, J.A.; Gostissa, M.; Roth, S.I.; Rodda, S.J.; Snay, E.; Dunning, P.; Fahey, F.H.; *et al.* Conditional mouse osteosarcoma, dependent on p53 loss and potentiated by loss of Rb, mimics the human disease. *Genes Dev* 2008, *22*, 1662–1676.

52. Rao, P.H.; Zhao, S.; Zhao, Y.J.; Yu, A.; Rainusso, N.; Trucco, M.; Allen-Rhoades, W.; Satterfield, L.; Fuja, D.; Borra, V.J.;*et al.* Coamplification of Myc/Pvt1 and homozygous deletion of Nlrp1 locus are frequent genetics changes in mouse osteosarcoma. *Genes Chromosomes Cancer* 2015, *54*, 796–808.

53. Mohseny, A.B.; Hogendoorn, P.C.; Cleton-Jansen, A.M. Osteosarcoma models: From cell lines to zebrafish. *Sarcoma*2012, *2012*, 417271.

54. Merchant, M.S.; Melchionda, F.; Sinha, M.; Khanna, C.; Helman, L.; Mackall, C.L. Immune reconstitution prevents metastatic recurrence of murine osteosarcoma. *Cancer Immunol. Immunother.* 2007, *56*, 1037–1046.

55. Olive, K.P.; Tuveson, D.A.; Ruhe, Z.C.; Yin, B.; Willis, N.A.; Bronson, R.T.; Crowley, D.; Jacks, T. Mutant p53 gain of function in two mouse models of Li-Fraumeni syndrome. *Cell* 2004, *119*, 847–860.

56. Angstadt, A.Y.; Thayanithy, V.; Subramanian, S.; Modiano, J.F.; Breen, M. A genome-wide approach to comparative oncology: High-resolution oligonucleotide aCGH of canine and human osteosarcoma pinpoints shared microaberrations. *Cancer Genet.* 2012, *205*, 572–587.

57. Chen, X.; Bahrami, A.; Pappo, A.; Easton, J.; Dalton, J.; Hedlund, E.; Ellison, D.; Shurtleff, S.; Wu, G.; Wei, L.; *et al.* Recurrent somatic structural variations contribute to tumorigenesis in pediatric osteosarcoma. *Cell Rep.* 2014, *7*, 104–112.

58. Scott, M.C.; Sarver, A.L.; Tomiyasu, H.; Cornax, I.; van Etten, J.; Varshney, J.; O'Sullivan, M.G.; Subramanian, S.; Modiano, J.F. Aberrant RB-E2F transcriptional regulation defines molecular phenotypes of osteosarcoma. *J. Biol. Chem.* 2015.

59. Ren, W.; Gu, G. Prognostic implications of RB1 tumour suppressor gene alterations in the clinical outcome of human osteosarcoma: A meta-analysis. *Eur. J. Cancer Care* 2015.

60. Sampson, V.B.; Yoo, S.; Kumar, A.; Vetter, N.S.; Kolb, E.A. MicroRNAs and potential targets in osteosarcoma: Review.*Front. Pediatr.* 2015, *3*, 69.

61. Zhang, J.; Yan, Y.G.; Wang, C.; Zhang, S.J.; Yu, X.H.; Wang, W.J. MicroRNAs in osteosarcoma. *Clin. Chim. Acta* 2015,*444*, 9–17.

62. Miao, J.; Wu, S.; Peng, Z.; Tania, M.; and Zhang, C. MicroRNAs in osteosarcoma: Diagnostic and therapeutic aspects.*Tumour Biol.* 2013, *34*, 2093–2098.

63. Zhou, G.; Shi, X.; Zhang, J.; Wu, S.; Zhao, J. MicroRNAs in osteosarcoma: From biological players to clinical contributors, a review. *J. Int. Med. Res.* 2013, *41*, 1–12.

64. Li, Y.; Zhang, J.; Zhang, L.; Si, M.; Yin, H.; Li, J. Diallyl trisulfide inhibits proliferation, invasion and angiogenesis of osteosarcoma cells by switching on suppressor microRNAs and inactivating of Notch-1 signaling. *Carcinogenesis* 2013,*34*, 1601–1610.

65. Sarver, A.L.; Thayanithy, V.; Scott, M.C.; Cleton-Jansen, A.M.; Hogendoorn, P.C.; Modiano, J.F.; Subramanian, S. MicroRNAs at the human 14q32 locus have

prognostic significance in osteosarcoma. *Orphanet J. Rare Dis.* 2013, *8*, 7.

66. Namlos, H.M.; Meza-Zepeda, L.A.; Baroy, T.; Ostensen, I.H.; Kresse, S.H.; Kuijjer, M.L.; Serra, M.; Burger, H.; Cleton-Jansen, A.M.; Myklebost, O. Modulation of the osteosarcoma expression phenotype by microRNAs. *PloS ONE* 2012, *7*, e48086.

67. Lulla, R.R.; Costa, F.F.; Bischof, J.M.; Chou, P.M.; de, F.B.M.; Vanin, E.F.; Soares, M.B. Identification of differentially expressed MicroRNAs in osteosarcoma. *Sarcoma* 2011, *2011*, 732690.

68. Varshney, J.; Subramanian, S. MicroRNAs as potential target in human bone and soft tissue sarcoma therapeutics.*Front. Mol. Biosci.* 2015, *2*, 31.

69. Sarver, A.L.; Phalak, R.; Thayanithy, V.; Subramanian, S. S-MED: Sarcoma microRNA expression database. *Lab. Investig. J. Tech. Methods Pathol.* 2010, *90*, 753–761.

70. Thayanithy, V.; Sarver, A.L.; Kartha, R.V.; Li, L.; Angstadt, A.Y.; Breen, M.; Steer, C.J.; Modiano, J.F.; Subramanian, S. Perturbation of 14q32 miRNAs-cMYC gene network in osteosarcoma. *Bone* 2012, *50*, 171–181.

71. Li, Y.; Choi, P.S.; Casey, S.C.; Dill, D.L.; Felsher, D.W. MYC through miR-17–92 suppresses specific target genes to maintain survival, autonomous proliferation, and a neoplastic state. *Cancer Cell* 2014, *26*, 262–272.

72. Schaap-Oziemlak, A.M.; Raymakers, R.A.; Bergevoet, S.M.; Gilissen, C.; Jansen, B.J.; Adema, G.J.; Kogler, G.; le Sage, C.; Agami, R.; van der Reijden, B.A.; *et al.* MicroRNA hsa-miR-135b regulates mineralization in osteogenic differentiation of human unrestricted somatic stem cells. *Stem. Cells Dev.* 2010, *19*, 877–885.

73. Wei, J.Q.; Chen, H.; Zheng, X.F.; Zhang, B.X.; Wang, Y.; Tang, P.F.; She, F.; Song, Q.; Li, T.S. Hsa-miR-654–5p regulates osteogenic differentiation of human bone marrow mesenchymal stem cells by repressing bone morphogenetic protein 2. *J. Southern Med. Univ.* 2012, *32*, 291–295. [Google Scholar]

74. Fang, S.; Deng, Y.; Gu, P.; Fan, X. MicroRNAs regulate bone development and regeneration. *Int. J. Mol. Sci.* 2015, *16*, 8227–8253.

75. Inose, H.; Ochi, H.; Kimura, A.; Fujita, K.; Xu, R.; Sato, S.; Iwasaki, M.; Sunamura, S.; Takeuchi, Y.; Fukumoto, S.; *et al.* A microRNA regulatory mechanism of osteoblast differentiation. *Proc. Natl. Acad. Sci. USA* 2009, *106*, 20794–20799.

76. Feng, Z.; Zhang, C.; Wu, R.; Hu, W. Tumor suppressor p53 meets microRNAs. *J. Mol. Cell Biol.* 2011, *3*, 44–50.

77. Wang, Y.; Jia, L.S.; Yuan, W.; Wu, Z.; Wang, H.B.; Xu, T.; Sun, J.C.; Cheng, K.F.; Shi, J.G. Low miR-34a and miR-192 are associated with unfavorable prognosis in patients suffering from osteosarcoma. *Am. J. Transl. Res.* 2015, *7*, 111–119.

78. Zhao, H.; Ma, B.; Wang, Y.; Han, T.; Zheng, L.; Sun, C.; Liu, T.; Zhang, Y.; Qiu, X.; Fan, Q. miR-34a inhibits the metastasis of osteosarcoma cells by repressing the expression of CD44. *Oncol. Rep.* 2013, *29*, 1027–1036.

79. He, C.; Xiong, J.; Xu, X.; Lu, W.; Liu, L.; Xiao, D.; Wang, D. Functional elucidation of MiR-34 in osteosarcoma cells and primary tumor samples. *Biochem. Biophys.*

Res. Commun. 2009, *388*, 35–40.

80. Pazzaglia, L.; Leonardi, L.; Conti, A.; Novello, C.; Quattrini, I.; Montanini, L.; Roperto, F.; del Piero, F.; di Guardo, G.; Piro, F.; *et al.* miR-196a expression in human and canine osteosarcomas: A comparative study. *Res. Vet. Sci.* 2015, *99*, 112–119.
81. Zhang, W.; Zhang, C.; Chen, H.; Li, L.; Tu, Y.; Liu, C.; Shi, S.; Zen, K.; Liu, Z. Evaluation of microRNAs miR-196a, miR-30a-5P, and miR-490 as biomarkers of disease activity among patients with FSGS. *Clin. J. Am. Soc. Nephrol.* 2014,*9*, 1545–1552.
82. Gardner, H.L.; Fenger, J.M.; London, C.A. Dogs as a model for cancer. *Annu. Rev. Anim. Biosci.* 2015. in print.
83. Xu, M.; Jin, H.; Xu, C.X.; Sun, B.; Song, Z.G.; Bi, W.Z.; Wang, Y. miR-382 inhibits osteosarcoma metastasis and relapse by targeting Y box-binding protein 1. *Mol. Ther.* 2015, *23*, 89–98.
84. Zhou, Y.; Huang, Z.; Wu, S.; Zang, X.; Liu, M.; Shi, J. miR-33a is up-regulated in chemoresistant osteosarcoma and promotes osteosarcoma cell resistance to cisplatin by down-regulating TWIST. *J. Exp. Clin. Cancer Res.* 2014, *33*, 12.
85. Xu, M.; Jin, H.; Xu, C.X.; Bi, W.Z.; Wang, Y. MiR-34c inhibits osteosarcoma metastasis and chemoresistance. *Med. Oncol.* 2014, *31*, 972.
86. Rosenblum, J.M.; Wijetunga, N.A.; Fazzari, M.J.; Krailo, M.; Barkauskas, D.A.; Gorlick, R.; Greally, J.M. Predictive properties of DNA methylation patterns in primary tumor samples for osteosarcoma relapse status. *Epigenetics* 2015,*10*, 31–39.
87. Kresse, S.H.; Rydbeck, H.; Skarn, M.; Namlos, H.M.; Barragan-Polania, A.H.; Cleton-Jansen, A.M.; Serra, M.; Liestol, K.; Hogendoorn, P.C.; Hovig, E.; *et al.* Integrative analysis reveals relationships of genetic and epigenetic alterations in osteosarcoma. *PLoS ONE* 2012, *7*, e48262.
88. Oh, J.H.; Kim, H.S.; Kim, H.H.; Kim, W.H.; Lee, S.H. Aberrant methylation of p14ARF gene correlates with poor survival in osteosarcoma. *Clin. Orthop. Relat. Res.* 2006, *442*, 216–222.
89. Park, Y.B.; Park, M.J.; Kimura, K.; Shimizu, K.; Lee, S.H.; Yokota, J. Alterations in the INK4a/ARF locus and their effects on the growth of human osteosarcoma cell lines. *Cancer Genet. Cytogenet.* 2002, *133*, 105–111.
90. Al-Romaih, K.; Sadikovic, B.; Yoshimoto, M.; Wang, Y.; Zielenska, M.; Squire, J.A. Decitabine-induced demethylation of 5′ CpG island in GADD45A leads to apoptosis in osteosarcoma cells. *Neoplasia* 2008, *10*, 471–480.
91. Badal, V.; Menendez, S.; Coomber, D.; Lane, D.P. Regulation of the p14ARF promoter by DNA methylation. *Cell Cycle*2008, *7*, 112–119.
92. Chen, W.; Cooper, T.K.; Zahnow, C.A.; Overholtzer, M.; Zhao, Z.; Ladanyi, M.; Karp, J.E.; Gokgoz, N.; Wunder, J.S.; Andrulis, I.L.; *et al.* Epigenetic and genetic loss of Hic1 function accentuates the role of p53 in tumorigenesis. *Cancer Cell* 2004, *6*, 387–398.

93. Lu, J.; Song, G.; Tang, Q.; Zou, C.; Han, F.; Zhao, Z.; Yong, B.; Yin, J.; Xu, H.; Xie, X.; *et al.* IRX1 hypomethylation promotes osteosarcoma metastasis via induction of CXCL14/NF-kappaB signaling. *J. Clin. Investig.* 2015, *125*, 1839–1856.

94. Li, Y.; Meng, G.; Huang, L.; Guo, Q.N. Hypomethylation of the P3 promoter is associated with up-regulation of IGF2 expression in human osteosarcoma. *Hum. Pathol.* 2009, *40*, 1441–1447.

95. Ulaner, G.A.; Vu, T.H.; Li, T.; Hu, J.F.; Yao, X.M.; Yang, Y.; Gorlick, R.; Meyers, P.; Healey, J.; Ladanyi, M.; *et al.* Loss of imprinting of IGF2 and H19 in osteosarcoma is accompanied by reciprocal methylation changes of a CTCF-binding site. *Hum. Mol. Genet.* 2003, *12*, 535–549.

96. Li, Y.; Meng, G.; Guo, Q.N. Changes in genomic imprinting and gene expression associated with transformation in a model of human osteosarcoma. *Exp. Mol. Pathol.* 2008, *84*, 234–239.

97. Lee, D.F.; Su, J.; Kim, H.S.; Chang, B.; Papatsenko, D.; Zhao, R.; Yuan, Y.; Gingold, J.; Xia, W.; Darr, H.; *et al.* Modeling familial cancer with induced pluripotent stem cells. *Cell* 2015, *161*, 240–254.

98. Thayanithy, V.; Park, C.; Sarver, A.L.; Kartha, R.V.; Korpela, D.M.; Graef, A.J.; Steer, C.J.; Modiano, J.F.; Subramanian, S. Combinatorial treatment of DNA and chromatin-modifying drugs cause cell death in human and canine osteosarcoma cell lines. *PLoS ONE* 2012, *7*, e43720.

99. Zhang, X.; Cruz, F.D.; Terry, M.; Remotti, F.; Matushansky, I. Terminal differentiation and loss of tumorigenicity of human cancers via pluripotency-based reprogramming. *Oncogene* 2013, *32*, 2249–2260.

100. Maniscalco, L. Canine osteosarcoma: Understanding its variability to improve treatment. *Vet. J.* 2015, *203*, 135–136.

101. Rodriguez, C.O., Jr. Using canine osteosarcoma as a model to assess efficacy of novel therapies: Can old dogs teach us new tricks? *Adv. Exp. Med. Biol.* 2014, *804*, 237–256.

102. Modiano, J.F.; Bellgrau, D.; Cutter, G.R.; Lana, S.E., Ehrhart, N.P.; Ehrhart, E.; Wilke, V.L.; Charles, J.B.; Munson, S.; Scott, M.C.; *et al.* Inflammation, apoptosis, and necrosis induced by neoadjuvant fas ligand gene therapy improves survival of dogs with spontaneous bone cancer. *Mol. Ther.* 2012, *20*, 2234–2243.

8

CHAPTER

KIDNEY ISCHAEMIA REPERFUSION INJURY IN THE RAT: THE EGTI SCORING SYSTEM AS A VALID AND RELIABLE TOOL FOR HISTOLOGICAL ASSESSMENT

Usman Khalid, Gilda Pino-Chavez, Prabhu Nesargikar, Robert H. Jenkins, Timothy Bowen, Donald J. Fraser and Rafael Chavez

Keywords: Ischaemia reperfusion injury (IRI), histology scoring system, EGTI scoring system, jablonski score

INTRODUCTION

Ischaemia reperfusion injury (IRI) is a complex pathological process characterized by initial restriction of blood supply to the organ followed by subsequent restoration of blood flow and oxygenation, and is an inevitable consequence of organ transplantation, causing significant morbidity and mortality. In kidney transplantation, IRI manifests as primary non-function and delayed graft function, leading to an increased risk of complications, acute allograft rejection and poorer long-term outcomes [1-3]. Due to the increasing donor shortage problem, expanded criteria donor organs' with the additional risk of increased IRI, are now increasingly used [4].

The pathophysiological processes involved in IRI are complex and include interactions between the endothelium, components of the immune system and cell death programs [3]. Briefly, ischaemia and resultant hypoxia cause an increase in vascular permeability and impaired endothelial cell barrier function. Cell death programs that consist of cell apoptosis, phagocytosis, and necrosis are activated. Apoptosis causes

Citation: Khalid U, Pino-Chavez G, Nesargikar P, Jenkins RH, Bowen T, Fraser DJ and Chavez R.Kidney ischaemia reperfusion injury in the rat: the EGTI scoring system as a valid and reliable tool for histological assessment. J Histol Histopathol. 2016; 3:1. http://dx.doi.org/10.7243/2055-091X-3-1.

nuclear fragmentation, loss of mitochondrial integrity and cell shrinkage. Activation of the innate and adaptive components of the immune system, such as complement, contributes significantly to injury [3,5].

In renal IRI, endothelial damage is the result of the initial ischaemia and hypoxia leading to impaired cell barrier function. This causes endothelial swelling and disruption, eventually leading to loss of endothelial integrity [6,7]. Tubular injury is a characteristic feature of kidney IRI since the tubules are most prone to ischaemic damage, and therefore potentially reversible acute tubular necrosis is a hallmark of kidney injury. Specifically, in IRI, hypoxia results in formation of plasma membrane blebs and loss of brush border membrane leading to loss of polarity and integrity of tight junctions. Cast formation occurs secondary to cell death and sloughing. As a result, cast formation and other debris lead to tubular obstruction. These changes, along with tubular necrosis, signify extensive tubular damage [8]. Interstitial damage is also seen in acute kidney injury, but may also result from chronic and progressive damage of varied aetiology. Inflammation, haemorrhage and necrosis are the hallmarks of acute ischaemic damage to the tubulo-interstitium [9]. Thickening of Bowman's capsule, retraction of the glomerular tuft and, in severe cases, glomerular fibrosis are the histological features of ischaemic glomerular damage [10].

Full and comprehensive documentation of these complex features of acute kidney injury is important, to facilitate determination of prognosis following biopsy, and to enable mechanistic studies in this area. The widely adopted 'gold standard' scoring system for reporting histological damage in kidney injury is the Jablonski scoring system [11]. This simple system is designed to give a rapid and objective assessment of kidney injury. In reality, however, it provides a limited score documenting predominantly the degree of necrosis within tubular cells only, ranging from 0 signifying 'no damage', to 4 'necrosis affecting all 3 segments of the proximal convoluted tubule'. It does not provide an assessment of the damage seen within the other cellular components, such as endothelial and glomerular cells. The Jablonski scoring system was originally described following a prolonged recovery period after ischaemic injury, and includes features of recovery (e.g., Tubular cell mitoses) that may not be evident in the typical recovery periods used experimentally, or in clinical samples.

The damage seen in IRI is not limited to tubular cells and includes also endothelial, glomerular and interstitial changes. Exclusive focus on the proximal tubule removes the possibility of detection of varied propensity for injury in these compartments, depending on clinical context and/or experimental therapeutic approach applied. There is a need, therefore, to develop a more detailed scoring system that is simple, reliable and more informative regarding the degree of tissue damage to the various cellular components of the kidney.

Here, we present the EGTI (Endothelial, Glomerular, Tubular, Interstitial) scoring system, and its analyisis in rat models of acute IRI, in comparison with the Jablonski scoring system. In addition, scores were correlated with established acute kidney injury markers neutrophil gelatinase-associated lipocalin (NGAL) and kidney injury molecule 1 (KIM-1), together with serum creatinine as a measure of excretory kidney function, in order to establish their inter-relationships in this model.

METHODS

Rat models of IRI

Adult (8 to 12 week old) male Lewis rats weighing 180-220g were used (Harlan Laboratories, UK). The rats were given a 7-day period of acclimatisation to their new environment and were housed and handled according to the local institutional policies and procedures licenced by the Home Office. Analgesia was provided 24 hours pre-op throughout until the time of retrieval in the form of 200mcg of buprenorphine dissolved in 500ml of drinking water. The animals were anaesthetized using Isoflurane and midline laparotomy incisions were made.

Two rat models were used: unilateral IRI and bilateral IRI. In the unilateral model, the left renal pedicle was identified and clamped for 45 minutes using a vascular clip (IRI group). In the bilateral model, both kidneys were identified and their pediclessimultaneously clamped for 45 minutes using vascular clips (IRI group). In both models, the kidneys were visually assessed for both ischaemia upon clamping and subsequent reperfusion upon release of the clamp. Sham controls underwent the same operation without the renal pedicle clamping. During the ischaemic period the abdominal cavity was covered with saline-soaked gauze. The kidneys were retrieved at 48 hours following terminal anaesthesia.

Histology

Kidney tissue was embedded in paraffin and 5 μm tissue sections obtained for Haemotoxylin and Eosin (H&E) staining. Histological damage was assessed by an experienced histopathologist blinded as to group allocation (sham versus IRI) and quantified using the EGTI scoring system devised specifically for animal research on kidney tissue in the context of injury (Table 1). The scoring system consists of histological damage in 4 individual components: Endothelial, Glomerular, Tubular, and Interstitial. The scoring was performed in both the preserved and damaged parts of the renal cortex. The Jablonski scorewas also recorded.

Table 1: The EGTI histology scoring system

Tissue type	Damage	Score
Tubular	No damage	0
	Loss of Brush Border (BB) in less than 25% of tubular cells. Integrity of basal membrane.	1
	Loss of BB in more than 25% of tubular cells, Thickened basal membrane	2
	(Plus) Inflammation, Cast formation, Necrosis up to 60% of tubular cells	3
	(Plus) Necrosis in more than 60% of tubular cells	4
Endothelial	No damage	0
	Endothelial swelling	1
	Endothelial disruption	2
	Endothelial loss	3
Glomerular	No damage	0
	Thickening of Bowman capsule	1
	Retraction of glomerular tuft	2
	Glomerular fibrosis	3
Tubulo/ Interstitial	No damage	0
	Inflammation, haemorrhage in less than 25% of tissue	1
	(Plus) necrosis in less than 25% of tissue	2
	Necrosis up to 60%	3
	Necrosis more than 60%	4

RT-qPCR

Total RNA was extracted using TRIzol reagent (Life technologies) according to manufacturer's instructions. Generation of cDNA was carried out using the High Capacity Reverse Transcription Kit (Life Technologies) with random primers, and RT-qPCR was performed on a ViiA7 Fast Real-Time PCR System (Life Technologies). NGAL and KIM-1 were quantified using the POWER SYBR® GREEN PCR Master Mix (Life technologies) with gene-specific primers and normalized to house keeping gene GAPDH. Changes in gene expression were analysed usingthe 2-DDCT method [12].

Primers› sequences used were:

GAPDH (forward, 5›-CCTCTGACTTCAACAGCGACAC-3′; reverse, 5′-TGTCATACCAGGAAATGAGCTTGA-3′)

NGAL (forward, 5›-GGGCTGTCCGATGAACTGAA-3›; reverse, 5›-CATTGGTCGGTGGGAACAGA-3›),

KIM-1 (forward, 5›-CGGCTAACCAGAGTGACTTGT-3›; reverse, 5›-TACAGAGCCTGGAAGAAGCAG-3›)

Serum Creatinine

Serum creatinine in mmol/l was measured using the Jaffe reaction before operation and at time of retrieval in the bilateral IRI model.

Statistical Analysis

Statistical analyses were performed using GraphPad Prism v6 software. Data were expressed as mean±SEM or median (and range) and assessed for statistical significance by unpaired Student's t test or Mann Whitney U test. The EGTI Histology score and the Jablonski score were correlated with serum ceatinine, NGAL and KIM-1. Correlation analysis was reported with significance levels as indicated, where appropriate, in the figures provided: *$p<0.05$, **$p<0.01$, ***$p<0.001$.

RESULTS

Histology

Ten rats were used for the unilateral model (5 IRI, 5 sham) and 17 for the bilateral model (9 IRI and 8 sham). Forty-five minutes of unilateral and bilateral IRI in the rat caused marked histological damage at 48 hours when compared with sham controls.

Figures 1A-1C show normal appearance of the renal cortex in a Sham rat. Figure 1A shows that the brush border of the tubular cells is intact with no thickening of the basal membrane. No inflammation or necrosis is seen (Tubular score 0). There is no visible interstitium signifying no damage/abnormality within the interstitial compartment (Interstitial score 0). Figure 1B shows a uniform endothelium with no swelling or disruption of the endothelial cells (Endothelial score 0). Figure 1C shows an intact glomerulus with thin walled Bowman's capsule and no tuft retraction (Glomerular score 0)

Figures 1D-1F show varying degrees of damage of the renal cortex in 45-minute bilateral IRI rats. Figure 1D shows inflammation and haemorrhage within the interstitium which is present in less than 25% of the tissue without any evidence of necrosis (Interstitial score 1). Figure 1E shows thickened basal membrane of the tubular cells with loss of the brush border in more than 25% of the tubular cells, without the presence of cast formation or necrosis (Tubular score 2). Figure 1F shows a glomerulus with evidence of thickened Bowman's capsule (Glomerular score 1), and glomerular tuft retraction (Glomerular score 2).

Figures 1G-1I show varying degrees of damage of the renal cortex in 45-minute unilateral IRI rats. Figure 1G shows inflammation and haemorrhage within the interstitial compartment, with necrosis in up to 60% of the cells (Interstitial score 3). Figure 1H shows complete necrosis in tubular and interstitial cellular compartments (Tubular score 4, Interstitial score 4). Figure 1I shows evidence of inflammation and cast formation within the tubules with evidence of necrosis in up to 60% of tubular cells (Tubular score 3), and endothelial cell disruption and loss (Endothelial score 3).

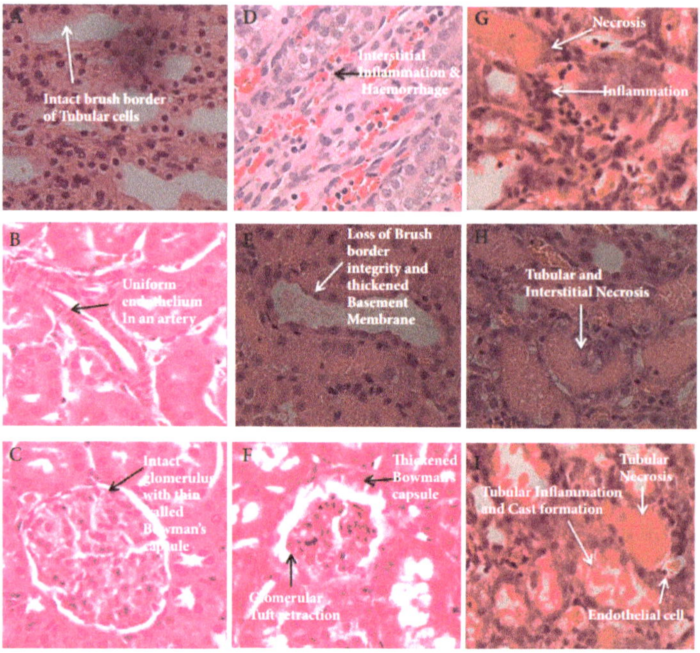

Figure 1: Histological images of rat renal cortex sections. Renal cortex H&E (x400) paraffin sections, from sham and 45-minute IRI in rats, at 48 hours after reperfusion (Bilateral sham n=8, Bilateral IRI n=9, Unilateral sham n=5, Unilateral IRI n=5) were assessed for Endothelial, Tubular, Glomerular and Interstitial cell damage. (A-C) Normal appearance of renal cortex ina sham rat. (D-F) Mild to moderate damage of the renal cortex in 45-minute bilateral IRI rats. (G-I) Moderate to significant damage of the renal cortex in unilateral 45-minute IRI rats.

Figure 2 shows mild damage of the renal cortex in a 45-minute bilateral IRI rat. There is endothelial swelling of the capillaries (A) and the vessel (B) without any disruption (Endothelial score 1).

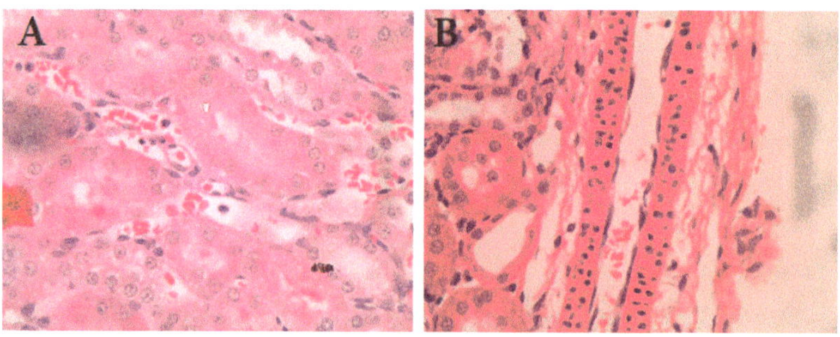

Figure 2: Histological images of endothelial cell swelling in rat renal cortex sections. Renal

cortex H&E (x400) paraffin sections, from sham and 45-minute IRI in rats, at 48 hours after reperfusion (Bilateral sham n=8, Bilateral IRI n=9, Unilateral sham n=5, Unilateral IRI n=5) were assessed for Endothelial, Tubular, Glomerular and Interstitial cell damage. Mild damage of the renal cortex in a 45-minute IRI rat.

Unilateral IRI

The median (and range) EGTI histology score was 10 (8-11) in the IRI group compared to 0 (0-1) in the sham group (p=0.0079). The mRNA expression of KIM-1 and NGAL was increased 300-fold and 30-fold in the IRI group respectively compared to sham group (p<0.0001) [13].

Bilateral IRI

The median (and range) EGTI histology score was 8 (6-9) in the IRI group compared to 0 (0-2) in the sham group (p<0.0001). Mean serum creatinine at 48 hours was 76.63(±13.36) mmol/l in the IRI group compared with 31.90(±0.25) mmol/l in the sham group (p=0.0067). The mRNA expression of KIM-1 and NGAL was increased 150-fold and 14-fold in the IRI group respectively (p<0.0001) (Figure 3). The individual components of the EGTI score were also significantly higher in the IRI group compared with sham (Figure 4).

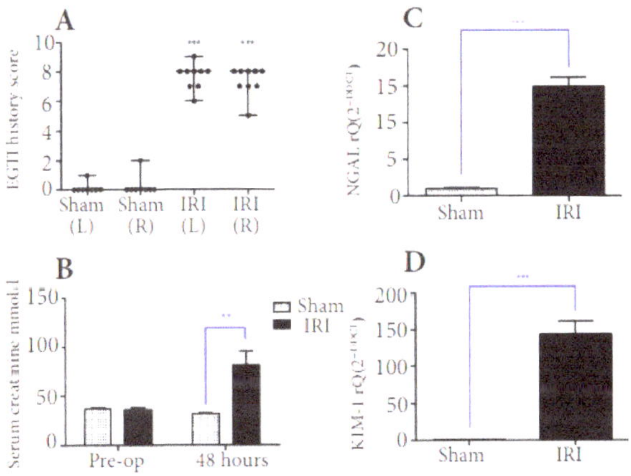

Figure 3: Effect of bilateral IRI on EGTIscore, serum creatinine and expression of NGAL and KIM-1. (A) Renal cortex sections from sham and 45-minute bilateral IRI in rats at 48 hours after reperfusion were stained with H&E and assessed using a comprehensive scoring system comprising of Endothelial, Glomerular, Tubular, and Interstitial cell damage (Sham n=8, IRI n=9). Histology scores are plotted as median and range, ***p<0.0001.

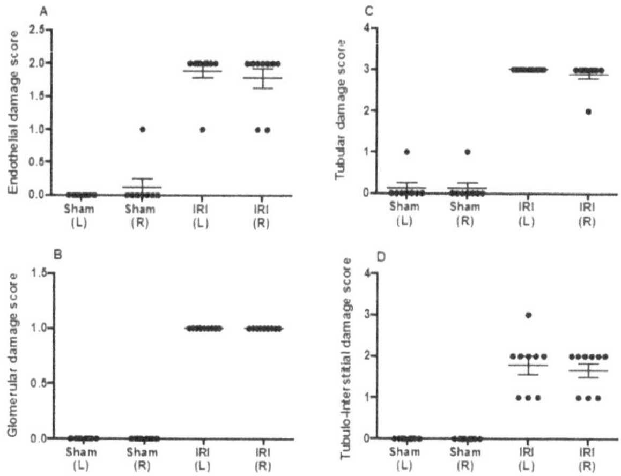

Figure 4: Effect of bilateral IRI on Endothelial, Tubular, Glomerular and Tubulo-Interstitial damages scores. Renal cortex sections from sham and 45-minute bilateral IRI in rats at 48 hours after reperfusion were stained with H&E and assessed using a comprehensive scoring system comprising of Endothelial, Glomerular, Tubular, and Interstitial cell damage (Sham n=8, IRI n=9). Individual cellular component scores are plotted as median and range for Tubular (A), Endothelial (B), Glomerular (C) TubuloInterstitial (D) components.

Correlation of EGTI Histology Scores and Jablonski Scores with Serum Creatinine, and AKI Markers

The EGTI and Jablonski scores both correlated significantly with serum creatinine at 48 hours, and expression of NGAL and KIM-1 (Figure 5). This suggests that both the EGTI score and the Jablonski score are highly predictive of kidney function and structural damage.

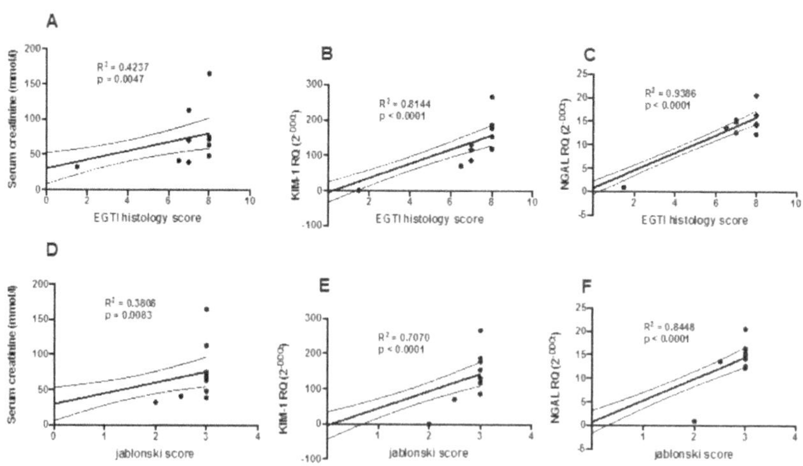

Figure 5: Correlation of EGTI and Jablonski scores with serum creatinine, NGAL and KIM-1.

Renal cortex sections from sham and 45-minute bilateral IRI in rats at 48 hours after reperfusion (Sham n=8, IRI n=9) were stained with H&E and scored using a comprehensive scoring system comprising of Endothelial, Glomerular, Tubular, and Interstitial cell damage, in addition to the Jablonski histology score. Serum creatinine was measured at 48 hours and RT-qPCR analysis of KIM-1 and NGAL was performed, with expression normalized to GAPDH. EGTI and Jablonski scores were both plotted and correlated with serum creatinine (A and D), KIM-1 (B and E), and NGAL (C and F).

In addition to this, the association between each component on the EGTI histology scoring system and serum creatinine at 48 hours, and expression of NGAL and KIM-1 was examined using univariate logistic regression analyses. Tubular, endothelial, glomerular, and tubulo-interstitial components were independently associated with serum creatinine at 48 hours ($p<0.05$), and NGAL and KIM-1 ($p<0.0001$).

DISCUSSION

This study used rat models of acute IRI to evaluate a new scoring system todocumentchanges in the histological architecture of the renal cortex, established acute kidney injury markers and renal function.

The rat models used in this study are well-established *in vivo* models of acute kidney injury [14,15]. Adult male rats are known to be more susceptible to injury, and so consistent sex selection is an important component [16]. The 45-minutes of cross-clamping of the renal pedicle produces significant but non-fatal, and potentially reversible, injury. The 48-hour reperfusion period is ample to assess the effects of a treatment modality on injury in the acute setting [17], and previous reports have shown that the 45-minute model of IRIused here allows robust and reproducible evaluation of treatment effects on IRI [18,19]. In kidney transplantation most damage occurs in the acute setting, therefore the model used in this study was chosen to reflect this. To ensure that the newly developed scoring system was robust in the presence of functional as well as structural changes as a consequence of IRI, bilateral as well as unilateral IRI models were employed.

The majority of studies investigating kidney IRI report the histological damage according to Jablonski›s acute tubular necrosis score [11]. This score is based solely on damage within the tubular cells. It does not document any damage seen to the other cellular components within the renal cortex. Tubular injury is arguably the most characteristic feature of kidney IRI but damage to other structural renal components is also important. The Jablonski scoring system is designed to give a rapid and objective assessment of kidney tubular injury, and is relatively straightforward to use. This system was originally described in a rat model of ischaemia followed by 7 or 14 days of reperfusion [11]. Such a prolonged reperfusion period results in the development of time-dependent morphological features in kidney tissue. For example, a score of ‹1› includes reference to the presence of mitoses. Mitoses are evident in the presence of tubular cell regeneration, which does not occur in acute models of IRI such as those used in the present study. For acute IRI models, the Jablonski scoring system must therefore be modified to exclude this mitotic criterion. Another significant limitation of the Jablonski system is the absence of brush border observations. One of the first tubular cell changes seen following iscahemic injury is loss of the brush border membrane, prior to cast formation or necrosis.

Kidney IRI is a complex pathophysiological process that causes structural damage to tubular, endothelial, glomerular and tubulo-interstitial cells. Loss of endothelial cell integrity, acute tubular necrosis, tubulo-interstitial damage and glomerular ischaemic damage are all hallmarks of kidney IRI thatare important to document fully and comprehensively. It is evident from Figures 1B-1D that there is some variation in IRI animals in terms of the damage to various cellular components. This supportsfurther the need for a histology scoring system that reports damage to all of these cellular components.

KIM-1 and NGAL were selected as accurate, robust and reliable biomarkers of acute kidney injury [14,20,21]. It is evident from the histological and acute kidney injury marker changes that the models of IRI used in this study led to significant injury to the kidney. Serum creatinine was selected as a marker of kidney function in the bilateral IRI model. It is the most widely usedmarker of excretory kidney function, reliablyestimating glomerular filtration rate in clinical practice [22]. In this study,changes in serum creatinine between bilateral sham and bilateral IRI rats suggest that this model of acute injury is robust.

The EGTI histology scoring system proposed in this study correlated significantly with established AKI markers and serum creatinine, demonstrating itsvalidity, reliability and sensitivity. Moreover, by reporting changes seen within all of the cellular components of the renal cortex, our new system offers a greater insight into the severity and range of damage than the Jablonski system. Similarly to the EGTI scores, the Jablonski scores correlated significantly with serum creatinine, NGAL, and KIM-1, although the correlation was slightly less pronounced.

CONCLUSION

The EGTI histology scoring system described in this paper is a reliable, sensitive and validtool to assess the degree of damage observed in kidney IRI. It is also more comprehensive than the widely used Jablonski scoring system.

AUTHORS' CONTRIBUTIONS

Authors' contributions	**UK**	**GPC**	**PN**	**RJ**	**TB**	**DF**	**RC**
Research concept and design	√	√	√	--	--	√	√
Collection and/or assembly of data	√	√	√	√	--	--	--
Data analysis and interpretation	√	√	√	√	√	√	√
Writing the article	√	--	--	--	--	--	--
Critical revision of the article	√	√	√	√	√	√	√
Final approval of article	√	√	√	√	√	√	√
Statistical analysis	√	--	--	√	--	--	--

ACKNOWLEDGEMENT AND FUNDING

We would like to thank Kidney Wales Foundation grant (for funding this project) and Department of Pathology, University Hospital of Wales, Cardiff (for their help with processing of kidney tissue specimens in formalin).

REFERENCES

1. Ojo AO, Wolfe RA, Held PJ, Port FK and Schmouder RL. **Delayed graft function: risk factors and implications for renal allograft survival**. *Transplantation*. 1997; 63:968-74.
2. Perico N, Cattaneo D, Sayegh MH and Remuzzi G. **Delayed graft function in kidney** transplantation.*Lancet*. 2004; 364:1814-27.
3. Eltzschig HK and Eckle T. **Ischemia and reperfusion--from mechanism to translation**. *Nat Med*. 2011;17:1391-401.
4. Transplant NBa. NHS Blood and Transplant Organ Donation and Transplantation Activity Report in the UK. 2014-15.
5. Godwin JG, Ge X, Stephan K, Jurisch A, Tullius SG and Iacomini J. **Identification of a microRNA signature of renal ischemia reperfusion injury**. *Proc Natl Acad Sci U S A*. 2010; 107:14339-44.
6. Bonventre JV and Yang L. **Cellular pathophysiology of ischemic acute kidney injury**. *J Clin Invest*. 2011; 121:4210-21.
7. Rabelink TJ, de Boer HC and van Zonneveld AJ. **Endothelial activation and circulating markers of endothelial activation in kidney disease**. *Nat Rev Nephrol*. 2010; 6:404-14.
8. Patschan D, Patschan S and Muller GA. **Inflammation and** microvasculopathy in renal ischemia reperfusion injury. *J Transplant*. 2012; 2012:764154.
9. Bonventre JV and Weinberg JM. **Recent advances in the pathophysiology of ischemic acute renal failure**. *J Am Soc Nephrol*. 2003; 14:2199-210.
10. Munshi R, Hsu C and Himmelfarb J. **Advances in understanding ischemic acute kidney injury**. *BMC Med*. 2011; 9:11.
11. Jablonski P, Howden BO, Rae DA, Birrell CS, Marshall VC and Tange J. **An experimental model for assessment of renal recovery from warm ischemia**. *Transplantation*. 1983; 35:198-204.
12. Livak KJ and Schmittgen TD. **Analysis of relative gene expression data using real-time quantitative PCR and the 2(-Delta** Delta C(T)) Method. *Methods*. 2001; 25:402-8.
13. Khalid U, Jenkins R, Pino-Chavez G, Bowen T, Fraser D and Chavez R. A Localized Ischemic Preconditioning Regimen Increases Tumor Necrosis α Expression in a Rat Model of Kidney Ischemia-Reperfusion Injury. *Experimental and Clinical Transplantation*. 2015.
14. Mishra J, Ma Q, Prada A, Mitsnefes M, Zahedi K, Yang J, Barasch J and Devarajan P. **Identification of neutrophil** gelatinase-associated lipocalin as a novel early

urinary biomarker for ischemic renal injury. *J Am Soc Nephrol*. 2003; 14:2534-43.

15. Kato J, Nakayama M, Zhu WJ, Yokoo T and Ito S. **Ischemia/reperfusion of unilateral kidney exaggerates aging-induced damage to the heart and contralateral kidney**. *Nephron Exp Nephrol*. 2014; 126:183-90.
16. Park KM, Kim JI, Ahn Y, Bonventre AJ and Bonventre JV. **Testosterone is responsible for enhanced susceptibility of males to ischemic renal injury**. *J Biol Chem*. 2004; 279:52282-92.
17. Dokuyucu R, Demir T, Yumrutas O, Erbagci AB, Orkmez M, Bahar AY, Bayraktar R, Bozgeyik I, Kaplan DS, Cengiz B and Bagci BC. **The role of** hepcidin and its related genes (BMP6, GDF-15, and HJV) in rats exposed to ischemia and reperfusion. *Turk J Med Sci*. 2014; 44:576-81.
18. Delbridge MS, Shrestha BM, Raftery AT, El Nahas AM and Haylor JL. **The effect of body temperature in a rat model of renal ischemia-reperfusion injury**. *Transplant Proc*. 2007; 39:2983-5.
19. Wystrychowski W, Wystrychowski G, Zukowska-Szczechowska E, Obuchowicz E, Grzeszczak W, Wiecek A and Wystrychowski A. Nephroprotective effect of pentoxifylline in renal ischemia-reperfusion in rat depends on the timing of its administration. *Transplant Proc*. 2014; 46:2555-7.
20. Vaidya VS, Ozer JS, Dieterle F, Collings FB, Ramirez V, Troth S, Muniappa N, Thudium D, Gerhold D, Holder DJ, Bobadilla NA, Marrer E, Perentes E, Cordier A, Vonderscher J, Maurer G, Goering PL, Sistare FD and Bonventre JV. **Kidney injury molecule-1 outperforms traditional biomarkers of kidney injury in preclinical biomarker qualification studies**. *Nat Biotechnol*. 2010; 28:478-85.
21. Mishra J, Dent C, Tarabishi R, Mitsnefes MM, Ma Q, Kelly C, Ruff SM, Zahedi K, Shao M, Bean J, Mori K, Barasch J and Devarajan P. **Neutrophil** gelatinase-associated lipocalin (NGAL) as a biomarker for acute renal injury after cardiac surgery. *Lancet*. 2005; 365:1231-8.
22. Suzuki Y, Matsushita K, Yoshida T, Sawabe Y and Nomura F. **[Clinical validity of renal function markers including serum** cystatin C on chronic kidney disease classification]. *Rinsho Byori*. 2011; 59:345-51.

9

CHAPTER

EFFECT OF HOMOCYSTEINE ON THE HISTOLOGICAL STRUCTURE OF FEMUR IN YOUNG MALE ALBINO RATS AND THE POSSIBLE PROTECTIVE ROLE OF FOLIC ACID

Rania A. Zidan and Heba M. Elnegris

Keywords: Homocysteine, femur, folic acid, growing rats

INTRODUCTION

Osteoporosis is a major health problem that is characterized by low bone mineral density, deterioration of bone microarchitecture and an increased risk of fracture [1].

Osteoporotic fractures are associated with increased level of morbidity and mortality and with substantial economic costs [2,3].

It has been hypothesized that the metabolism of homocysteine is involved in osteoporosis [4]. Homocystinuria, a rare autosomal recessive disease characterized by markedly elevated levels of plasma homocysteine, has several clinical manifestations involving the eyes, the vasculature, and the central nervous system. The presence of homocystinuria is associated with the early onset of generalized osteoporosis [5,6]. The underlying pathophysiological mechanism for the occurrence of early osteoporosis in patients who have homocystinuria is not completely understood [7].

Several studies confirmed an association between homocysteine and bone mineral density in postmenopausal women [8,9], in patients with Crohn's disease [10], primary

Citation: Rania A. Zidan and Heba M. Elnegris, Effect of homocysteine on the histological structure of femur in young male albino rats and the possible protective role of folic acid, DOI : http://dx.doi.org/10.7243/2055-091X-2-16.

billiary cirrhosis [11], and hyperparathyroidism [12]. A high circulating homocysteine concentration has also been mentioned as an independent risk factor for several chronic conditions, including cardiovascular and Alzheimer disease [13]. It has been proved that the administration of homocysteine caused osteopenia in newborn rats [14]. Whereas, other studies failed to confirm such an association [15].

Homocysteine (HCY) is a sulfur-containing amino acid formed in the metabolic pathway between methionine and cysteine [16]. Elevated levels of homocysteine known as hyperhomocysteinemia (HHCY) are associated with various bone abnormalities, such as osteopenia and osteoporosis [17,18]. The thiol groups in Hcy undergo auto-oxidation, thus triggering oxidative stress. Methionine is condensed with ATP to form S-adenosylmethionine, the universal methyl donor in transmethylation reactions and the direct precursor of HCY *in vivo* [19].

Folate, vitamin B_6 and vitamin B_{12} are important enzymatic cofactors in the synthesis of methionine from homocysteine (Hcy), and an elevation of Hcy can be caused by insufficiency of folate, vitamin B_6 or vitamin B_{12}[20,21].

Numerous studies have linked high circulating Hcy levels and low concentrations of folate or vitamin B_{12} with increased risk of low bone mineral density (BMD) in non-diabetic subjects [22,23].

Supplementation with vitamin B_{12} and folate has recently been shown to decrease fracture risk in stroke patients [24].

Folic acid (FA) is a naturally occurring dietary component [25]. A lack of dietary folic acid leads to a folate deficiency [26].

Folic acid is essential to numerous body functions ranging from nucleotide biosynthesis to the remethylation of homocysteine [27,28]. Children and adults both require folic acid in order to produce healthy red blood cells and prevent anemia. Folic acid can be used to treat Alzheimer's disease, depression, and certain types of cancer [29].

Previous data indicated a higher bone turnover (resorption and formation) leading to decreased bone mineral density (BMD) among individuals with high Hcy levels. A high bone turnover may lead to lower BMD and is also a risk factor for fracture [30].

Osteoclasts are specialized cells that resorb bone, whereas osteoblasts are cells that synthesize new bone. The RANK ligand (RANKL), a protein expressed by the osteoblasts, plays an important role in osteoclast formation, function, and survival through its interaction with RANK on the osteoclast [31]. Osteoprotegerin (OPG), a natural inhibitor of RANKL, interferes with RANKL and RANK association and thereby regulates osteoclast activity and resorption in the bone [32,33]. Despite this considerable evidence that identifies homocysteine as a risk factor for osteoporosis, the molecular mechanisms of how bone remodeling is hampered during hyperhomocysteinemia still remain ambiguous.The aim of the present work is to investigate the structural changes that occur in the bone and epiphyseal plate of femur in young male albino rats after being treated with oral HCY and the possible protective role of folic acid.

MATERIALS AND METHODS

Experimental animals

Thirty six young male albino rats (aged 3 weeks, weighing 50-60gm at the beginning of experiment) were housed in stainless steel cages at Animal House, Faculty of Medicine, Zagazig University at room temperature, fed standard balanced diet and allowed water ad libitum. The experiment was performed in accordance with the "Guide for the Care and Use of Laboratory Animals" [34]. The experimental protocol was approved by the Ethical Committee of Zagazig University.

Chemicals

Homocysteine (HCY)

Was obtained from Sigma-Aldrich, USA. The drug was dissolved in distilled water as a vehicle.

Folic acid

Was obtained from El Nasr Pharmaceutical Chemicals Co. And was dissolved in normal saline to give a suspension.

Groups

Rats were classified into three equal groups (12 animals each).

Group I (Control)

Rats were further subdivided into three equal subgroups.

Subgroup IA (negative control group)

Rats were gavaged with 1 ml of distilled water once daily for 6 weeks.

Subgroup IB (saline positive control group)

Rats were gavaged with 1 ml of normal saline {solution of 0.90%w/v of NaCl, isotonic saline} (the solvent of folic acid) once daily for 6weeks [35].

Subgroup IC (folic acid positive control group)

Rats were gavaged with folic acid at a dose of 2 mg/kg dissolved in 1 ml of normal saline for 6weeks [35].

Group II (homocysteine treated group)

In which rats received daily Hcys at a dose of 0.6 mg/kg b.wt. dissolved in 1 ml distilled water [36] for 6 weeks through oral gavage [37].

Group III: (homocysteine+folic acid group) (protected group)

The animals in this group received concomitant administration of homocysteine at the same dose and duration as group II plus folic acid at the same dose and duration as group IC.

At the end of experiment, rats of all studied groups were anesthetized with 35mg/kg body weight sodium pentobarbital intraperitoneally [38].

Biochemical study

Blood samples were collected to undergo estimation of serum homocysteine by enzyme-linked immuno sorbent assay (ELISA) test.

With the use of a commercial enzyme-linked immunosorbent assay (ELISA kit) (Automated Chemiluminescent System, AUS: 180®, Bayer HealthCarc). Total HCY concentration was determined after protein-bound HCY was converted to free HCY, which was then enzymatically converted to S-adenosyl- L-HCY (SAH) by S-adenosylhomocysteine hydrolase enzyme. The enzyme is specific for the L-form of homocysteine, which is the only form present in the blood.

Histological study

Specimen preparation for light microscope examination

The right femurs were carefully dissected free of soft tissue. The distal part of each bone (including the diaphysis with distal metaphysis were obtained using a sharp blade) was immediately fixed in 10% neutral buffered formaldehyde for 2 days. After fixation, preparation of decalcified specimens was performed using the chelating agent ethylene diamine tetra acetic acid (EDTA) in the form of its disodium salt (5.5 g ethylene diamine tetra acetic acid in 90 ml distilled water and 10 ml formaldehyde 37-40%). Decalcification was carried out for 3 weeks, during this time the decalcifying solution was changed every day [39]. The decalcified specimens were dehydrated and processed to form paraffin blocks. Serial coronal sections (6 um thick) parallel to the long axis of the femur and extending from one-third to one-half the thickness of each bone were prepared and stained with hematoxylin and eosin (H&E) and Mallory trichrome stains [39].

The immunohistochemical staining for localization of osteoprotegerin protein was carried out by means of the avidin biotin-peroxidase complex method following the manufacturer's instructions. The slides were incubated with mouse monoclonal anti-OPG antibody 1:250, (MAb 8051, R&D Systems, Abingdon, UK) for 1 h, washed and incubated for 30 min with antimouse biotin-conjugated secondary antibody (30 μl/2 ml of casein solution diluted 1:50) (Vector Laboratories, Peterborough, UK). Slides were washed and developed using ABC Elite kit (Vector Laboratories), followed by diaminobenzidine (DAB) and a 20 sec counterstain with haematoxylin. Negative control sections were incubated with PBS instead of the primary antibody [40].

Positive reaction appeared as brownish granules mainly in the cytoplasm of cells of osteoblastic cell lineage and sometimes areas of the trabecular surface [41]. Positive reaction was also detected in maturative/hypertrophic chondrocytes, and early osteocytes [42].

Specimen preparation for electron microscope examination

Small pieces from shaft of femur were immediately fixed in 2.5% glutaraldehyde buffered with 0.1 M phosphate buffer at pH 7.4 for 2 hours at 4°C and then washed with phosphate buffer, postfixed in 1% osmium tetraoxide in the same buffer for one hour at 4°C. The postfixed specimens were decalcified by EDTA solution in buffer for 3 successive days at 4°C. Then the specimens were washed in phosphate buffer and were dehydrated with ascending grades of ethanol. They were put in propylene oxide for 30 minutes at room temperature, impregnated in a mixture of propylene oxide and resin (1:1) for 24 hours and in a pure resin for another 24 hours. Then, the specimens were embedded in Embed-812 resin in BEEM capsules at 60°C for 24 hours [43].

Ultra-thin sections were obtained using Leica ultra cut UCT and stained with uranyl acetate and lead citrate [43] and were examined with JEOL JEM 1010 electron microscope in Electron Microscope Research Laboratory (EMRL) of Histology and Cell Biology Department, Faculty of Medicine, Zagazig University.

Morphometric and statistical study

The following parameters 'of the femur bone were quantified:

- Outer cortical bone thickness (um) of diaphysis; (mean width of outer cortical bone). This was measured by drawing a perpendicular line from just beneath the periosteum to the endosteum. Cortical bone thickness or width (μm) were determined at five levels (0.5mm apart), starting 0.2 mm below the lowest point of the growth plate [44].
- Trabecular bone thickness (um): the thickness of trabeculae in cancellous bone of distal metaphysis were measured at their midpoint away from their branching areas [45]. For estimation of outer cortical bone thickness and trabecular bone thickness, the mean values of ten non overlapping fields (at magnificationx200) from each of five different sections at different femur levels of 4 animals from each group were taken.
- The number of osteoclasts was estimated/high power field (hpf). Osteoclasts were counted in ten random high power non overlopping fields in five sections obtained from each animal of 4animals in each group.

The standard deviation was calculated and statistical analysis was carried out. The image analyzer computer system Leica Qwin 500 (Leica Ltd, Cambridge, UK) at the Image Analyzing Unit of the Pathology Department, Faculty of Dentistry, Cairo University (Egypt), was used. using SPSS statistical program version 17.

Data were evaluated by using the one-way analysis of variance test. The probability values (P) less than 0.05 was considered significant and highly significant when the P values were less than 0.001.

RESULTS

Light microscopic observations

The light and electron microscopic examinations of subgroups Ia, Ib and Ic of the control group revealed similar morphological results; hence, we chose the results of subgroup Ia (negative control) to represent the control group.

Observations of H&E stained sections

The distal metaphysis of control femur showed a network of irregular bone trabeculae and bone marrow spaces between them. The osteocytes surrounded by their lacunae were present in the bone matrix (Figure 1A).

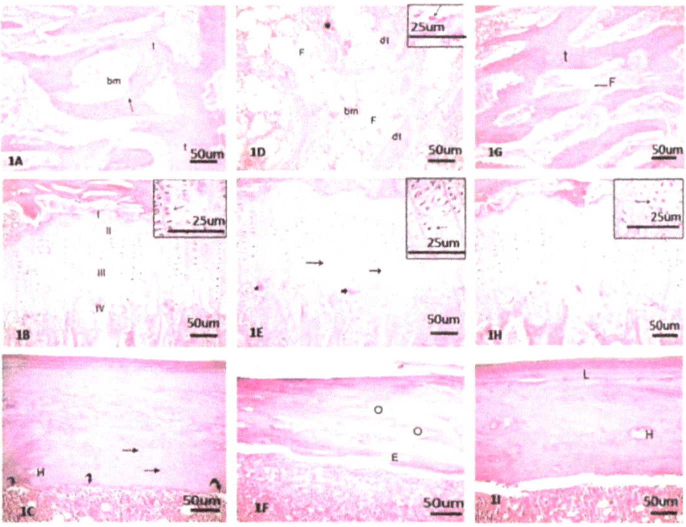

Figure 1: H&E stained sections of rat femur. Control group showing (A): A network of bone trabeculae (t) at the distal metaphysis separated by bone marrow spaces (bm). Osteocytes (arrows) surrounded by their lacunae are seen in the bone matrix. (B): Distal epiphyseal plate; showing the four well distinct zones of the epiphyseal plate; resting (I), proliferative (II), hypertrophied (III) and calcified (IV) Inset: highly organized chondrocytes (arrow). (C): Cortical bone of femur diaphysis with haversian canals (H) and osteocytes in their lacunae (arrows) Cuboidal basophilic osteoblasts on smooth endosteal bone surface (curved arrow) are also observed. Treated group showing (D): Thin widely separated disconnected trabeculae (dt) of distal metaphysis and wide bone marrow spaces in between trabeculae (bm) filled with many fat cells (F). Notice the congest-

ed blood sinusoids (*). Inset: is showing an acidophilic osteoclast (arrow) housed in the eroded bone surface. (E): Epiphyseal plate with disorganized chondrocyte column arrangement (arrow). Note the presence of many acidophilic oosteoclast (short thick arrow). Inset: most chondrocytes appear shrunken and atrophied with deeply stained nuclei. (F): Osteoporotic cavities (O) and multiple eroded (E) areas at the endosteal surface of the cortical bone. Protected group showing (G): The cancellous bone trabeculae (t) of femur metaphysis almost attaining their normal architecture as compared to group I with few fat cells (F) in marrow spaces. (H): The epiphyseal plate is almost identical with the control group in thickness. Inset: nearly preserved structure of chondrocytes. (I): Cortical bone of femur diaphysis: with observed reversal lines (L) and disappearance of osteoporotic cavities. (scale bar=50μm, inset scale bar=25μm).

The distal epiphyseal plate of control femur showed the four distinct zones of the epiphyseal growth plate with regular chondrocyte column arrangement. The growth plate showed columns of resting zone, proliferative zone, the prominent hypertrophic zone and the calcification zone, (Figure 1B). The cortical bone of femur diaphysis of the same group showed many haversian systems with well observed haversian canals and osteocytes in their lacunae. Basophilic osteoblasts on smooth endosteal bone surface were also noticed (Figure 1C).

Examination of H&E stained sections at the distal metaphysis of treated femur revealed thin widely separated disconnected trabeculae, wide bone marrow spaces filled with many fat cells and congested blood sinusoids (Figure 1D). Osteoclasts housed in the eroded bone surface were also seen (inset, Figure 1D).

Examination of H&E epiphyseal plate sections obtained from homocysteine treated rats revealed disorganized chondrocyte column arrangement, chondrocytes appeared shrunken atrophied with deeply stained nuclei. Also, many acidophilic osteoclasts were noticed (Figure 1E). As regard, sections of the femur diaphysis of this group; osteoprotic cavities (Resorption cavities) were observed in the cortical bone. Moreover, the endosteal surface of the cortical bone appeared irregularly eroded (Figure 1F).

Examination of H&E stained sections at the distal metaphysis of femur of protected group showed bone trabeculae almost attaining their normal architecture as compared with group I. Scattered adipocytes in marrow spaces were noticed. (Figure 1G). Whereas, the epiphyseal plate was almost identical with the control group in thickness and chondrocytes attain nearly preserved structure (Figure 1H). The femur diaphysis of this group showed cortical bone with disappearance of osteoporotic cavities and appearance of many reversal lines (Figure 1I).

Observations of mallory trichrome stained sections

Ttrabecular bone of control group showed high content of blue collagen fibers (Figure 2A). As regard the epiphyseal plate; the highly organized chondrocytes were embedded in an abundant bluish extracellular matrix (Figure 2B). Whereas; Cortical bone of femur diaphysis had many regularly arranged blue stained collagen fibers (Figure 2C). Mallory trichrome stained sections of treated group showed; few collagen fibers in the trabecular bone that appeared widely separated by bone marrow rich in fat cells (Figure 2D). The epiphyseal plate extracellular matrix had weak staining affinity so it appeared faint basophilic (Figure 2E). Femur diaphysis showed cortical bone with osteoporotic cavities, and few blue-stained collagen fibers. Note. Non homogenous matrix (Figure 2F).

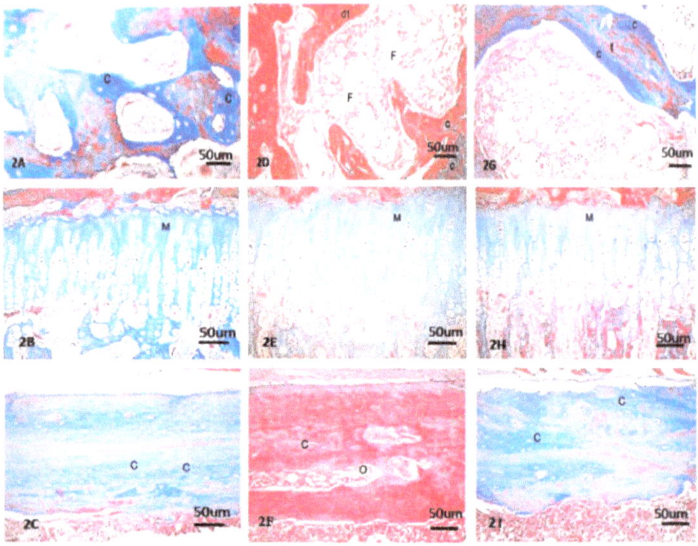

Figure 2: Mallory trichrome stained sections of rat femur. Control group showing. (A): High content of collagen fibers (C) in bone trabeculae of distal metaphysis. (B): Distal epiphyseal plate showing an abundant bluish extracellular matrix (M). (C): Cortical bone of femur diaphysis with many regularly arranged blue stained collagen fibers (C). Treated group showing. (D): Few collagen fibers (C) in the trabecular bone (dt) that appeared widely separated by bone marrow rich in fat cells (F). (E): Extracellular matrix (M) of epiphyseal plate has a weak staining affinity and appeared faint basophilic. (F): Cortical bone with osteoporotic cavities (O), and few blue-stained collagen fibers (C). Note: Non homogenous matrix. Protected group (as compared with control group) showing. (G): Nearly normal content and distribution of collagen fibers (C) in the trabecular bone (t). (H): Eepiphseal plate matrix (M) with a little reduced staining affinity in comparison with control group. (I): Cortical bone with nearly normal content and distribution of bluestained collagen fibers (C) with no cavity formation. (scale bar=50μm).

Mallory trichrome stained sections of protected group retained about normal content and distribution of collagen fibers in the trabecular bone in comparison with control group (Figure 2G). The epiphyseal plate matrix showed a little reduced staining affinity in comparison with control group (Figure 2H). Whereas, the cortical bone showed nearly normal content and distribution of blue-stained collagen fibers with no cavity formation (Figure 2I).

Osteoprotegerin immunohistochemistry

Control group of distal femur metaphysic revealed; osteoproteosteoprotegerin positive expression in the cytoplasm of most osteoblasts of endosteum. Some osteoprotegerin expression is also observed on the trabecular bone surface (Figure 3A). Examination of distal epiphyseal plate showed most hypertrophic chondrocytes and cartilage-bone interfaces are osteoprotegerin positive (Figure 3B). Whereas, cortical bone of diaphysis of the same group showed that most osteocytes were osteoprotegerin negative while few osteocytes were osteoprotegerin positive (Figure 3C).

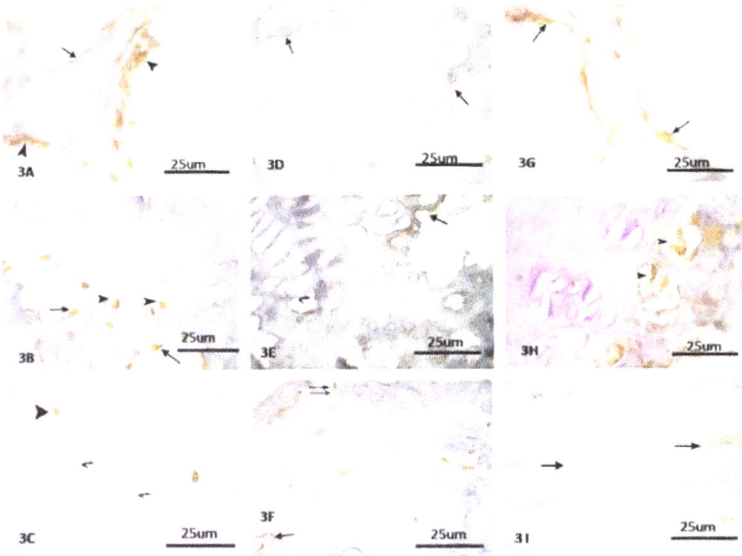

Figure 3: Osteoprotegerin stained sections of rat femur. Control group. (A): Distal metaphysis; showing the cytoplasm of most osteoblasts of endosteum are osteoprotegerin positive (arrowhead). Some osteoprotegerin expression is also observed on the trabecular bone surface (arrow) of distal metaphysis. (B): Epiphyseal plate showing most hypertrophic chondrocytes (arrow head) and cartilage-bone interfaces (arrow) are osteoprotegerin positive. (C): Cortical bone of diaphysis showing most osteocytes (curved arrow) are osteoprotegerin negative. Few osteocytes are osteoprotegerin positive (arrowhead). Treated group. (D): Trabecular bone showing weak osteoprotegerin expression in most of the cells covering the trabecular surface (arrow). (E): Epiphyseal plate revealing empty lacunae (curved arrow) and few cartilage-bone interfaces (arrow) are osteoprotegerin positive. (3): Cortical bone showing; few lining cells of osteoprotic cavities (arrow) and surface cells (double arrow) are osteoprotegerin positive. Protected group. (G): Trabecular bone showing some of the cells covering the trabecular surface are osteoprotegerin positive (arrow). (H). Epiphysal plate:a positive immunoreaction is observed in some hypertrophic chondrocytes (arrow head). (I): Cortical bone, revealing extracellular osteoprotegerin expression observed in bone matrix (arrow). (scale bar=25μm).

Examination of osteoprotegrin stained sections of treated group showed trabecular bone having weak osteoprotegerin expression in most of the cells covering the trabecular surface (Figure 3D). Examination of epiphyseal plate sections revealed empty lacunae with negative expression of osteoprotegerin whereas few cartilage-bone interfaces were osteoprotegerin positive (Figure 3E). As regard sections at femur diaphysis, lining cells of osteoprotic cavities were osteoprotegerin positive (Figure 3F).

Examination of osteoprotegrin stained sections of protected group: showed some of the cells covering the trabecular surface were osteoprotegerin positive (Figure 3G).

The epiphysal plate sections of the same group showed a positive immunoreaction observed in some hypertrophic chondrocytes (Figure 3H). Whereas; cortical bone revealed extracellular osteoprotegerin expression observed in bone matrix (Figure 3I).

Electron microscopic results

Considering examination of ultrathin sections from cortical bone of femur diaphysis of control rats revealed osteoprogenitor cells on bone surface, they contained euchromatic indented nuclei. The osteoblasts were present on the surface side by side, each cell showed many rough endoplasmic reticulum, and euochromatic nucleus with periphral heterochromatin (Figure 4A).

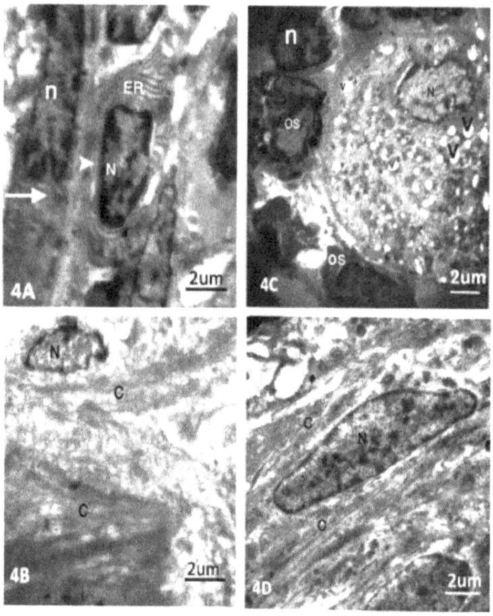

Figure 4: Electron micrographs of ultrathin sections of femur cortical bone (A) control group showing an osteoprogenitor cell (arrow) with euchromatic indented nucleus (n). An osteoblast (arrow head) is also seen having euchromatic nucleus (N) with peripheral heterochromatin and many rough endolasmic reticulum (ER). Treated group (B): Showing an osteocyt with irregular nucleus (N) containing condensed peripheral chromatin, and surrounded with many irregular collagen fibrils (C). (C): Showing an osteoclast with irregular nucleus (N). The cytoplasm contains many membrane bound-vacuoles (v) of different sizes. A row of osteoblasts, (OS) with heterochromatic nuclei (n) surrounding themselves within their osteoid product are also seen. (D): protected group showing an osteocyte with an oval nucleus (N). It is surrounded by few collagenous fibrils (C) in regular lamellae. (Scale bar=2 μm).

In treated group; osteocytes had irregular nuclei. They were surrounded by many irregular collagen fibrils (Figure 4B). The osteoclasts had irregular nuclei and many membrane bound vacuoles of different sizes. The cells were surrounded with row of osteoblasts within their osteoid product (Figure 4C). In protected group; osteocytes showed oval nuclei and were surrounded by few collagen fibrils in regular lamellae

(Figure 4D).

Biochemical results

There was no significant difference between the biochemical results of group IA, group IB and IC.

There was a significant increase in the levels of serum homocysteine in treated group in comparison with the control group. On the other hand, the protected group showed a significant decrease in homocysteine level when compared with treated group. There was no significant change between the protected group and the control group (Table 1, Figure 5A).

Table 1: Mean values of serum homocysteine (**μmol**/l) in different groups

	Mean±SD				
	Group IA	**Group IB**	**Group IC**	**Group II** (**HCY treated**)	**Group III** (**HCY+folic acid**) (**protected**)
Serum homocysteine (μmol/l)	6.4±2.36	5.9±1.2[n]	6.3±1.25[n]	11.5±3.23[a]	7.2±2.26[b]

[n]non significant as compared with group IA
[a]significant as compared with group IA
[b]significant as compared with group II

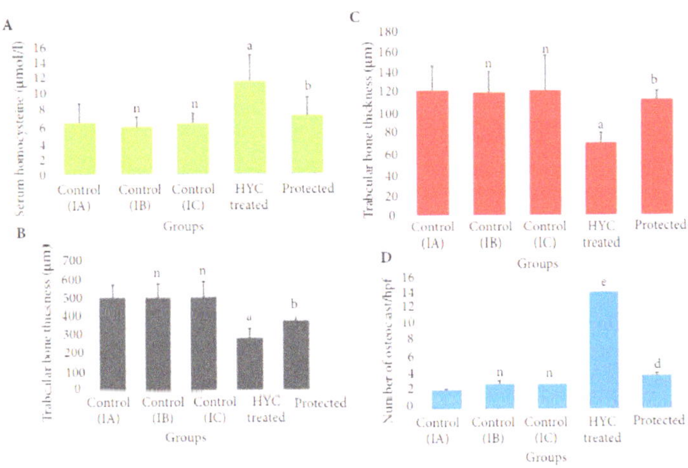

Figure 5: Histogram showing (A) the mean serum homocysteine (μmol/l), (B) outer cortical bone thickness (μm), (C) trabecular bone thickness (μm), (D) number of osteoclasts/hpf in different studied groups.

Morphometric results

There was no significant difference between the morphometric results of group IA, group IB and IC.

The mean cortical and trabecular bone thickness in group II (treated group) presented a significant decrease, ($p<0.05$) in comparison with the control group. both parameters showed a significant increase when comparing group III with group II (Table 2, Figures 5B and 5C). As regard the number of osteoclasts, there was a highly significant increase in treated group in comparison with the control group. whereas; there was a highly significant reduction in the number of osteoclasts ($P<0.001$) in protected group (III) as compared to group (II) (Table 2, Figure 5D).

Table 2: Showing the mean outer cortical bone thickness, the mean bone trabecular thickness and the number of osteoclasts/hpf in different groups

	Mean±SD				
	Group IA	**Group IB**	**Group IC**	**Group II (HCY treated)**	**Group III (HCY+folic acid) (protected)**
Outer cortical bone thickness(μm)	499.98±67.86	498±75.7[n]	501±83.2[n]	279.42±48.87[a]	370.47±20.75[b]
trabecular bone thickness(μm)	121.43±24.1	119.3±21.3[n]	121.4±34.2[n]	70.13±9.85[a]	112.52±8.4[b]
number of osteoclasts/hpf	2±0.1	3±0.37[n]	3±0.32[n]	14±0.26[c]	4±0.27[d]

[n]non significant as compared with group IA
[a]significant as compared with group IA
[b]significant as compared with group II
[c]highly significant as compared with group IA
[d]highly significant as compared with group II

DISCUSSION

Recent reports have indicated a higher risk of fractures among men and women with high levels of serum homocysteine (HCY) [46].

However, the mechanistic role of Hcy in osteoporosis is still unknown.

Regarding, the present histomorphometric results HCY treated group showed a significant reduction of cortical bone thickness with multiple cavity formation as well as a significant reduction in the trabecular bone thickness when compared with that of control rats of group I.

Previous researchers [48] have described osteoporosis as a syndrome of excessive skeletal fragility that results from both the loss of trabecular bone mass and trabecular bone connectivity.

Regarding the epiphyseal plate of HCy treated rats of the present study showed abnormal chondrocyte column cavity, shrunken atrophied chondrocytes with deeply stained nuclei. The extracellular matrix had weak staining affinity.

The observed results were in accordance with previous researcher findings [1] who demonstrated that homocysteine promoted growth in hypophysectomized rats, a finding, associated with increased thickness of epiphyseal plate.

In addition, other investigators [49] stated that HCY induced endoplasmic reticulum stress and reduced the secretion and expression of extracellular superoxide dismutase leading to an increase in the production of extracellular reactive oxygen species in vascular smooth muscle cells, leading to increased oxidative stress in the vascular wall [50,51].

In the present study, there was an accumulation of fat cells in the bone marrow of group II, Whereas, the protected group showed a decrease in marrow fat accumulation with the use of folic acid. Previous researchers [52] had reported an inverse relationship between fat and bone volume. This inverse relationship has been documented in bone obtained from animal models with high levels of marrow fat infiltration, such as osteoporosis and senescence-accelerated mouse. The mechanism suggested is through shifting of mesenchymal stem cells into fat cells at the expense of osteoblasts [53].

In the current work, osteoclasts of the treated group exhibited an increase in number as proved statitistically with subsequent bone erosions. Coinciding with these results, clinical studies have shown that adding homocysteine to chick-bud mesenchymal micromass culture caused matrix disorganization, decreased the ability of matrix to support mineralization, increased alkaline phosphatase activity, and abnormalities in collagen cross link formation [54]. Inhibition of collagen cross-linking [55], disturbance of osteoblast function [56], and increased osteoclast activity [57], were also observed in hyperhomocysteinemia.

Osteoprotegerin (OPG), is a member of the tumor necrosis factor receptor gene superfamily [58].

Osteoprotegerin (OPG) is secreted by stromal and osteoblastic lineage cells and inhibits osteoclastogenesis by preventing the interaction of receptor activator of nuclear factor-κB ligand (RANKL) with receptor activator of nuclear factor-κB (RANK) [41].

Ablation of OPG by targeted gene deletion in mice leads to early onset osteoporosis, demonstrating for the first time a critical requirement for endogenous OPG in the maintenance of normal postnatal bone mass and skeletal architecture [59].

In the current study, positive immunohistochemical expression of osteoprotegerin protein in control animals appeared mainly in the cytoplasm of the osteogenic cells and osteoblasts lining the trabecular surface, whereas epiphyseal plates showed positive reaction in maturative/hypertrophic chondrocytes. Most osteocytes of cortical bone appeared negative for osteoprotegerin. The distribution f OPG was previously demonstrated by previous studies [42].

In treated animals of the current work; the trabecular bone showed weak osteoprotegerin expression in most of the cells covering the trabecular surface. Whereas, negative expression of osteoprotegerin was demonstrated in maturative/hypertrophic chondrocytes of epiphyseal plate while treated cortical bone showed positive expression of OPG in few lining cells of osteoprotic cavities.

Similar observations were detected by previous studies [42] who also observed an extracellular immunolocalization of osteoprotegerin in the cement lines. The presence of osteoprotegerin in these site-specific areas of the trabecular bone matrix could be related to its protective action against the resorbing activity of osteoclasts.

An additional role for OPG in regulating remodeling within the cortical shafts of long bones and within bones of the skull was recorded in OPG-deficient mice [59].

It was found that osteoprotegerin administration inhibited trabecular bone loss and maintained the internal trabecular bone structure and volume in osteoprotegerin deficient mice [60].

In addition, osteoprotegerin administration in mice resulted in a decrease in the number of ostcoclasts together with absence of the ruffled border denoting reduced activity. The positive effect of osteoprotegerin on bone was most probably related to its antiosteoclastogenic capacity [61]. With reference to rats treated with HCY in the current study, electron microscopic examination revealed many degenerative changes in osteoblasts and osteocytes in the form of irregular nuclei with condensation of their chromatin. The matrix appears highly affected and its fibrils were irregularly arranged. On the other hand, the osteoclasts became more active, their cytoplasm contained many membrane-bound vesicles of various sizes that represent many lysosomes or ruffled border cut in many planes. Therefore, the osteoclasts were more active while osteoblasts and osteocytes were degenerated; reflecting that the bone resorption was more than bone formation with an inaccurate bone remdeling.

Previous experimental data have suggested that high HCY levels affected both osteoclasts and osteoblasts. It was suggested a dysbalance between osteoblasts and osteoclasts in favor of osteoclasts as a major mechanism for HCY-induced bone loss and reduced bone quality *in vivo* [4,6].

The ultrastructural results of the current work also showed that HCY treatment resulted in an irregular deposition of collagen fibrils in the extracellular compartment. This could be attributed to disruption of collagen cross-links with other agents which prevent the orderly arrangement of the extracellular matrix. The abnormal deposition of collagen in the extracellular matrix may lead to abnormal cell-matrix interactions [54].

In our study, rats of group III (protected with folic acid) had shown significant lower levels of homocysteine, histologically, these animals were protected from bone loss as compared with treated rats. However, it is not clear whether folic acid directly prevents bone loss or acts via its homocysteine lowering effect. This needs to be clarified in the next studies.

Prevention of bone loss and hyperhomocysteinemia by folic acid supplements in the present study are consistent with previous studies [62,63] which stated that the serum homocysteine level is inversely associated with folate level, and that folate supplements therapy can lower homocysteine level effectively.

Previous data suggested a role of folic acid in modulating the expression of the redox enzymes (Trx-1/NOX-4) disrupted by increased levels of HCY. These results also suggested that folic acid alleviates the oxidative stress [37].

CONCLUSION

The results of this study showed that hyperhomocysteinemia induced marked structural changes in the epiphyseal plate, trabecular and cortical bone of femur in young rats. These changes confirmed the association between increased homocysteine level and fracture risk. The suggested mechanism for these changes could be related to decreased osteoprotegerin expression as proved in our work.

Moreover, folic acid provided significant protection against bone changes induced by increased homocysteine levels. However, it is not clear whether folic acid directly prevents bone loss or acts via its homocysteine lowering effect. We recommend further research to clarify this point in the next studies. In addition, future research studies are needed to evaluate the potential clinical utility of folic acid as a therapeutic agent to prevent osteoporosis associated with hyperhomocysteinemia.

AUTHORS' CONTRIBUTIONS

Authors' contributions	RAZ	HMV
Research concept and design	√	√
Collection and/or assembly of data	√	√
Data analysis and interpretation	√	√
Writing the article	√	--
Critical revision of the article	--	√
Final approval of article	--	√
Statistical analysis	√	--

ACKNOWLEDGEMENT

We would like to thank Dr. Mona AboElkhair. For her aid in statistical results.

REFERENCES

1. Ray NF, Chan JK, Thamer M and Melton LJ, 3rd. **Medical expenditures for the treatment of osteoporotic fractures in the United States in 1995: report from the National Osteoporosis Foundation**. *J Bone Miner Res*. 1997; 12:24-35.
2. Center JR, Nguyen TV, Schneider D, Sambrook PN and Eisman JA. **Mortality after all major types of osteoporotic fracture in men and women: an observational study**. *Lancet*. 1999; 353:878-82.
3. Melton LJ, 3rd. Adverse outcomes of osteoporotic fractures in the general population. *J Bone Miner Res*. 2003; 18:1139-41.
4. van Meurs JB, Dhonukshe-Rutten RA, Pluijm SM, van der Klift M, de Jonge R, Lindemans J, de Groot LC, Hofman A, Witteman JC, van Leeuwen JP, Breteler MM, Lips P, Pols HA and Uitterlinden AG. Homocysteine levels and the risk of osteoporotic fracture. *N Engl J Med*. 2004; 350:2033-41.
5. Aubin JE, Liu F, Malaval L and Gupta AK. **Osteoblast and** chondroblast differentiation. *Bone*. 1995;17:77S-83S.
6. McLean R.R, Jacques P.F, Selhub J, Tucker K.L, Samelson E.J, Broe K.E and Kiel D.P. Homocysteine as a predictive factor for hip fracture in older persons. *N Engl J Med*. 2004; 350:2042-2049.
7. Sakamoto W, Fujie K, Isomura S, Kaga M, Kohgo T, Yamada N and Nishihira J. **Secretion of macrophage migration inhibitory factor differs from interleukin-6 in hydrogen peroxide- and LPS-stimulated human fibroblasts**. *Int Immunopharmacol*. 2002; 2:1123-31.
8. Cagnacci A, Baldassari F, Rivolta G, Arangino S and Volpe A. **Relation of** homocysteine, folate, and vitamin B12 to bone mineral density of postmenopausal women. *Bone*. 2003; 33:956-9.
9. Bucciarelli P, Martini G, Martinelli I, Ceccarelli E, Gennari L, Bader R, Valenti

R, Franci B, Nuti R and Mannucci PM. **The relationship between plasma** homocysteine levels and bone mineral density in post-menopausal women. *Eur J Intern Med.* 2010; 21:301-5.

10. Roblin X, Phelip JM, Genevois M, Ducros V and Bonaz B. Hyperhomocysteinaemia is associated with osteoporosis in patients with Crohn›s disease. *Aliment Pharmacol Ther*. 2007; 25:797-804.

11. Biagini MR, Tozzi A, Bongini E, Capanni M, Galli A, Milani S and Surrenti C. **Association of plasma** homocysteine with bone mineral density in postmenopausal women with osteoporosis or osteopenia affected by primary biliary cirrhosis. *J Clin Gastroenterol.* 2007; 41:635.

12. Alley RA, Chen EL, Beyer TD and Prinz RA. **Does** homocysteine contribute to bone disease in hyperparathyroidism? *Am J Surg*. 2008; 195:374-7.

13. Seshadri S, Beiser A, Selhub J, Jacques PF, Rosenberg IH, D›Agostino RB, Wilson PW and Wolf PA. **Plasma** homocysteine as a risk factor for dementia and Alzheimer›s disease. *N Engl J Med.* 2002; 346:476-83.

14. Azizi ZA, Zamani A, Omrani LR, Omrani L, Dabaghmanesh MH, Mohammadi A, Namavar MR and Omrani GR. **Effects of** hyperhomocysteinemia during the gestational period on ossification in rat embryo.*Bone*. 2010; 46:1344-8.

15. McLean RR, Jacques PF, Selhub J, Fredman L, Tucker KL, Samelson EJ, Kiel DP, Cupples LA and Hannan MT. **Plasma B vitamins,** homocysteine, and their relation with bone loss and hip fracture in elderly men and women. *J Clin Endocrinol Metab*. 2008; 93:2206-12.

16. Dhonukshe-Rutten RA, Pluijm SM, de Groot LC, Lips P, Smit JH and van Staveren WA. Homocysteine and vitamin B12 status relate to bone turnover markers, broadband ultrasound attenuation, and fractures in healthy elderly people. *J Bone Miner Res*. 2005; 20:921-9.

17. Eberhardt RT, Forgione MA, Cap A, Leopold JA, Rudd MA, Trolliet M, Heydrick S, Stark R, Klings ES, Moldovan NI, Yaghoubi M, Goldschmidt-Clermont PJ, Farber HW, Cohen R and Loscalzo J. **Endothelial dysfunction in a murine model of mild** hyperhomocyst(e)inemia. *J Clin Invest*. 2000; 106:483-91.

18. Dworakowski R, Anilkumar N, Zhang M and Shah AM. **Redox** signalling involving NADPH oxidase-derived reactive oxygen species. *Biochem Soc Trans*. 2006; 34:960-4.

19. Satta E, Perna A.F, Lombardi C, Acanfora F, Violetti E, Romano M.M, Capasso R, Pisano M, Paduano F and De Santo N.G. Hyperhomocyteinemia in chronic renal failure. *G. Ital. Nefrol*. 2006; 23:480-489.

20. Golbahar J, Hamidi A, Aminzadeh MA and Omrani GR. **Association of plasma folate, plasma total** homocysteine, but not methylenetetrahydrofolate reductase C667T polymorphism, with bone mineral density in postmenopausal Iranian women: a cross-sectional study. *Bone*. 2004; 35:760-5.

21. Morris MS, Jacques PF and Selhub J. **Relation between** homocysteine and B-vitamin status indicators and bone mineral density in older Americans. *Bone*.

2005; 37:234-42.

22. Stead LM, Brosnan ME and Brosnan JT. **Characterization of** homocysteine metabolism in the rat liver.*Biochem J*. 2000; 350 Pt 3:685-92.
23. Boushey CJ, Beresford SA, Omenn GS and Motulsky AG. **A quantitative assessment of plasma** homocysteine as a risk factor for vascular disease. Probable benefits of increasing folic acid intakes. *JAMA*. 1995; 274:1049-57.
24. Sato Y, Honda Y, Iwamoto J, Kanoko T and Satoh K. **Effect of folate and** mecobalamin on hip fractures in patients with stroke: a randomized controlled trial. *JAMA*. 2005; 293:1082-8.
25. Woo KS, Chook P, Lolin YI, Sanderson JE, Metreweli C and Celermajer DS. **Folic acid improves arterial endothelial function in adults with** hyperhomocystinemia. *J Am Coll Cardiol*. 1999; 34:2002-6.
26. Herrmann M, Taban-Shomal O, Muller S, Gunter L, Hubner U, Bohm M and Herrmann W.Hyperhomocysteinemia--the biochemical link between a weak heart and brittle bones? *Clin Lab*. 2006; 52:137-47.
27. Matte C, Scherer EB, Stefanello FM, Barschak AG, Vargas CR, Netto CA and Wyse AT. **Concurrent folate treatment prevents** Na+,K+-ATPase activity inhibition and memory impairments caused by chronic hyperhomocysteinemia during rat development. *Int J Dev Neurosci*. 2007; 25:545-52.
28. Bazzano LA. **Folic acid supplementation and cardiovascular disease: the state of the art**. *Am J Med Sci*. 2009; 338:48-9.
29. Zhu X, Smith MA, Honda K, Aliev G, Moreira PI, Nunomura A, Casadesus G, Harris PL, Siedlak SL and Perry G. **Vascular oxidative stress in Alzheimer disease**. *J Neurol Sci*. 2007; 257:240-6.
30. Gerdhem P, Ivaska KK, Isaksson A, Pettersson K, Vaananen HK, Obrant KJ and Akesson K. **Associations between** homocysteine, bone turnover, BMD, mortality, and fracture risk in elderly women. *J Bone Miner Res*. 2007; 22:127-34.
31. Boyce BF and Xing L. **Biology of RANK, RANKL, and** osteoprotegerin. *Arthritis Res Ther*. 2007; 9 Suppl 1:S1.
32. Hofbauer LC and Schoppet M. **Clinical implications of the** osteoprotegerin/RANKL/RANK system for bone and vascular diseases. *JAMA*. 2004; 292:490-5.
33. Boyce BF and Xing L. **Functions of RANKL/RANK/OPG in bone modeling and remodeling**. *Arch Biochem Biophys*. 2008; 473:139-46.
34. Institute of Laboratory Animal Resources. Guide for the Care and Use of Laboratory Animals. *National Academy Press*. Washington, DC. 1996.
35. Ajeigbe KO, Olaleye SB, Oladejo EO and Olayanju AO. **Effect of folic acid supplementation on oxidative gastric mucosa damage and acid secretory response in the rat**. *Indian J Pharmacol*. 2011; 43:578-81.
36. Masse PG, Boskey AL, Ziv I, Hauschka P, Donovan SM, Howell DS and Cole DE. **Chemical and biomechanical characterization of** hyperhomocysteinemic bone disease in an animal model. *BMC Musculoskelet Disord*. 2003; 4:2.

37. Tyagi N, Kandel M, Munjal C, Qipshidze N, Vacek JC, Pushpakumar SB, Metreveli N and Tyagi SC.Homocysteine mediated decrease in bone blood flow and remodeling: role of folic acid. *J Orthop Res*. 2011; 29:1511-6.

38. Waynforth HB. Experimental and **surgical** techniques in the rat. London: Academic Press. 1980.

39. Bancroft JD and Gamble M. Theory and practice of histological techniques. 6th ed. London, NewYork, Philadelphia: Churchill Livingstone. 2008.

40. Cross SS, Yang Z, Brown NJ, Balasubramanian SP, Evans CA, Woodward JK, Neville-Webbe HL, Lippitt JM, Reed MW, Coleman RE and Holen I. Osteoprotegerin (OPG)--a potential new role in the regulation of endothelial cell phenotype and tumour angiogenesis? *Int J Cancer*. 2006; 118:1901-8.

41. Hofbauer LC and Heufelder AE. **Clinical review 114: hot topic. The role of receptor activator of nuclear factor**-kappaB ligand and osteoprotegerin in the pathogenesis and treatment of metabolic bone diseases. *J Clin Endocrinol Metab*. 2000; 85:2355-63.

42. Silvestrini G, Ballanti P, Patacchioli F, Leopizzi M, Gualtieri N, Monnazzi P, Tremante E, Sardella D and Bonucci E. **Detection of** osteoprotegerin (OPG) and its ligand (RANKL) mRNA and protein in femur and tibia of the rat. *J Mol Histol*. 2005; 36:59-67.

43. Singh D. Principle **and** Techniques. In Histology, Microscopy and Photography., 2003. 1st ed., CBS Puplishers and Distributers. New Delhy, Bangalore (India). 2003; 679-699.

44. Surve VV, Andersson N, Lehto-Axtelius D and Hakanson R. **Comparison of osteopenia after** gastrectomy, ovariectomy and prednisolone treatment in the young female rat. *Acta Orthop Scand*. 2001; 72:525-32.

45. Balena R, Toolan BC, Shea M, Markatos A, Myers ER, Lee SC, Opas EE, Seedor JG, Klein H, Frankenfield D and et al. **The effects of 2-year treatment with the** aminobisphosphonate alendronate on bone metabolism, bone histomorphometry, and bone strength in ovariectomized nonhuman primates. *J Clin Invest*. 1993; 92:2577-86.

46. Sato Y, Iwamoto J, Kanoko T and Satoh K. Homocysteine as a predictive factor for hip fracture in elderly women with Parkinson›s disease. *Am J Med*. 2005; 118:1250-5.

47. Gerdhem P, Ivaska KK, Alatalo SL, Halleen JM, Hellman J, Isaksson A, Pettersson K, Vaananen HK, Akesson K and Obrant KJ. **Biochemical markers of bone metabolism and prediction of fracture in elderly women**. *J Bone Miner Res*. 2004; 19:386-93.

48. Lane NE, Yao W, Kinney JH, Modin G, Balooch M and Wronski TJ. **Both** hPTH(1-34) and bFGF increase trabecular bone mass in osteopenic rats but they have different effects on trabecular bone architecture. *J Bone Miner Res*. 2003; 18:2105-15.

49. Nonaka H, Tsujino T, Watari Y, Emoto N and Yokoyama M. Taurine prevents

the decrease in expression and secretion of extracellular superoxide dismutase induced by homocysteine: amelioration of homocysteine-induced endoplasmic reticulum stress by taurine. *Circulation*. 2001; 104:1165-70.

50. Zhang Q, Zeng X, Guo J and Wang X. **Effects of** homocysteine on murine splenic B lymphocyte proliferation and its signal transduction mechanism. *Cardiovasc Res*. 2001; 52:328-36.

51. Zhang Q, Zeng X, Guo J and Wang X. **Oxidant stress mechanism of** homocysteine potentiating Con A-induced proliferation in murine splenic T lymphocytes. *Cardiovasc Res*. 2002; 53:1035-42.

52. Pei L and Tontonoz P. **Fat's loss is bone's gain**. *J Clin Invest*. 2004; 113:805-6.

53. Ng A and Duque G. Osteoporosis **as** a lipotoxic disease. *IBMS BoneKEy*. 2010; 7:108-123.

54. Khan M, Yamauchi M, Srisawasdi S, Stiner D, Doty S, Paschalis EP and Boskey AL. Homocysteine decreases chondrocyte-mediated matrix mineralization in differentiating chick limb-bud mesenchymal cell micro-mass cultures. *Bone*. 2001; 28:387-98.

55. Lubec B, Fang-Kircher S, Lubec T, Blom HJ and Boers GH. **Evidence for** McKusick›s hypothesis of deficient collagen cross-linking in patients with homocystinuria. *Biochim Biophys Acta*. 1996;1315:159-62.

56. Sakamoto W, Isomura H, Fujie K, Deyama Y, Kato A, Nishihira J and Izumi H. Homocysteine attenuates the expression of osteocalcin but enhances osteopontin in MC3T3-E1 preosteoblastic cells. *Biochim Biophys Acta*. 2005; 1740:12-6.

57. Herrmann M, Widmann T, Colaianni G, Colucci S, Zallone A and Herrmann W. **Increased osteoclast activity in the presence of increased** homocysteine concentrations. *Clin Chem*. 2005; 51:2348-53.

58. Simonet WS, Lacey DL, Dunstan CR, Kelley M, Chang MS, Luthy R, Nguyen HQ, Wooden S, Bennett L and Boone T et al. Osteoprotegerin: a novel secreted protein involved in the regulation of bone density.*Cell*. 1997; 89:309-19.

59. Bucay N, Sarosi I, Dunstan CR, Morony S, Tarpley J, Capparelli C, Scully S, Tan HL, Xu W, Lacey DL, Boyle WJ and Simonet WS. osteoprotegerin-deficient mice develop early onset osteoporosis and arterial calcification. *Genes Dev*. 1998; 12:1260-8.

60. Yamazaki H and Sasaki T. **Effects of** osteoprotegerin administration on osteoclast differentiation and trabecular bone structure in osteoprotegerin-deficient mice. *J Electron Microsc (Tokyo)*. 2005; 54:467-77.

61. Gruber HE and Rude RK. **Alterations in osteoclast morphology following** osteoprotegerin administration in the magnesium-deficient mouse. *Biotech Histochem*. 2003; 78:231-6.

62. Manolagas SC. **Birth and death of bone cells: basic regulatory mechanisms and implications for the pathogenesis and treatment of osteoporosis**. *Endocr Rev*. 2000; 21:115-37.

63. Claes L, Schmalenbach J, Herrmann M, Olku I, Garcia P, Histing T,

Obeid R, Schorr H, Herrmann W, Pohlemann T, Menger MD and Holstein JH. Hyperhomocysteinemia is associated with impaired fracture healing in mice. *Calcif Tissue Int*. 2009; 85:17-21.

10
CHAPTER

EFFECT OF TOPICAL ALOE VERA ON THE PROCESS OF HEALING OF FULL-THICKNESS SKIN BURN: A HISTOLOGICAL AND IMMUNOHISTOCHEMICAL STUDY

Ahmed A.M. Abdel Hamid and Mona FM Soliman

Keywords: Full-thickness skin burn, aloe vera, pericytes, inflammation, healing

INTRODUCTION

Skin burn wound injury is ranked fourth in all injuries [1]. It can severely affect not only the skin but the whole body according to their depth and extension [2]. Although there are advances in its treatment the incidence of scarring remains high [3] and the deaths are over 300,000 each year throughout the world [1].

Healing of burn wound is essentially dependent on the angiogenesis which is the mainstay in the granulation tissue formation [4]. Apart from that they are considered as progenitor/stem cells, pericytes are bone marrow-derived cells (BMDC) embedded within the basement membrane of capillaries [5,6]. During the process of angiogenesis, there is a very intimate interaction between endothelial cells and pericytes [7,8]. Furthermore, pericytes play a key role not only in the proliferation and migration of the endothelium and but also in their stabilization [5]. In addition, the transmigrated inflammatory cells interact with the endothelial basement membrane to enter the site of injury [4]. Several natural substances had been tried to improve burn healing; honey is claimed to delay healing in both partial- and full-thickness burns [9]. On the other hand,

Citation: Ahmed A.M. Abdel Hamid and Mona FM Soliman, Effect of topical aloe vera on the process of healing of full-thickness skin burn: a histological and immunohistochemical study, DOI : http://dx.doi.org/10.7243/2055-091X-2-3.

topical application of curcumin showed beneficial effects in the acceleration of partial-thickness burns healing [10].

Aloe vera (AV) is a cactus-like perennial succulent that belongs to the Liliaceae Family that is usually cultivated in tropical areas [11]. It is the one of oldest medicinal substances that was used in wound healing [12]. AV has a potentially significant anti-inflammatory effect, therefore it could be used in treating: gingivitis [12-14], skin wound [15-17] and first to second degree burns [18,19]. Topical application of AV has been demonstrated to have a promising effect on the wound healing process [15]. It might have greater efficacy over silver sulfadiazine cream for treating second-degree burns [18]. However, other study claimed that AV did not increase burn healing [11] or even delayed the healing process of the burn compared with silver sulfadiazine cream [20]. In addition, it might increase production of human fibroblasts 6-8 folds faster than conventional, improve their structure and accelerate their collagen production [21].

The aim of this study was to explore the effect of AV on the process of healing specially angiogenesis in full thickness (FT) skin burn and to find out whether it improves this healing or not and the mechanism by which it acts.

MATERIAL AND METHODS

Animals

In the current study, 70 adult male albino rats weighing 180-200 gm were provided by Animal Housing of the Mansoura Faculty of Pharmacy. The animals were placed in standard plastic cages (2 animals per cage) for 12 days under 12/12 hours light/dark cycle with 23-25°C room temperature. All animals were received standard laboratory animal's chow and water ad labitum during the whole period of experiment. The experiment was performed according to the guide for the care and use of laboratory animals (Institute for Laboratory Animal Research, National Research Council, Washington, DC: National Academy Press, no. 85-23, revised 1996).

Experimental procedure

For the experiment, animals received general anesthesia by intramuscular injection of Ketamine hydrochloride (Ketalar®, Parke-Davis), 85 mg/kg of body weight, and Xylazine hydrochloride (Rompun®, Bayer), 6 mg/kg of body weight each. Then the hair on the back of the dorsal region was removed. FT skin burns were produced to each animal by using a cone-shaped, stainless steel specially-made metal instrument (purchased from Hisham Medical Company, Mansoura, Egypt), equipped with a control thermometer and heated to 1000C in a pot of boiling water for 5 seconds. Then this instrument was applied on the upper back of the rat to produce a FT burn of an area of about 2-3 cm^2. A dry dressing was applied to the wound of each, after inducing the burn, Daily monitoring of the animals and the burned wound were done.

Aloe vera gel preparation Plant leaves of AV were obtained from and processed in the Department of Pharmacognosy and Medicinal Plants, Mansoura Faulty of Pharmacy. After cleaning and disinfection, the gel was extracted by an incision in the plant leaves, which then was exposed to heat at 50°C and filtered. Glycerin and triethanolamine were added to achieve purity of AV gel of 95% which was administrated at a concentration of 200 mg/kg [22,23].

Experimental design

Group A: control group contained 10 animals. Group B: 30 animals were left to spontaneous healing. The animals were randomly divided into three subgroups of 10 animals each. Under general anesthesia, from each subgroup the burnt skin area was collected, at 4, 8, 12 days postburn. Group C: 30 animals had topical AV gel application once daily at a concentration of 200 mg/kg on the burnt skin. Then animals were randomly divided into three subgroups of ten animals each. Under general anesthesia, from each subgroup the burnt skin area was collected at 4, 8, 12 days postburn.

Histological study

Specimens were taken from the burnt skin of spontaneouslyhealed animals as well as from AV treated ones. Specimens were processed for light microscopic examination and fixed in 10% neutral-buffered formalin. They were then processed for preparation of serial paraffin sections (5 µm thick). Then, these sections were stained with H&E and MT stains [24].

Immunohistochemical study

Sections of 3 µm-thick were cut and collected on poly-L-lysine coated slides for the immunohistochemical study. Then the slides were left for 24 hours to dry at 37°C for ideal adhesion of the specimens to the surface of the slide. Following deparaffinization, hydration and antigen retrieval, sections were cooled down to room temperature. Next, they were incubated for 30 minutes in 1% H_2O_2 solution and washed in PBS, then followed by blocking in 2% skim milk for 30 minutes. The slides were incubated with the primary antibodies at 40°C for a night, and the next day, a peroxidase polymer-based secondary detection system (Dako, Heliopolis, Cairo, Egypt) was used for 30 minutes for signal amplification. 3, 3'-diaminobenzidine (DAB) (Dako, Egypt) was used for signal detection and the slides were counterstained by Hematoxylin then coverslipped. The mouse anti-α-SMA primary antibodies (Dako, Egypt) were used at dilution 1:100 for the immunohistochemical study according to the standard guidelines. They stain pericytes of blood capillaries, meanwhile the endothelium cells do not show α-SMA positivity [25,26].

Morphometric study

The sections were imaged with a microscope (Olympus, Japan) equipped with a digital camera connected to a computer and were randomly evaluated by two 8-year experience histologists under blindfold conditions.

Qualitative assessment of the phases of healing was done by employing a scoring system (0–3) for each section in various groups. This system is basically dependent on specific selected parameters which are: the inflammatory cells, the collagen deposition, the angiogenesis and the granulation tissue (Table 1) [10,27,28]. The extent of collagen deposition was qualitatively evaluated by MT stain, while the other parameters were qualitatively assessed using H&E stained sections.

Table 1: Histological scoring system for skin burn healing evaluation according to the listed specific parameters

	0	1	2	3
Inflammatory cells	None	Minimal	Mild	Evident
Collagen deposition	None	Minimal	Mild	Evident
Angiogenesis	None	Minimal	Mild	Evident
Granulation tissue	None	Minimal	Mild	Evident

Quantitative assessment of the neovascularization during the healing process in the GT was carried out. Four images from areas of maximum density of vessels(NFC) were captured in each specimen that stained by anti-α-SMA (with an x20 objective) in each group. Then, they were digitally imported to a professional image analyzer software (Image Pro Plus 6.0, Media Cybernetics, Bethesda, MD). Both the areas and numbers (densities) of the neovascularization in the GT in the specimens of each group were assessed.

The average of all values measured from images of the same slide was used, and the results were expressed as average vascular areas/1000 μm^2, and average vessel numbers/1 mm^2 respectively [7].

Statistical analysis

All statistical data analysis and graphs were carried out using SPSS 16.0 (SPSS, Chicago, IL, USA) and Microsoft Excel 13. Data were presented in mean(±)standard deviations (SD) by using ANOVA test for dual comparisons between groups, except the scoring system of healing which was evaluated by Mann–Whitney U test. The differences were considered significant when probability (P) was less than 0.05.

RESULTS

By H&E stain in the control group, the skin was formed of dermis and epidermis. The dermis was divided into papillary layer and reticular layer. The papillary layer contained dermal papillae, blood vessels and loose connective tissue (CT) with fine collagen fibers, while the reticular layer contained dense CT with coarse collagen fibers which stained blue by MT (Figures 1A-1C). Minimal α-SMA expression could be detected in the capillaries of the papillary layer of the dermis (Figure 1D).

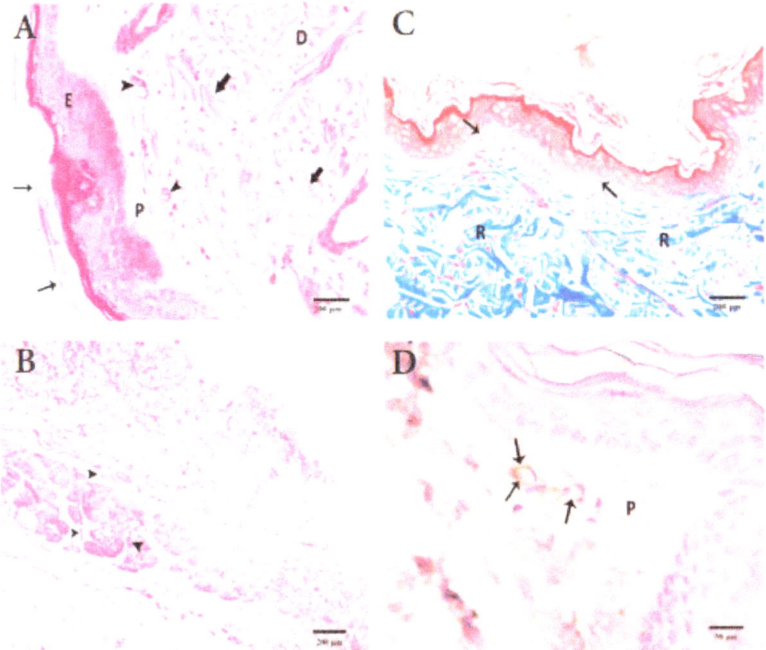

Figure 1: Photomicrographs of thin skin sections. (A) A section in thin skin of control group showing the two layers of the skin; epidermis (E) and dermis (D). The epidermis is formed of stratified squamous keratinized epithelium (arrows) covered by a thin layer of keratin. The dermis is formed of papillary layer containing abundant blood vessels (arrowheads) surrounded fine collagen while the reticular layer is formed mainly of coarse collagen (thick arrows). (H&E, x200, Scale bar=200 **μm**). (B) A section in thin skin 4 days post burn involving the whole layers of the skin in the form of tissue loss of the epidermis and coagulation necrosis of the dermis with infiltration of the deep dermis with mononuclear cell infriltrate (arrowheads) extending to the muscle layer. (H&E, x200, Scale bar=200 **μm**). (C) A section in thin skin of control group showing fine collagen fibers in the papillary layer stained light blue (arrows) while the reticular layer (R) contains more dense collagen bundles stained deep blue. (MT, x200, Scale bar=200 **μm**) (D) A section in thin skin of control group showing negative to weak positive α-SMA expression (arrows) in the blood capillaries in the papillary layer (P) of the dermis. (**α-SMA** immunostaining, x1000, Scale bar=50 **μm**).

After 4 days from inducing FT burn, sections in the skin stained by H&E stain showed coagulative necrosis involving the whole thickness of the skin with tissue loss of the epidermis and superficial layer of dermis fibers (Figure 1B). By higher magnification, there were severely congested blood vessels and marked infiltration of the dermis by significant mononuclear inflammatory cells in the GT appeared at base of the burnt area. This GT was formed of collagen fibers and NFC. Fibroblasts were the predominant cells between the collagen fibers (Figure 2A). On the other hand, in sections of 4 days skin burn treated with AV, there were less inflammatory cells infiltrate in the GT deposited at the base of the burnt area (Figure 2B).

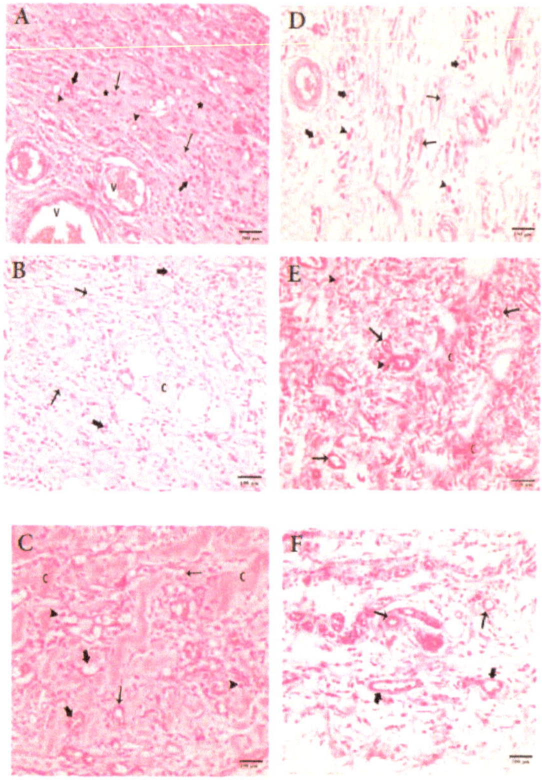

Figure 2: Photomicrographs of a H&E (x400) sections. (A) A section in thin skin 4 days post burn showing inflitration of the deep dermis with GT contining both collagen fibres (*) and NFC (arrowheads). Larger sized blood vessels (V) appear congested and surrounded by mononuclear inflammatory cells (thick arrows) together with other CT cells mainly fibroblasts (arrows). (H&E, x400, Scale bar=100 **μm**). (B) A section in thin skin 4 days post burn treated with AV showing GT containing abundant less coarse collagen bundles (C) with abundant CT cells specially fibroblasts (arrows) in between. Fewer inflammatory cells (thick arrows) are seen compared with 4-d skin burn per se group. (H&E, x400, Scale bar=100 **μm**). (C): A section in thin skin 8 days post burn showing increased number of immature NFC (arrows) which have sometimes incomplete wall (thick arrows) with a relatively decreased number of inflammatory cells (arrowheads) lying between the coarse collagen bundles (C). (H&E, x400, Scale bar=100 **μm**). (D) A section in thin skin 8 days post burn treated with AV showing increased number of NFC (thick arrows) and marked decrease in the inflammatory cells (arrowheads) lying in fine collagen fibers (arrows). (H&E, x400, Scale bar=100 **μm**). (E) A section in thin skin 12 days post burn showing increased GT formation in the form of increased density of the numerous NFC (arrows) lying in the abundant irregular collagen fibers (C) which enclose less mononuclear inflammatory cells (arrowheads). (H&E, x400, Scale bar=100 **μm**). (F) A section in thin skin 12 days post burn treated with AV showing increase of the NFC (arrows) with appearance of larger-sized blood vessels (thick arrows) in the GT. (H&E, x400, Scale bar=100 **μm**).

After 8 and 12 days from inducing FT burn, in sections of the skin stained by H&E stain, the GT showed porgessive significant increase in the vascularity by appearance of more NFC toghther with deposition of significantly more collagen rather than inflammatory cells (Figures 2C and 2E) (Histograms 2 and 3). On the other hand, in skin sections of 8,12 days skin burn treated with AV, the inflammatory cells infiltrate were decreased significantly in the deposited GT compared with burn per se group (Figures 2D and 2F); (Histogram 1).

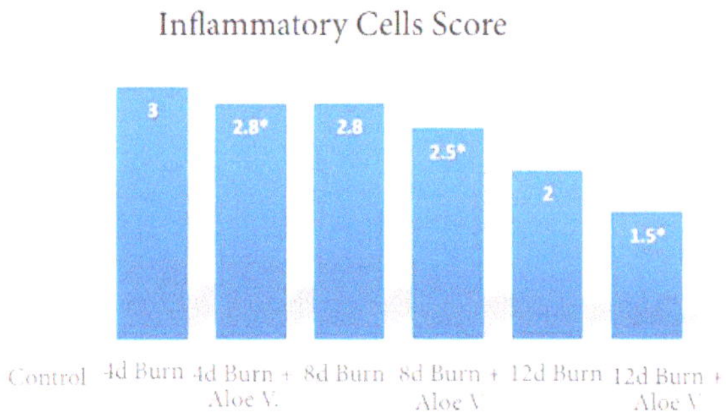

Histogram 1: Inflammatory cells score. It shows qualitative assessment of healing taking the inflammatory cells as one parameter of this assessment. *Significant difference between the means of all the groups ($p<0.05$).

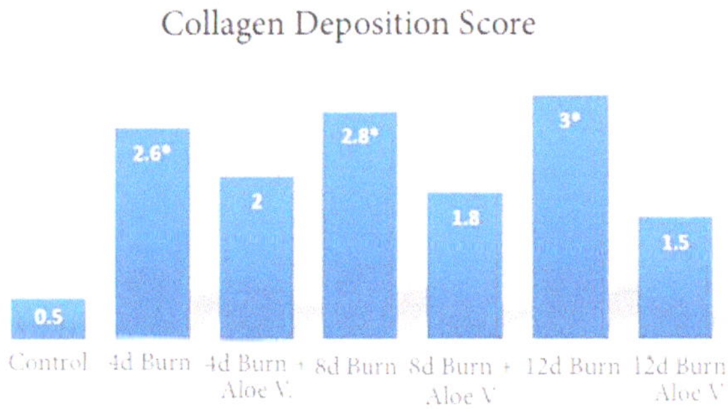

Histogram 2: Collagen deposition score. It shows qualitative assessment of healing taking the-collagen deposition as one parameter of this assessment. *Significant difference between the means of all the groups ($p<0.05$).

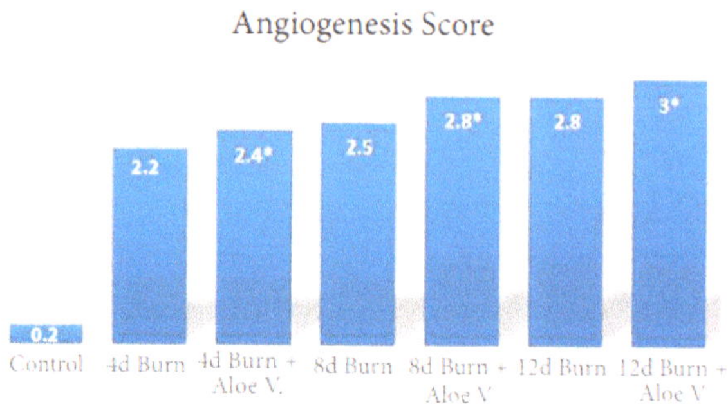

Histogram 3: Angiogenesis score. It shows qualitative assessment of healing taking the degree of angiogenesis as one parameter of this assessment. *Significant difference between the means of all the groups ($p<0.05$).

By MT stain, after 4 days of the burn, skin sections showed collagen deposition which appeared blue in color which progressively increased on 8th and 12th day sections (Figures 3A, 3C and 3E). On the other hand, in the groups treated with AV after 4, 8 and 12 days of the burn, skin sections showed much fine, less dense and more well-remodeled bluish collagen fibers compared with burn per se groups (Figures 3B, 3D and 3F); (Histograms 2 and4).

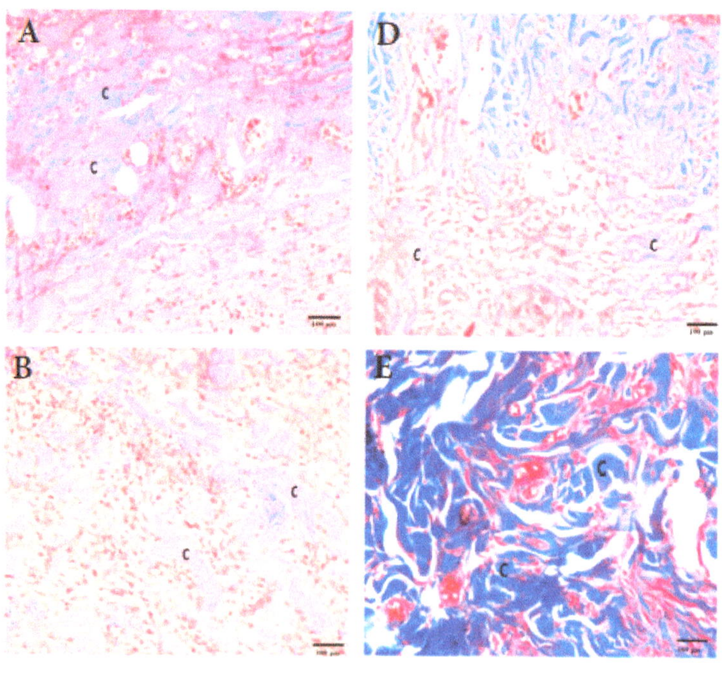

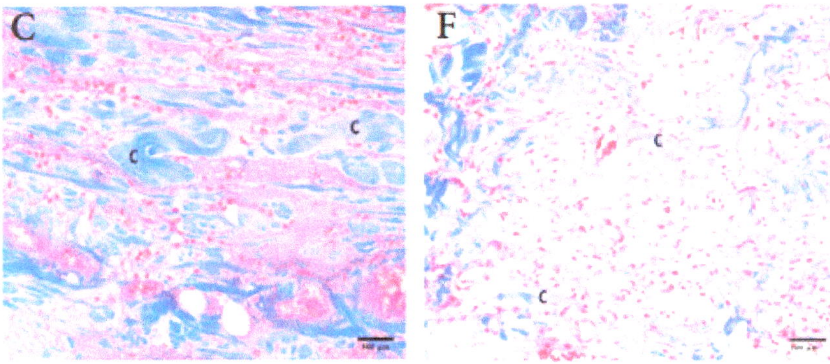

Figure 3: Photomicrographs of MT (x400) sections. (A) A section in thin skin 4 days post burn showing coarse thick bundles of collagen (C) stained blue. (MT, x400, Scale bar=100 **µm**). (B) A section in thin skin 4 days post burn treated with AV showing much more fine collagen bundles (C) compared with A. (MT, x400, Scale bar=100 **µm**). (C) A section in thin skin 8 days post burn showing excessive irregular dense collagen deposition (C). (MT, x400, Scale bar=100 **µm**). (D) A section in thin skin 8 days post burn treated with AV showing finer and more regular collagen fibers (C) in the GT compared with C. (MT, x400, Scale bar=100 **µm**). (E) A section in thin skin 12 days post burn showing increased the deposition of coarse collagen fibers (C) in the GT of the dermis. (MT, x400, Scale bar=100 **µm**). (F) A section in thin skin 12 days post burn treated with AV showing well-formed collagen deposition (c) in the dermis. (MT, x400, Scale bar=100 **µm**).

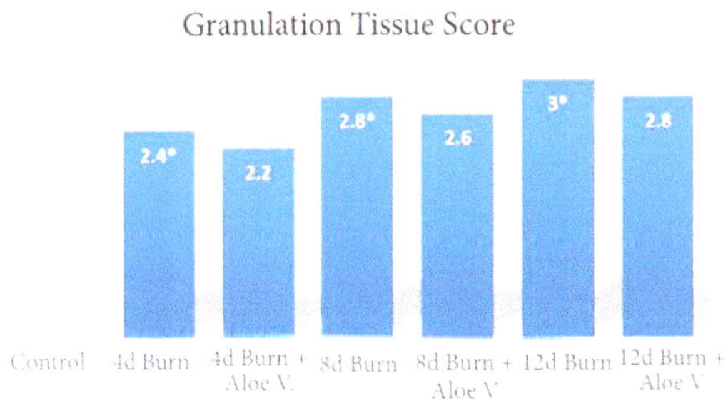

Histogram 4: Granulation tissue score. It shows qualitative assessment of healing taking the granulation tissue as one parameter of this assessment. * Significant difference between the means of all the groups ($p<0.05$).

By α-SMA immunostain, in the 4 and 8 days burn per se group, skin sections showed progressive increase in the α-SMA expression in the pericytes surrounding the immature variable size NFC in the GT. This expression become less detected on 12th day sections postburn per se. The immaturity of NFC appeared both in their size and shape; some of these NFC were small in size while the other are larger. Many of the NFC were multilayered and their lumen sometimes ranged from obliterated to partially- to fully-lumenized NFC. This NFC immaturity appeared on 4th and reached maximum on 8th day postburn per se then they become more mature in both size and shape on the 12th day sections as most these NFC were luminized with disappearance of the multilayered wall. In addition, the endothelium lining of these NFC showed always negative α-SMA expression in all sections (Figures 4A, 4C and4D).

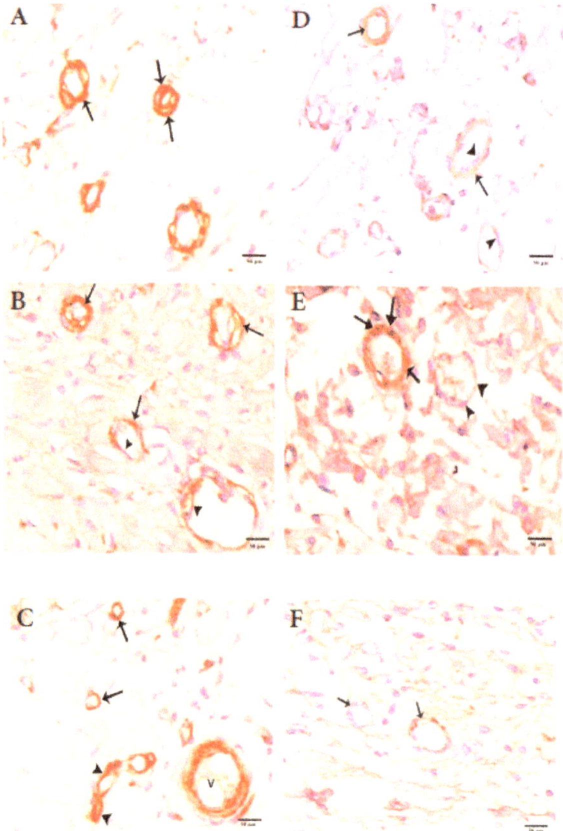

Figure 4: Photomicrographs of α-SMA immune-stained (x1000) sections. (A) A section in thin skin 4 days post burn showing increased number of immature multilayered NFC with strong positive α-SMA-stained pericytes (arrows). (**α-SMA** immunostaining, x1000, Scale bar=50 **μm**). (B) A section in thin skin 4 days post burn treated with AV showing immature variable size NFC made up of two rows of cells: internal negative α-SMAstained endothelial cell (arrowheads) and external positive α-SMA-stained pericytes (arrows) surrounding the lumen which appears partially obliterated in some and fully canalized in others. (**α-SMA** immunostaining, x1000, Scale bar=50 **μm**). (C) A section in thin skin 8 days post burn showing increased density of the immature variable-sized NFC surrounded by positive α-SMA-stained pericytes (arrows). Blood vessels sometimes appear as partially erupted cord (arrowheads) and occasionally acquire more layers to form a larger vessel (V). (**α-SMA** immunostaining, x1000, Scale bar=50 **μm**). (D) A section in thin skin 8 days post burn treated with AV showing more mature NFC with patent lumen lined by negative α-SMA-stained endothelium (arrowheads) surrounded by moderately positive α-SMA-stained pericytes (arrows). (**α-SMA** immunostaining, x1000, Scale bar=50 **μm**). (E) A section in thin skin 12 days post burn showing two NFC; one shows a moderately positiveα-SMA expres-

sion (arrows)while in the other no α-SMA expression could be detected (arrowheads). (**α-SMA** immunostaining, x1000, Scale bar=50 **μm**). (F) A section in thin skin 12 days post burn treated with AV showing more mature NFC with negative α-SMA immunostaining in most of the pericytes (arrows). (**α-SMA** immunostaining, x1000, Scale bar=50 **μm**).

In sections of 4, 8 and 12 days skin burn treated with AV, the α-SMA expression was less detected and moderate in intensity compared with burn per se groups, then this expression decreased progressively on the 8th day till it became minimally detected in most of the pericytes on the 12th day postburn (Figure 4B). Moreover, in sections of 8 and 12 days skin burn treated with AV, NFC size as well as lumen was relatively more uniform, reflecting more mature NFC compared with burn per se groups (Figures 4B, 4E and 4F). In addition, there was a significant increase in vascular numbers (densities) as well as areas on 4th , 8th and 12th day postburn groups treated with AV compared with non treated groups (Tables 2 and 3).

Table 2: Average vascular areas in different groups. Average vascular areas/1000 μm²

	FT Burn per se	FT Burn+AV
4d	42±4	48±3*
8d	71±5	78±2*
12d	87±4	96±1*

*Significant difference between the means of all the groups ($p<0.05$).

Table 3: Average vascular numbers (densities) in different groups/mm²

	FT Burn per se	FT Burn+AV
4d	86±4	94±2*
8d	154±6	168±3*
12d	189±6	197±5*

*Significant difference between the means of all the groups ($p<0.05$).

DISCUSSION

After 4 days from inducing FT skin burn, there was coagulative necrosis which is healed by GT appeared at base of the burnt area. On 8th and until 12th day from inducing the FT skin burn, the vascularity of the GT is increased by appearance of more NFC together with deposition of more collagen rather that inflammatory cells. These results were in agreement with previous studies [7,29]. Fibroblasts were always the predominant CT cells in the GT regardless the stage of healing. The core function of fibroblasts is the formation of collagen, which is a supportive protein that responsible for the skin to be firm [21]. Therefore, these non-inflammatory BMDCs are essential for homeostasis and healing of the skin [30]. Moreover, fibroblasts crosstalk with monocytes/macrophages that infiltrate the site of injury and orchestrate the healing process and tissue repair.

Monocytes dynamically react with selected extracellular matrix (ECM) components secreted by the fibroblasts. In addition, monocytes decreased fibroblast interleukin (IL)-1α and transforming growth factor-alpha (TGF)-α, however they highly increased fibroblast matrix metalloproteinase (MMP)-2 and granulocyte-macrophage colony-stimulating factor (GM-CSF) [31].

In this study, there was heavy infiltration mononuclear inflammatory cells especially initially after 4 days of inducing the burn which became milder later, when the GT acquired collagen rather than inflammatory cells. This was in agreement with other researchers [2], who claimed that macrophages initially increased by about 3 folds, then decreased gradually with maturation of the GT. Monocytes/macrophages are crucial regulatory inflammatory cells as well as the immediate arm of the innate immunity [32-34], therefore their influx into the tissue plays a critical role in the healing process. In addition, it was demonstrated that depletion of macrophages in early inflammatory phase of the healing, significantly reduced GT formation [35].

In the present study, there was significant progressive increase in the number as well as area of NFC. Macrophages, which are also BMDC, secrete proangiogenic cytokines, ECMremodeling proteases and provide physical support to the growing NFC [6,36]. Therefore, they could be responsible for the increased angiogenesis more than 10% in severe inflammatory reactions as in FT burns [2]. This may explain the significant increase in the vascularity from 4th to 12th in this study and its induction by the severity of the inflammation especially in the early reparatory phase of the burn healing.

In this experiment, in the 4 days burn per se group, skin sections showed α-SMA positive expression in the pericytes surrounding the immature variable size NFC in the GT. Then after 8 days from inducing the burn there was increase of the α-SMA expression in the pericytes. This might indicate increased immaturity of the NFC till 8 days post burn, then became less detected 12 days post burn specimens. These results were in agreement with previous studies [7] which demonstrated that during the process of angiogenesis, there was an intimate relationship between pericytes (α-SMApositive) and endothelial cells. These BMDCs, stimulated by PDGFR (platelet-derived growth factor receptors)-β, can promote mechanical support and signaling to maintain the NFC by direct interaction with endothelial cells [6]. Moreover, they could transdifferentiate into other mesenchymal cell types, including fibroblasts, smooth muscle cells or even osteoblasts. Furthermore, the increased expression of these α-SMA-positive investing pericytes could mediates sprouting as well as remodeling new vessels [37]. This might explain how essential the abundant expression of these α-SMA-positive progenitor cells specially early in 4th to 8th day post-burn rather than 12th day post-burn as they might transdifferentiate into a rather mature clone of cells in the wall of the vessel.

In skin sections of 4, 8 and 12 days skin burn treated with AV there were a significantly less inflammatory cells infiltrate in the GT compared with 4, 8 and 12 skin burn per se specimens respectively. These might be attributed to the potentially significant anti-inflammatory effect of AV [12-14]. Other researchers reported that in addition to its anti-inflammatory effect, AV acts as immunomodulator as well as scavenger of free radicals [38]. Moreover, previous studies demonstrated that AV inhibited the cyclooxygenase pathway and reduced prostaglandin E2 which might be attributed to an anti-inflammatory compound called C-glucosyl chromone isolated from AV [38,39]. In addition, recent studies suggest that a bradykinase isolated from AV could break down bradykinin, an inflammatory substance that induces pain and inflammation [21] and this might disclose the mechanisms by which AV acts as anti-inflammatory.

The collagen fibers in skin sections of 4, 8 and 12 days skin burn treated with AV there were less dense, thinner and more remodeled compared with 4, 8 and 12 skin burn per se specimens respectively. This was in agreement with previous studies, which postulated that AV induced more rapid maturation of collagen [40]. Some researchers attributed this action to glucomannan, a mannose-rich polysaccharide [41,42]. On the other hand, other researchers claimed that gibberellin, a growth hormone, interacts with receptor on the fibroblasts, thereby stimulating its activity and proliferation, which in turn accelerated collagen synthesis after topical or oral application of AV [43]. Other studies suggest that AV is an inhibitor of collagenase which might be responsible for the better remodeled collagen in the AV-treated groups [38].

In the present study, in skin sections of 4, 8 and 12 days treated with AV there were gradual decrease in α-SMA expression together with gradual significant increase in density and area as well as the maturity of NFC compared with specimens of 4, 8 and 12 d skin burn without AV respectively. This was in concurrence with other researchers who postulated that AV improved healing by increasing angiogenesis and thereby oxygenation [44,45]. This could be attributed to acemannan, a polysaccharide in AV, which was shown to activate macrophages, an effect that improved healing in a rat model [46,47]. In addition, it was reported that AV stimulated blood vessel formation in the vascular chorioallantoic membrane in chicken by a glycoprotein which could promote the stimulation of endothelial cells proliferation *in vitro* and induced them to interact with collagen [48]. However, other studies postulated that AV reduced both the vascularity and mast cells number of inflamed synovial membrane to about the half [49].

Therefore, the neovascularization effect of AV might be multifactorial from tissue to other, affected not only by the hypoxia but also by the cellular interactions and molecular alterations promoted by the injury.

CONCLUSION

In full-thickness skin burn, aloe vera shows a beneficial effect by reducing the inflammation significantly and providing a more mature granulation tissue which could accelerate healing and might produce a sound well-remodeled scar. Based on the significantly positive results of this study, it is recommended to carry out further experimental research as well as clinical trials to standardize aloe vera as a biological treatment in skin burn.

AUTHORS' CONTRIBUTIONS

Authors contributions	AAMAH	MFMS
Research concept and design	√	--

Collection and/or assembly of data	√	--
Data analysis and interpretation	√	--
Writing the article	√	√
Critical revision of the article	√	√
Final approval of article	√	√
Statistical analysis	√	--

REFERENCES

1. Peck MD. Epidemiology of burns throughout the world. Part I: Distribution and risk factors. *Burns.*2011; 37:1087-100.
2. Busuioc CJ, Popescu FC, Mogosanu GD, Parvanescu H, Streba L and Mogoanta L. Histological and immunohistochemical study of cutaneous angiogenesis process in experimental third-degree skin burns treated with allograft. *Rom J Morphol Embryol.* 2012; 53:1061-7.
3. Penn JW, Grobbelaar AO and Rolfe KJ. The role of the TGF-beta family in wound healing, burns and scarring: a review. *Int J Burns Trauma.* 2012; 2:18-28.
4. Li J, Zhang YP and Kirsner RS. Angiogenesis in wound repair: angiogenic growth factors and the extracellular matrix. *Microsc Res Tech.* 2003; 60:107-14.
5. Ribatti D, Nico B and Crivellato E. The role of pericytes in angiogenesis. *Int J Dev Biol.* 2011; 55:261-8.
6. Ding Y, Song N and Luo Y. Role of bone marrow-derived cells in angiogenesis: focus on macrophages and pericytes. *Cancer Microenviron.* 2012; 5:225-36.
7. Busuioc CJ, Popescu FC, Mogosanu GD, Lascar I, Pirici I, Pop OT and Mogoanta L. Angiogenesis assessment in experimental third degree skin burns: a histological and immunohistochemical study.*Rom J Morphol Embryol.* 2011; 52:887-95.
8. Siemerink MJ, Klaassen I, Vogels IM, Griffioen AW, Van Noorden CJ and Schlingemann RO. CD34 marks angiogenic tip cells in human vascular endothelial cell cultures. *Angiogenesis.* 2012; 15:151-63.
9. Jull AB, Rodgers A and Walker N. Honey as a topical treatment for wounds. *Cochrane Database Syst Rev.* 2008; CD005083.
10. Kulac M, Aktas C, Tulubas F, Uygur R, Kanter M, Erboga M, Ceber M, Topcu B and Ozen OA. The effects of topical treatment with curcumin on burn wound healing in rats. *J Mol Histol.* 2013; 44:83-90.
11. Dat AD, Poon F, Pham KB and Doust J. Aloe vera for treating acute and chronic wounds. *Cochrane Database Syst Rev.* 2012; 2:CD008762.
12. Ajmera N, Chatterjee A and Goyal V. Aloe vera: It›s effect on gingivitis. *J Indian Soc Periodontol.* 2013;17:435-8.
13. Karim B, Bhaskar DJ, Agali C, Gupta D, Gupta RK, Jain A and Kanwar A. Effect of Aloe vera mouthwash on periodontal health: triple blind randomized control trial. *Oral Health Dent Manag.* 2014; 13:14-9.

14. Gupta RK, Gupta D, Bhaskar DJ, Yadav A, Obaid K and Mishra S. Preliminary antiplaque efficacy of aloe vera mouthwash on 4 day plaque re-growth model: randomized control trial. *Ethiop J Health Sci.* 2014;24:139-44.

15. Khan AW, Kotta S, Ansari SH, Sharma RK, Kumar A and Ali J. Formulation development, optimization and evaluation of aloe vera gel for wound healing. *Pharmacogn Mag.* 2013; 9:S6-S10.

16. Feily A and Namazi MR. Aloe vera in dermatology: a brief review. *G Ital Dermatol Venereol.* 2009; 144:85-91.

17. Mendonca FA, Passarini Junior JR, Esquisatto MA, Mendonca JS, Franchini CC and Santos GM. Effects of the application of Aloe vera (L.) and microcurrent on the healing of wounds surgically induced in Wistar rats. *Acta Cir Bras.* 2009; 24:150-5.

18. Khorasani G, Hosseinimehr SJ, Azadbakht M, Zamani A and Mahdavi MR. Aloe versus silver sulfadiazine creams for second-degree burns: a randomized controlled study. *Surg Today.* 2009; 39:587-91.

19. Maenthaisong R, Chaiyakunapruk N, Niruntraporn S and Kongkaew C. The efficacy of aloe vera used for burn wound healing: a systematic review. *Burns.* 2007; 33:713-8.

20. Kaufman T, Kalderon N, Ullmann Y and Berger J. Aloe vera gel hindered wound healing of experimental second-degree burns: a quantitative controlled study. *J Burn Care Rehabil.* 1988; 9:156-9.

21. Ahmadi A. Potential prevention: Aloe vera mouthwash may reduce radiation-induced oral mucositis in head and neck cancer patients. *Chin J Integr Med.* 2012; 18:635-40.

22. Rajasekaran S, Sivagnanam K, Ravi K and Subramanian S. Hypoglycemic effect of Aloe vera gel on streptozotocin-induced diabetes in experimental rats. *J Med Food.* 2004; 7:61-6.

23. Daburkar M, Lohar V, Rathore AS, Bhutada P and Tangadpaliwar S. An in vivo and in vitro investigation of the effect of Aloe vera gel ethanolic extract using animal model with diabetic foot ulcer. *J Pharm Bioallied Sci.* 2014; 6:205-12.

24. Bancroft JD and Layton C. The Hematoxylin and eosin. In: Suvarna SK, Layton C and Bancroft JD editors. Theory & Practice of histological techniques. 7th ed., Churchill Livingstone of El Sevier. Philadelphia. Ch.10 and 11. 2013; 173-214.

25. Jackson P and Blythe D. Immunohistochemical techniques. In: Suvarna SK, Layton C and Bancroft JD editors. Theory & Practice of histological techniques. 7th ed., Churchill Livingstone of El Sevier. Philadelphia. Ch. 18. 2013; 381-434.

26. Busuioc CJ, Mogosanu GD, Popescu FC, Lascar I, Parvanescu H and Mogoanta L. Phases of the cutaneous angiogenesis process in experimental third-degree skin burns: histological and immunohistochemical study. *Rom J Morphol Embryol.* 2013; 54:163-71.

27. Schlager A, Oehler K, Huebner KU, Schmuth M and Spoetl L. Healing of burns after treatment with 670-nanometer low-power laser light. *Plast Reconstr*

Surg. 2000; 105:1635-9.

28. Karadag CA, Birtane M, Aygit AC, Uzunca K and Doganay L. The efficacy of linear polarized polychromatic light on burn wound healing: an experimental study on rats. *J Burn Care Res.* 2007;28:291-8.

29. Nassar MA, Eldien HM, Tawab HS, Saleem TH, Omar HM, Nassar AY and Hussein MR. Time-dependent morphological and biochemical changes following cutaneous thermal burn injury and their modulation by copper nicotinate complex: an animal model. *Ultrastruct Pathol.* 2012; 36:343-55.

30. Wu Y, Zhao RC and Tredget EE. Concise review: bone marrow-derived stem/progenitor cells in cutaneous repair and regeneration. *Stem Cells.* 2010; 28:905-15.

31. Chung AS and Kao WJ. Fibroblasts regulate monocyte response to ECM-derived matrix: the effects on monocyte adhesion and the production of inflammatory, matrix remodeling, and growth factor proteins. *J Biomed Mater Res A.* 2009; 89:841-53.

32. Geissmann F, Manz MG, Jung S, Sieweke MH, Merad M and Ley K. Development of monocytes, macrophages, and dendritic cells. *Science.* 2010; 327:656-61.

33. Popescu FC, Mogosanu GD, Busuioc CJ, Parvanescu H, Lascar I and Mogoanta L. Macrophage response in experimental third-degree skin burns treated with allograft. Histological and immunohistochemical study. *Rom J Morphol Embryol.* 2012; 53:1027-36

34. Mannon RB. Macrophages: contributors to allograft dysfunction, repair, or innocent bystanders?*Curr Opin Organ Transplant.* 2012; 17:20-5.

35. Lucas T, Waisman A, Ranjan R, Roes J, Krieg T, Muller W, Roers A and Eming SA. Differential roles of macrophages in diverse phases of skin repair. *J Immunol.* 2010; 184:3964-77.

36. Nucera S, Biziato D and De Palma M. The interplay between macrophages and angiogenesis in development, tissue injury and regeneration. *Int J Dev Biol.* 2011; 55:495-503.

37. Gerhardt H and Betsholtz C. Endothelial-pericyte interactions in angiogenesis. *Cell Tissue Res.* 2003;314:15-23.

38. Hutter JA, Salman M, Stavinoha WB, Satsangi N, Williams RF, Streeper RT and Weintraub ST.Antiinflammatory C-glucosyl chromone from Aloe barbadensis. *J Nat Prod.* 1996; 59:541-3.

39. Yagi A, Kabash A, Mizuno K, Moustafa SM, Khalifa TI and Tsuji H. Radical scavenging glycoprotein inhibiting cyclooxygenase-2 and thromboxane A2 synthase from aloe vera gel. *Planta Med.* 2003;69:269-71.

40. Reynolds T and Dweck AC. Aloe vera leaf gel: a review update. *J Ethnopharmacol.* 1999; 68:3-37.

41. Tai-Nin Chow J, Williamson DA, Yates KM and Goux WJ. Chemical characterization of the immunomodulating polysaccharide of Aloe vera L. *Carbohydr Res.* 2005; 340:1131-42.

42. Gupta VK and Malhotra S. Pharmacological attribute of Aloe vera: Revalidation through experimental and clinical studies. *Ayu.* 2012; 33:193-6.

43. Heggers JP, Kucukcelebi A, Listengarten D, Stabenau J, Ko F, Broemeling LD, Robson MC and Winters WD.Beneficial effect of Aloe on wound healing in an excisional wound model. *J Altern Complement Med.*1996; 2:271-7.

44. Yagi A, Egusa T, Arase M, Tanabe M and Tsuji H. Isolation and characterization of the glycoprotein fraction with a proliferation-promoting activity on human and hamster cells in vitro from Aloe vera gel. *Planta Med.* 1997; 63:18-21.

45. Davis RH and Maro NP. Aloe vera and gibberellin. Anti-inflammatory activity in diabetes. *J Am Podiatr Med Assoc.* 1989; 79:24-6.

46. Rodriguez Rodriguez E, Darias Martin J and Diaz Romero C. Aloe vera as a functional ingredient in foods. *Crit Rev Food Sci Nutr.* 2010; 50:305-26.

47. Jittapiromsak N, Sahawat D, Banlunara W, Sangvanich P and Thunyakitpisal P. Acemannan, an extracted product from Aloe vera, stimulates dental pulp cell proliferation, differentiation, mineralization, and dentin formation. *Tissue Eng Part A.* 2010; 16:1997-2006.

48. Davis RH, Donato JJ, Hartman GM and Haas RC. Anti-inflammatory and wound healing activity of a growth substance in Aloe vera. *J Am Podiatr Med Assoc.* 1994; 84:77-81.

49. Davis RH, Stewart GJ and Bregman PJ. Aloe vera and the inflamed synovial pouch model. *J Am Podiatr Med Assoc.* 1992; 82:140-8.

11

CHAPTER

CYTOGENOMICS OF FELINE CANCERS: ADVANCES AND OPPORTUNITIES

Rachael Thomas

Keywords: Cat, feline, genomics, chromosome, cytogenomics, cancer; comparative, fibrosarcoma, lymphoma, mammary carcinoma

INTRODUCTION

The domestic cat offers a diverse range of opportunities to contribute to the "One Health" concept, which capitalizes on the integration of complementary human and veterinary biomedical research efforts for synergistic gain. Cats continue to grow in popularity as family-owned pets and benefit from increasingly comprehensive medical surveillance [1]. It has been estimated that one in three U.S. households owns at least one cat, equating to a total U.S. cat population of approximately 74 million and a total annual expenditure of approximately $7.4 billion on veterinary services [2]. Cats exhibit approximately 200 genetic diseases that are considered analogous to human disorders, many of which are rarely encountered in any other widely studied species [3]. The cat has served as a particularly powerful model system for studying facets of neuroscience, reproduction and both heritable and infectious disease, and the field of feline oncology offers several novel angles to the comparative medicine arena. The ability to explore these attributes from a molecular standpoint has become possible only relatively recently through intensive efforts to characterize domestic cat genome organization in detail. The combination of data from complementary approaches now allows us to explore the cat genome directly in context with that of humans and other key players in comparative biomedical research. In turn we may now begin to investi-

Citation: Rachael Thomas, Cytogenomics of Feline Cancers: Advances and Opportunities, doi:10.3390/vetsci2030246.

gate in earnest the causes and consequences of genomic abnormalities associated with heritable and spontaneous disease in our feline companions.

GROSS KARYOTYPIC ORGANIZATION IN THE DOMESTIC CAT

The genome of the domestic cat (*Felis catus*, FCA) is organized into 18 pairs of autosomes and two sex chromosomes. Unlike in other mammals, where autosomes are numbered consecutively in descending order of size, standardized nomenclature in the cat takes into account both chromosome size and morphology. The karyotype comprises six autosomal subgroups termed A-F, with between two and four members in each. All but two autosomal pairs, cat chromosomes (FCA) F1 and F2, are biarmed, as are both sex chromosomes. There is substantial variation in chromosome size throughout the karyotype, from the largest (FCA A1, 240Mb) to the smallest (FCA E3, 43Mb) [4,5]. This marked diversity in size and morphology, broadly comparable to that of the human karyotype, means that chromosome identification in the cat is generally less challenging than in other key model species that exhibit more limited karyotypic variation. Gross similarity in the architecture of the human and domestic cat karyotypes has long been evident through direct comparison of their chromosome banding patterns [6,7]. These observations were reinforced by a series of molecular cytogenetic studies that indicated a remarkably limited degree of divergent evolution between the human and domestic cat genomes over the 92 million years since they shared a common ancestor, compared to the more extensive reshuffling evident in other model species [4,8,9,10,11]. The passage towards development of whole genome sequence assemblies for diverse mammals has since provided a far more comprehensive appreciation of conserved genome organization and potential mechanisms for karyotypic evolution.

GENERATION OF A REFERENCE CAT GENOME SEQUENCE ASSEMBLY

The potential role of the domestic cat in comparative biomedical research was boosted substantially by the generation of a light (~two-fold) coverage feline genome sequence assembly of "Cinnamon", a female Abyssinian, which captured ~65% of euchromatic sequence [12]. This formed part of a broader initiative funded by the National Human Genome Research Institute (NHGRI) to aid interpretation of the human genome sequence assembly, and to investigate patterns of sequence conservation, divergence and rearrangement between rodents, primates and other carnivores [13]. These studies showed that genome evolution in canine, ursine and murine lineages was driven strongly by interchromosomal translocation events, while intrachromosomal inversions were predominant in felids and also most primates [10,12]. A ~14x coverage whole genome assembly has recently become available for "Cinnamon", spanning 2.35 Gb, with sequence annotation for almost 22,000 putative protein-coding cat genes [4,5]. This resource affords a fascinating insight into the genomic factors that provide the unique phenotypic attributes of the domestic cat, and firmly equips the cat to contribute to, and benefit from, a "One Health" approach to biomedical research. Among the most rapid and exciting advances in feline molecular medicine are now being made in the area of oncology.

FUNDAMENTALS OF CANCER CYTOGENOMICS

It is well established that the onset of a malignant phenotype is associated with the accumulation of both random and non-random genomic abnormalities [14,15]. Molecular characterization of numerous diverse human cancers has identified vast numbers of recurrent somatic abnormalities, of which a proportion have been shown to correlate with discrete clinicopathologic criteria [16]. The ability to screen individual patients for these genomic markers has revolutionized diagnostic and prognostic capabilities, refining historically broad tumor classifications into clinically predictive subcategories and paving the way towards personalized disease management strategies. "Genomic profiling" also provides insight into the molecular pathogenesis of disease, identifying gene dosage imbalances associated with functional disruption of regulatory pathways, revealing key mechanistic processes underlying neoplastic transformation and progression and highlighting opportunities for targeted therapeutics.

Techniques for molecular cytogenomic evaluation of tumors fall broadly into two categories (see [17] for a detailed review). Direct techniques, such as fluorescence *in situ* hybridization (FISH) analysis, enable both structural and numerical assessment of small numbers of discrete genomic loci (typically < five) within individual cells. In contrast, indirect methods, such as comparative genomic hybridization (CGH) analysis, permit semi-quantitative measurement of mean DNA copy number within a tumor cell population at many thousands of defined intervals selected throughout the genome, but cannot detect balanced structural rearrangements. Since cancers typically exhibit a combination of both structural and numerical aberrations coupled with cell-to-cell heterogeneity, these highly complementary approaches are often used in tandem. Modified protocols allow their application to challenging specimens, such as those where the availability of clinical material is limited, or where the integrity of the sample is compromised, such as archived histologic specimens. This opens up a multitude of possibilities for retrospective studies of case materials for which detailed clinical histories are available.

The concepts of cancer cytogenomics are well established in human medicine, and enormous strides have been made in translating the same fundamental principles to domestic dog cancers. This has revealed remarkable conservation of discrete molecular alterations in human and canine counterparts of the same cancer (reviewed in [18,19]), providing strong evidence in support of a shared pathogenesis. Progress in the feline field is now gaining momentum, particularly in those areas in which the cat offers a novel perspective that has not been explored in other model species.

INJECTION-SITE SARCOMA

It is now 25 years since concerns were first raised over the increasing number of reports of malignant lesions arising at routine vaccination sites in cats [20]. The masses, predominantly fibrosarcomas, were observed most commonly in association with inflammatory reactions following the use of adjuvanted vaccines against rabies and feline leukemia virus. Vaccine-site sarcomas typically exhibit a rapid, aggressive clinical course and a bleak long-term prognosis. Treatment often involves radical surgical intervention due to the highly invasive nature of the disease, despite which localized post-surgical recurrence is common [21]. Since wide surgical margins markedly reduce the risk of tumor regrowth, there has been widespread encouragement for a transition away from traditional interscapular and femoral vaccination sites where adequate resection is highly challenging. The introduction of non-adjuvanted vaccines has also gone some way to limit the impact of vaccine-site sarcoma; however it remains a substantial clinical concern in feline medicine [22].

Interestingly, histopathologically similar tumors have also been described, infrequently, in dogs, ferrets and rabbits [23,24]. Furthermore, this phenomenon is not restricted to vaccination, since there are reports, albeit rare, of apparently related tumors manifesting in conjunction with injection of other fluids, in response to non-absorbable suture materials and even following microchipping procedures [21]. This has led to increased usage of the term "injection-site sarcoma" (ISS). Additionally, ISS shares many features with lesions occurring following ocular trauma in cats, and also with tumors arising in people in response to prolonged contact with foreign materials, such as artificial implants [22,25]. Taken in combination, these observations provide intriguing evidence for an association between persistent inflammation and malignant transformation. More than two decades after the first description of ISS, however, there remains no solid, detailed explanation for their underlying etiology, and they remain somewhat of an enigma [26,27].

Recognition of the etiology, incidence and impact of feline ISS has been challenged by difficulty in conclusive distinction between these sarcomas and those arising spontaneously without an apparent underlying injection-related origin. ISS typically are more locally invasive and prone to local recurrence than fibrosarcomas of spontaneous origin (non-ISS). Consequently, ISS generally warrant highly extensive surgical margins followed by regular and meticulous monitoring for recurrence, while non-ISS tumors may respond favorably to more conservative clinical management [27,28]. The ability to distinguish ISS from non-ISS at diagnosis therefore has far-reaching implications for patient, owner and clinician; however their extensive clinicopathologic similarity often confounds prompt and unequivocal identification. Distinction between these subtypes currently involves combinatorial consideration of multiple histopathologic features in context with clinical history and anatomical location, and often remains subjective and inconclusive. Currently there are no robust and broadly consistent diagnostic features for distinction between these subtypes. Advances in feline genomics now offer a potential molecular means to address this need and comprehend the factors that underlie the differences in their biological behavior.

Prior to the genomics era, conventional cytogenetic studies identified highly disrupted karyotypic organization in feline fibrosarcomas, with frequent hyperdiploidy and broad cell-to-cell heterogeneity [29,30,31,32]. A putative link has since been reported between amplification of feline satellite DNA sequences and the onset of genomic instability in fibrosarcomas, likely through disruption of normal centromere activity and the formation of aberrant marker chromosomes [33]. A subsequent study of five established ISS cell lines by classical enumeration of banded chromosome preparations also showed tremendously complex karyotypic reorganization, with a range of 19 to 155 chromosomes per cell, as compared to the normal 2n = 38 [34]. None of these studies, however, included detailed assessment of the composition of these aberrant chromosome structures.

Towards this goal, a microarray platform was developed to permit CGH-based identification of recurrent genomic DNA copy number aberrations (CNAs) in feline tumors [35]. This "aneuploidy array" comprised 210 large-insert clones representing loci anchored at ~15 Mb intervals throughout the initial 2x-coverage cat genome sequence assembly. Microarray-based profiling of 46 retrospective primary feline fibrosarcomas identified an extensive range of highly recurrent CNAs, consistent with the high level of genomic instability identified in earlier chromosome-based studies. Targeted FISH analysis of tumor chromosome preparations demonstrated broad heterogeneity in the patterns of structural and numerical aberrations evident both within and between cases. Remarkably, combined CGH and FISH analyses showed that a subset of genomic regions exhibited in excess of 30 copies within individual tumor cells, which were distributed across as many as ten different chromosome structures. Also of note, ISS cases showed non-random reorganization of FCA E1 in conjunction with copy number amplification of a discrete region on FCA E1p12 [35], consistent with the location of a nucleolar organizing region (NOR) [36]. Elevated argyrophilic nucleolar organizing region (AgNOR) scores, as defined by silver staining analysis, are common indicators of increased cellular proliferation, and have been associated with decreased overall survival for canine soft tissue sarcomas [37]. It is tempting to consider that this may reflect the inferior outcome that is typically associated with ISS. Statistical comparison of genomic profiles across the cohort identified two subchromosomal regions that showed significant differences in DNA copy number status in ISS *versus* non-ISS cases. While providing support for molecular discrimination, the limited resolution capabilities of the aneuploidy array confounded the ability to refine the boundaries of these regions and in turn to assess their gene content [35].

A higher-density second-generation cat CGH microarray platform has since been developed utilizing the 14x coverage cat genome sequence assembly, comprising ~110,000 oligonucleotide probes distributed at mean intervals of ~21kb. This provides a >300-fold increase in resolution over the aneuploidy array, bringing feline resources closely in line with those of other model systems for the first time. Evaluation of the same cohort of feline fibrosarcomas with this more comprehensive platform [38] identified homozygous deletions of the tumor-suppressor gene *PTEN* and recurrent amplifications of the *KIT*proto-oncogene. Elevated *KIT* protein expression has been reported as a persistent finding in both ISS and non-ISS tumors [39]; however it is not yet clear whether upregulation is a direct consequence of increased *KIT* gene dosage, nor whether this confers potential for utilizing targeted therapies directed towards this receptor tyrosine kinase. ISS and non-ISS tumors showed grossly comparable profiles of DNA copy number imbalance; however ISS cases exhibited elevated levels of global genomic disruption, consistent with their typically more aggressive behavior and poorer outcome. Among these lay a subset of discrete regions with promise as discriminatory markers [38]. With focus on the most clinicopathologically compelling genomic regions, in combination with assessment of transcriptional and translational status, there is great promise for a more detailed definition of the molecular pathogenesis of feline fibrosarcomas, and in turn, for refinement of diagnostic and therapeutic modalities for both subtypes. In a broader sense, genomic characterization of ISS also may aid elucidation of molecular mechanisms involved in the passage from chronic inflammation to neoplastic transformation, which continues to challenge human medicine.

LYMPHOMA

Lymphoma is the most common hematopoietic malignancy of cats and the third most common feline cancer overall, comprising approximately one third of all cancer diagnoses. Moreover, cats are considered to show the highest relative incidence of lymphoma among all species studied to date (reviewed in [40]), offering another promising angle for comprehending key facets of tumor biology. Historically, cytogenetic studies of feline lymphomas have focused heavily on established cell lines, primarily those developed from tumors associated with infection by feline leukemia virus, which often are nodal or mediastinal in origin. Common observations from these reports include hyperdiploidies resulting from low amplitude copy number increases of a variety of chromosomes, with no strongly recurrent features. These investigations have greatly expanded our understanding of the mechanisms by which clonal proviral integration into a host genome can initiate tumorigenesis and genomic instability through oncogenic activation [41,42]. With the diminished incidence of retrovirus-associated feline lymphoma since the 1980's, as a result of increased testing, vaccination and global vigilance, the focus has since shifted toward subtypes that offer opportunities for a more comparative approach. Extensive volumes of clinically predictive cytogenomic data are accumulating for nodal lymphomas in human patients, and more recently also in dogs [43,44]. In contrast, gastrointestinal (GI) lymphoma, which represents the most common extranodal form in people and comprises more than 50% of all feline lymphomas, remains vastly understudied at the molecular level [45,46,47,48]. Given the high incidence of the disease in cats there is an opportunity for feline studies to pave the way forward for mutual benefit. In cats, the overall survival time for low-grade small-cell GI-lymphomas is generally four-fold greater than for high-grade large-cell tumors, following standard of care chemotherapy [45,49]. The relative frequency of these histologic subtypes in different anatomical locations varies widely in prior reports [40,45,50,51,52], in part due to the logistical challenges of performing diagnostic evaluation of GI lesions by surgical biopsy [40,53]. This invites assessment of a genomic approach for comprehensive DNA-based subclassification. Initial observations from microarray-based CGH analysis have indicated that feline GI-lymphoma exhibits a relatively subtle degree of genomic copy number instability, with no evidence for recurrent high-level amplifications or homozygous deletions. The majority of aberrations are shared by fewer than 30% of cases, and include defects involving key cancer-associated genes, such as elevated copy number of the *MYC* proto-oncogene and deletion of *PTEN*. Efforts to identify candidates for molecular distinction between histologic and immunophenotypic subtypes are now underway [54].

MAMMARY CARCINOMA

Mammary tumors represent the third most commonly diagnosed feline neoplasm, the vast majority of which (in contrast to dogs) are malignant, primarily simple carcinomas. Feline mammary carcinomas (FMCs) generally are highly aggressive, infiltrative and metastatic and show extensive heterogeneity in outcome that is not readily predicted at the time of diagnosis [55]. FMC shares extensive clinicopathologic, demographic and epidemiological similarity with human breast carcinoma (HBC), the most frequently diagnosed cancer in women [56]. While there is evidence for steroid hormone involvement in some FMCs, 80%–90% are estrogen- and progesterone-receptor negative [57,58,59]. FMC therefore offers a particularly powerful spontaneous model of the ~30% of "basal-like" late-stage HBCs that are highly aggressive and unresponsive to hormone-antagonist therapies, with a lack of targeted treatments and a poor prognosis.

Diagnostic and prognostic descriptions for FMC frequently are limited in detail since there is little evidence to associate specific histomorphologic subtypes with outcome. In HBC histologic grade, typically defined using the Elston and Ellis scoring system, is one of the most robust prognostic factors [60]. Although inconclusive in dogs, it has been shown recently, using this same grading system, that invasive FMC also shows a significant incremental association between histologic grade and outcome [61]. In both human and feline patients, intermediate grade tumors show the lowest concordance in routine diagnosis and the broadest heterogeneity in outcome [60,61], and thus the greatest need for improved subclassification.

Genome-wide surveys of HBC have identified discrete genomic signatures that define clinically predictive subtypes, leading to effective treatment strategies based on molecular pathogenesis [62]. Assessment of evidence for corresponding molecular subtypes in FMC may confer potential to extrapolate these advances rapidly to feline patients. To date, the search for prognostic factors for FMC from a molecular perspective has been targeted to individual candidate genes known to be associated with HBC. Of particular note, approximately 25% of HBCs exhibit upregulation of the *ERBB2* gene encoding the receptor tyrosine kinase HER2/neu, of which >90% exhibit DNA copy number amplification of this region [63]. This aberration, historically considered to be an indicator of poor prognosis, also confers susceptibility to Trastuzamab (Herceptin®), a monoclonal antibody targeted against the HER2/neu receptor. Published estimates of HER2-positive FMCs by immunohistochemistry show tremendous variation between studies, largely due to the use of diverse patient cohorts and contrasting analytical techniques [64]. Consequently the true frequency of HER2-positive FMC, and the relationship between protein expression and gene copy number, is yet to be determined.

At the genome-wide level, early conventional chromosome banding studies of FMC identified highly disrupted karyotypes, including recurrent deletions of FCA B2 and gains of FCA E3 [65,66]. These long predated the "genomics era", precluding detailed interpretation in terms of their significance in disease pathogenesis. Microarray-based molecular profiling of FMC is now yielding more substantial insight. Preliminary results with the second-generation CGH array have demonstrated moderate DNA copy number instability in FMC that is distributed broadly throughout the genome, with very few CNAs shared by more than 50% of cases surveyed [67]. Overall, higher-grade tumors exhibit an elevated incidence of genomic imbalance, suggesting that increased chromosome instability may itself represent an indicator of inferior outcome. Interestingly, copy number gain of *ERBB2* was >3-fold more common in high-grade *versus* intermediate-grade tumors. The incidence of *PTEN* deletion was also increased in high-grade tumors, correlating with an earlier study that showed inferior outcome in FMC cases with decreased PTEN protein expression [68]. Gain of *ERBB2* and deletion of *PTEN* are among the most recurrent genomic imbalances in HBC and are associated with concomitant disregulation of gene expression and anti-apoptotic activity, and in turn with inferior outcome [69]. Continued efforts should offer new insight into the degree to which the clinicopathologic similarities between HBC and FMC are recapitulated at the genomic level, highlighting disrupted pathways and potential therapeutic targets for FMC.

CONCLUSIONS

The domestic cat is becoming increasingly well placed to stimulate new advances in molecular medicine. The unique range and distribution of cancers diagnosed in our feline companions fills a series of critical niches that have confounded progress in human medicine. Included among this diverse spectrum are those with direct human counterparts that have remained understudied due to their rarity in people, while others offer a means to study discrete facets of tumor biology that are largely peculiar to the cat. We are now in a position to perform rapid and comprehensive interrogation of normal and aberrant feline genomes and to interpret our observations directly in terms of gene content and potential dysfunction. In turn we have the ability to extrapolate with relative ease between the genomes of different species in the search for conserved molecular features that suggest a common disease mechanism. Given the gross similarity in the structural organization and evolutionary history of the human and cat genomes, it is conceivable that an integrated cytogenomic approach may help to reveal as yet unrecognized mechanisms of tumor-associated chromosome instability.

The field of personalized medicine continues to make tremendous strides in the human field, and opportunities to integrate similar concepts into the veterinary arena are gradually becoming a reality. Cytogenomic techniques are continuing to evolve, with increases in resolution, sensitivity, flexibility, throughput and cost-effectiveness, coupled with the ability to combine related techniques into single platforms that allow synergistic acquisition of data from complementary approaches in a single experiment. In the human field, cancer cytogenomic discovery is gradually transitioning from chromosome- and microarray-based techniques toward the use of next generation sequencing approaches [17]. These strategies provide substantially increased resolution capabilities and have the advantage of permitting concomitant assessment of both structural and numerical aberrations in conjunction with detection of sequence mutations. At the present time, however, their integration into the veterinary arena is constrained by high costs and intensive computational needs, and limited access to dedicated reagents and analytical tools for non-human species. Ten years ago, the same limitations applied to the use of microarray-based technologies such as those described here. Given that the field of veterinary molecular oncology is now well established, and its comparative and translational value is continually being proven, one must hope that the delay in widespread introduction of next generation sequencing strategies for use in companion animal medicine will be less profound.

REFERENCES

1. Cannon, C. Cats, cancer and comparative oncology. *Vet. Sci.* 2015, *2*, 111–126.
2. American Veterinary Medical Association (AVMA). *U.S. Pet Ownership and Demographics Sourcebook*; AVMA: Schaumburg, IL, USA, 2012.
3. Online Mendelian Inheritance in Animals (OMIA). Faculty of Veterinary Science, University of Sydney. Available online: http://omia.angis.org.au (accessed on 28 May 2015).
4. Montague, M.J.; Li, G.; Gandolfi, B.; Khan, R.; Aken, B.L.; Searle, S.M.; Minx, P.; Hillier, L.W.; Koboldt, D.C.; Davis, B.W.; *et al.* Comparative analysis of the domestic cat genome reveals genetic signatures underlying feline biology and domestication. *Proc. Natl. Acad. Sci. USA* 2014, *111*, 17230–17235.
5. Tamazian, G.; Simonov, S.; Dobrynin, P.; Makunin, A.; Logachev, A.; Komissarov, A.; Shevchenko, A.; Brukhin, V.; Cherkasov, N.; Svitin, A.; *et al.* Annotated features of domestic cat-*Felis catus* genome. *Gigascience* 2014, *3*.
6. Nash, W.G.; O'Brien, S.J. Conserved regions of homologous G-banded chromosomes between orders in mammalian evolution: Carnivores and primates. *Proc. Natl. Acad. Sci. USA* 1982, *79*, 6631–6635.
7. Yang, F.; Graphodatsky, A.S.; O'Brien, P.C.; Colabella, A.; Solanky, N.; Squire, M.; Sargan, D.R.; Ferguson-Smith, M.A. Reciprocal chromosome painting illuminates the history of genome evolution of the domestic cat, dog and human. *Chromosome Res.* 2000, *8*, 393–404.
8. Rettenberger, G.; Klett, C.; Zechner, U.; Bruch, J.; Just, W.; Vogel, W.; Hameister, H. Zoo-FISH analysis: Cat and human karyotypes closely resemble the putative ancestral mammalian karyotype. *Chromosome Res.* 1995, *3*, 479–486.
9. Stanyon, R.; Yang, F.; Cavagna, P.; O'Brien, P.C.; Bagga, M.; Ferguson-Smith, M.A.; Wienberg, J. Reciprocal chromosome painting shows that genomic rearrangement between rat and mouse proceeds ten times faster than between humans and cats. *Cytogenet. Cell Genet.* 1999, *84*, 150–155.
10. O'Brien, S.J.; Johnson, W.; Driscoll, C.; Pontius, J.; Pecon-Slattery, J.; Menotti-Raymond, M. State of cat genomics.*Trends Genet.* 2008, *24*, 268–279.
11. Graphodatsky, A.S.; Trifonov, V.A.; Stanyon, R. The genome diversity and karyotype evolution of mammals. *Mol. Cytogenet.* 2011, *4*.
12. Pontius, J.U.; Mullikin, J.C.; Smith, D.R.; Lindblad-Toh, K.; Gnerre, S.; Clamp, M.; Chang, J.; Stephens, R.; Neelam, B.; Volfovsky, N.; *et al.* Initial sequence and comparative analysis of the cat genome. *Genome Res.* 2007, *17*, 1675–1689.
13. Lindblad-Toh, K.; Garber, M.; Zuk, O.; Lin, M.F.; Parker, B.J.; Washietl, S.; Kheradpour, P.; Ernst, J.; Jordan, G.; Mauceli, E.; *et al.* A high-resolution map of

human evolutionary constraint using 29 mammals. *Nature* 2011, *478*, 476–482.

14. Bernheim, A. Cytogenomics of cancers: From chromosome to sequence. *Mol. Oncol.* 2010, *4*, 309–322.
15. Sandberg, A.A.; Meloni-Ehrig, A.M. Cytogenetics and genetics of human cancer: Methods and accomplishments.*Cancer Genet. Cytogenet.* 2010, *203*, 102–126.
16. Mitelman, F.; Johansson, B.; Mertens, F. Mitelman Database of Chromosome Aberrations and Gene Fusions in Cancer. Available online: http://cgap.nci.nih.gov/chromosomes/mitelman (accessed on 31 May 2015).
17. Le Scouarnec, S.; Gribble, S.M. Characterising chromosome rearrangements: Recent technical advances in molecular cytogenetics. *Heredity (Edinb)* 2012, *108*, 75–85.
18. Breen, M. Comparative Cytogenetics. Available online: http://www.els.net (accessed on 22 July 2015).
19. Schiffman, J.D.; Breen, M. Comparative oncology: What dogs and other species can teach us about humans with cancer. *Phil. Trans. Roy. Soc. B-Biol. Sci.* 2015, *370*.
20. Hendrick, M.J.; Goldschmidt, M.H. Do injection site reactions induce fibrosarcomas in cats? *J. Amer. Vet. Med. Assoc.*1991. Avaiable online: http://europepmc.org/abstract/med/1748617 (accessed 28 August 2015).
21. Martano, M.; Morello, E.; Buracco, P. Feline injection-site sarcoma: Past, present and future perspectives. *Vet. J.* 2011,*188*, 136–141.
22. Woodward, K.N. Origins of injection-site sarcomas in cats: The possible role of chronic inflammation—A review.*ISRN Vet. Sci.* 2011, *2011*.
23. Munday, J.S.; Stedman, N.L.; Richey, L.J. Histology and immunohistochemistry of seven ferret vaccination-site fibrosarcomas. *Vet. Pathol.* 2003, *40*, 288–293.
24. Vascellari, M.; Melchiotti, E.; Bozza, M.A.; Mutinelli, F. Fibrosarcomas at presumed sites of injection in dogs: Characteristics and comparison with non-vaccination site fibrosarcomas and feline post-vaccinal fibrosarcomas. *J. Vet. Med. A-Physiol. Pathol. Clin. Med.* 2003, *50*, 286–291.
25. Moizhess, T.G. Carcinogenesis induced by foreign bodies. *Biochemistry (Mosc.)* 2008, *73*, 763–775.
26. Hendrick, M.J. Musings on feline injection site sarcomas. *Vet. J.* 2011, *188*, 130–131.
27. Ladlow, J. Injection site-associated sarcoma in the cat: Treatment recommendations and results to date. *J. Feline Med. Surg.* 2013, *15*, 409–418.
28. Dobson, J.M.; Demetriou, J.; Seguin, B. Chapters 20: Skin tumors and 22: Injection site sarcomas. In *Feline Soft Tissue and General Surgery*, 1st ed.; Langley-Hobbs, S., Demetriou, J., Ladlow, J., Eds.; Saunders Elsevier: Philadelphia, PA, USA, 2013; pp. 209–242.
29. Kalat, M.; Mayr, B.; Schleger, W.; Wagner, B.; Reifinger, M. Chromosomal hyperdiploidy in a feline sarcoma. *Res. Vet. Sci.* 1991, *51*, 227–228.

30. Mayr, B.; Bockstahler, B.; Loupal, G.; Reifinger, M.; Schleger, W. Cytogenetic variation between four cases of feline fibrosarcoma. *Res. Vet. Sci.* 1996, *61*, 268–270.

31. Mayr, B.; Eschborn, U.; Kalat, M. Near triploidy in a feline fibrosarcoma. *Zentralbl. Veterinarmed. A* 1991, *38*, 617–620.

32. Mayr, B.; Hofstadler, E.; Schleger, W.; Reifinger, M.; Eisenmenger, E. Trisomy D1, marker F1: New cytogenetic findings in two cases of feline fibrosarcoma. *Zentralbl. Veterinarmed. A* 1994, *41*, 197–201.

33. Santos, S.; Chaves, R.; Adega, F.; Bastos, E.; Guedes-Pinto, H. Amplification of the major satellite DNA family (FA-SAT) in a cat fibrosarcoma might be related to chromosomal instability. *J. Hered.* 2006, *97*, 114–118.

34. von Erichsen, J.; Hecht, W.; Lohberg-Gruene, C.; Reinacher, M. Cell lines derived from feline fibrosarcoma display unstable chromosomal aneuploidy and additionally centrosome number aberrations. *Vet. Pathol.* 2012, *49*, 648–657.

35. Thomas, R.; Valli, V.E.; Ellis, P.; Bell, J.; Karlsson, E.K.; Cullen, J.; Lindblad-Toh, K.; Langford, C.F.; Breen, M. Microarray-based cytogenetic profiling reveals recurrent and subtype-associated genomic copy number aberrations in feline sarcomas. *Chromosome Res.* 2009, *17*, 987–1000.

36. Szczerbal, I.; Michalak, E. FISH-localization of the nucleolar organizer region on the feline E1p12 chromosome. *Anim. Genet.* 2003, *34*, 386–387.

37. Ettinger, S.N.; Scase, T.J.; Oberthaler, K.T.; Craft, D.M.; McKnight, J.A.; Leibman, N.F.; Charney, S.C.; Bergman, P.J. Association of argyrophilic nucleolar organizing regions, Ki-67, and proliferating cell nuclear antigen scores with histologic grade and survival in dogs with soft tissue sarcomas: 60 cases (1996–2002). *J. Am. Vet. Med. Assoc.* 2006, *228*, 1053–1062.

38. Thomas, R.; Pontius, J.; Borst, L.; Lamm, C.; Breen, M. Development Of A Genome-Anchored Microarray Platform for Identification of Clinically Predictive Somatic DNA Copy Number Aberrations in Feline Cancers. In Proceedings of the 7th International Conference on Advances in Canine and Feline Genomics and Inherited Diseases, Cambridge, MA, USA, 23–27 September 2013.

39. Smith, A.J.; Njaa, B.L.; Lamm, C.G. Immunohistochemical expression of c-KIT protein in feline soft tissue fibrosarcomas. *Vet. Pathol.* 2009, *46*, 934–939.

40. Moore, P.F.; Rodriguez-Bertos, A.; Kass, P.H. Feline gastrointestinal lymphoma: Mucosal architecture, immunophenotype, and molecular clonality. *Vet. Pathol.* 2011, *49*, 658–668.

41. Wu, F.Y.; Iijima, K.; Tsujimoto, H.; Tamura, Y.; Higurashi, M. Chromosomal translocations in two feline T-cell lymphomas. *Leuk. Res.* 1995, *19*, 857–860.

42. Fujino, Y.; Ma, Z.; Satoh, H.; Mizuno, T.; Hisasue, M.; Baba, K.; Masuda, K.; Ohno, K.; Onishi, T.; Tsujimoto, H. Characterization of a newly established nonproducer lymphoma cell line for feline leukemia virus. *Vet. Immunol. Immunopathol.* 2004, *102*, 429–439.

43. Breen, M.; Modiano, J.F. Evolutionarily conserved cytogenetic changes in

hematological malignancies of dogs and humans—Man and his best friend share more than companionship. *Chromosome Res.* 2008, *16*, 145–154.

44. Thomas, R.; Seiser, E.L.; Motsinger-Reif, A.; Borst, L.; Valli, V.E.; Kelley, K.; Suter, S.E.; Argyle, D.; Burgess, K.; Bell, J.;*et al.* Refining tumor-associated aneuploidy through "genomic recoding" of recurrent DNA copy number aberrations in 150 canine non-Hodgkin lymphomas. *Leuk. Lymphoma* 2011, *52*, 1321–1335.
45. Wilson, H.M. Feline alimentary lymphoma: Demystifying the enigma. *Top. Companion Anim. Med.* 2008, *23*, 177–184.
46. Vail, D.M. Chapter 324: Hematopoetic tumors. In *Textbook of Veterinary Internal Medicine*, 7th ed.; Ettinger, S.N., Feldman, E.C., Eds.; Saunders: Philadelphia, PA, USA, 2009; p. 2148.
47. Rissetto, K.; Villamil, J.A.; Selting, K.A.; Tyler, J.; Henry, C.J. Recent trends in feline intestinal neoplasia: An epidemiologic study of 1129 cases in the veterinary medical database from 1964 to 2004. *J. Am. Anim. Hosp. Assoc.*2011, *47*, 28–36.
48. Jasdanwala, S.; Pitchumoni, C. Epidemiological spectrum of gastrointestinal lymphoma. *Pract. Gastroenterol.* 2014, *38*, 8–28.
49. Moore, P.F.; Woo, J.C.; Vernau, W.; Kosten, S.; Graham, P.S. Characterization of feline T cell receptor gamma (TCRG) variable region genes for the molecular diagnosis of feline intestinal T cell lymphoma. *Vet. Immunol. Immunopathol.*2005, *106*, 167–178.
50. Waly, N.E.; Gruffydd-Jones, T.J.; Stokes, C.R.; Day, M.J. Immunohistochemical diagnosis of alimentary lymphomas and severe intestinal inflammation in cats. *J. Comp. Pathol.* 2005, *133*, 253–260.
51. Briscoe, K.A.; Krockenberger, M.; Beatty, J.A.; Crowley, A.; Dennis, M.M.; Canfield, P.J.; Dhand, N.; Lingard, A.E.; Barrs, V.R. Histopathological and immunohistochemical evaluation of 53 cases of feline lymphoplasmacytic enteritis and low-grade alimentary lymphoma. *J. Comp. Pathol.* 2011, *145*, 187–198.
52. Pohlman, L.M.; Higginbotham, M.L.; Welles, E.G.; Johnson, C.M. Immunophenotypic and histologic classification of 50 cases of feline gastrointestinal lymphoma. *Vet. Pathol.* 2009, *46*, 259–268.
53. Scott, K.D.; Zoran, D.L.; Mansell, J.; Norby, B.; Willard, M.D. Utility of endoscopic biopsies of the duodenum and ileum for diagnosis of inflammatory bowel disease and small cell lymphoma in cats. *J. Vet. Intern. Med.* 2011, *25*, 1253–1257.
54. Thomas, R.; *et al.* Genomic profiling of feline gastrointestinal lymphoma (To be submitted).
55. Hughes, K.; Dobson, J.M. Prognostic histopathological and molecular markers in feline mammary neoplasia. *Vet. J.*2012, *194*, 19–26.
56. Siegel, R.; Naishadham, D.; Jemal, A. Cancer statistics, 2013. *CA Cancer J. Clin.* 2013, *63*, 11–30.

57. Burrai, G.P.; Mohammed, S.I.; Miller, M.A.; Marras, V.; Pirino, S.; Addis, M.F.; Uzzau, S.; Antuofermo, E. Spontaneous feline mammary intraepithelial lesions as a model for human estrogen receptor- and progesterone receptor-negative breast lesions. *BMC Cancer* 2010, *10*.

58. Gimenez, F.; Hecht, S.; Craig, L.E.; Legendre, A.M. Early detection, aggressive therapy: Optimizing the management of feline mammary masses. *J. Feline Med. Surg.* 2010, *12*, 214–224.

59. Zappulli, V.; De Zan, G.; Cardazzo, B.; Bargelloni, L.; Castagnaro, M. Feline mammary tumours in comparative oncology. *J. Dairy Res.* 2005, *72*, 98–106.

60. Rakha, E.A.; Reis-Filho, J.S.; Baehner, F.; Dabbs, D.J.; Decker, T.; Eusebi, V.; Fox, S.B.; Ichihara, S.; Jacquemier, J.; Lakhani, S.R.; *et al.* Breast cancer prognostic classification in the molecular era: The role of histological grade. *Breast Cancer Res.* 2010, *12*, 207.

61. Seixas, F.; Palmeira, C.; Pires, M.A.; Bento, M.J.; Lopes, C. Grade is an independent prognostic factor for feline mammary carcinomas: A clinicopathological and survival analysis. *Vet. J.* 2011, *187*, 65–71.

62. Curtis, C.; Shah, S.P.; Chin, S.F.; Turashvili, G.; Rueda, O.M.; Dunning, M.J.; Speed, D.; Lynch, A.G.; Samarajiwa, S.; Yuan, Y.; *et al.* The genomic and transcriptomic architecture of 2000 breast tumours reveals novel subgroups. *Nature*2012, *486*, 346–352.

63. Kiyose, S.; Igarashi, H.; Nagura, K.; Kamo, T.; Kawane, K.; Mori, H.; Ozawa, T.; Maeda, M.; Konno, K.; Hoshino, H.; *et al.* Chromogenic *in situ* hybridization (CISH) to detect HER2 gene amplification in breast and gastric cancer: Comparison with immunohistochemistry (IHC) and fluorescence *in situ* hybridization (FISH). *Pathol. Int.* 2012, *62*, 728–734.

64. Rasotto, R.; Caliari, D.; Castagnaro, M.; Zanetti, R.; Zappulli, V. An immunohistochemical study of HER-2 expression in feline mammary tumours. *J. Comp. Pathol.* 2011, *144*, 170–179.

65. Mayr, B.; Jugl, M.; Brem, G.; Reifinger, M.; Loupal, G. Cytogenetic variation in six cases of feline mammary tumours.*Zentralbl. Veterinarmed. A* 1999, *46*, 367–377.

66. Mayr, B.; Ortner, W.; Reifinger, M.; Loupal, G. Loss of chromosome B2-material in three cases of feline mammary tumours. *Res. Vet. Sci* 1995, *59*, 61–63.

67. Thomas, R.; Seixas, F.; Borst, L.; Breen, M. Landscapes of Genomic Copy Number Aberrations in Feline Mammary Cancer. In Proceedings of the 8th International Conference on Advances in Canine and Feline Genomics and Inherited Diseases, Cambridge, UK; Available online: http://www.caninefelinegenomicsconference.org/ (accessed on 22–26 June 2015).

68. Ressel, L.; Millanta, F.; Caleri, E.; Innocenti, V.M.; Poli, A. Reduced pten protein expression and its prognostic implications in canine and feline mammary tumors. *Vet. Pathol.* 2009, *46*, 860–868.

69. Curtis, C.; Lynch, A.G.; Dunning, M.J.; Spiteri, I.; Marioni, J.C.; Hadfield, J.; Chin,

S.F.; Brenton, J.D.; Tavare, S.; Caldas, C. The pitfalls of platform comparison: DNA copy number array technologies assessed. *BMC Genom.* 2009, *10*.

12
CHAPTER

FROM "ONE HEALTH" TO "ONE COMMUNICATION": THE CONTRIBUTION OF COMMUNICATION IN VETERINARY MEDICINE TO PUBLIC HEALTH

Micaela Cipolla, Luigi Bonizzi and Alfonso Zecconi

Keywords: Communication, One Health, public health, antimicrobial resistance, food safety, food-producing animals, risk communication, companion animal practice

INTRODUCTION

Health Communication is a discipline only recently developed, and it is "The study of how health information is generated and disseminated and how that information affects individuals, community groups, institutions and public policy" [1].

The aim of health communication is to inform and influence people's behaviour and attitude in order to improve health [2,3,4]. This is possible because it concerns all aspects of health, including, *i.e.*, research, clinical practice, public health, global health and policy making [5,6]. Different approaches are available to investigate all of the aspects, *i.e.*, health campaigns, risk communication and patient-provider communication.

An effective communication is essential to public health. It can be written and verbal, taking many forms and using various channels such as physicians and other health professionals, family, friends and mass media, Internet, advertisement. For its growing importance, the World Health Organization (WHO) includes health communication in its activities and provides several guides supporting communication strategies development for different situations, such as health emergencies and disease prevention [7,8,9,10,11,12,13]. Moreover, WHO considers communication expertise as

Citation: Micaela Cipolla, Luigi Bonizzi and Alfonso Zecconi, From "One Health" to "One Communication": The Contribution of Communication in Veterinary Medicine to Public Health, doi:10.3390/vetsci2030135.

essential to outbreak control as well as epidemiological training and laboratory analysis, and demonstrated a significant reduction of cases during an outbreak when applied a proactive communication [14,15]. Many other institutions, such as UNICEF, FAO, CDC, Johns Hopkins University and others agree that communication is a necessary tool for public health [16,17,18,19,20,21,22,23,24,25,26,27,28].

Any advice aiming to enhance health by changing people's behaviour is a communicative act. Health communication allows to identify contexts, channels, messages and factors having the potential to motivate individuals to use correctly health information. Therefore, health communication supports health professionals in their daily work, educates patients and helps policy makers; it has a powerful role in disease prevention and health promotion. It is part of health management, even in settings with limited resources, helping to use information and interacting with the community or other partners.

Due to its pivotal importance, health communication became part of the curriculum in several Medicine and Veterinary Medicine Schools worldwide, but usually health communication refers to human health and it is generally less considered in veterinary medicine. The intended outcome of this article is to describe this new aspect of veterinary medicine—the health communication—and its contribution to public health. With our paper we highlight the role of communication in the main branches of veterinary activity, to help veterinarians to find their role in the "One communication" perspective. Indeed, communication in veterinary medicine has the potential to contribute to public health and should be considered in a One Health perspective.

One Health

The One Health concept links human, animal and environmental health, it is "a worldwide strategy for expanding interdisciplinary collaborations and communications in all aspects of health care for humans, animals and the environment. The synergism achieved will advance health care for the 21st century and beyond by accelerating biomedical research discoveries, enhancing public health efficacy, expeditiously expanding the scientific knowledge base, and improving medical education and clinical care."[29]. This approach considers all global health threats to gain cross-disciplinary collaboration, especially between physicians and veterinarians. The result is a collaborative effort to enhance human and animal health between the health professions.

One Health has its origins in the 1800s, when Rudolf Virchow, the German physician who coined the term "zoonosis", highlighted the linkages between human and veterinary medicine [30]. In the following years, other physicians and veterinarians recognized the importance of good animal health for the public health. One of them, Calvin Schwabe, made important contributions to epidemiology, zoonoses, tropical health and public health. He coined the term "One medicine", emphasizing the close interdependence and similarities between human and veterinary medicine [31]. More recently, the Wildlife Conservation Society promoted a symposium to discuss the movements of diseases among human, domestic animal and wildlife populations. The symposium set twelve priorities—the Manhattan Principles—for an interdisciplinary strategy to combat diseases and maintain the ecosystem integrity. These principles considered, with human and animal health, also environment health [32].

The One Health approach has been endorsed by the main global health organizations, such as WHO, CDC, EFSA, OIE, FAO [33,34,35,36,37]. The collaborative effort between human and veterinary medicine should be applied not only at global level but also at local level, where it could be a new paradigm of health management [38]. This will result in a more effective and sustainable organization of public health, reducing the risk of zoonotic diseases such as rabies, H5N1 avian influenza, West Nile disease, TBC and diseases caused by E. coli STEC, *Staphylococcus aureus* MRSA, Nipah and Hendra viruses, Hantaviruses, Filovirus such as Ebola and Marburg viruses.

VETERINARY MEDICINE AND PUBLIC HEALTH

The purpose of veterinary medicine is to protect public health, through the promotion of animal health and food safety. To fulfil this objective, veterinary medicine has many arenas of activity in public health, including (Figure 1):

- Institutions (health authority, healthcare system)
- Food safety and nutrition
- Clinical practice
    - companion animals
    - food-producing animals
- Pharmacology and drugs
- Wildlife fauna
- Environment

In all these fields, communication has a key role and can contribute to public health by influencing people's behaviour and attitude.

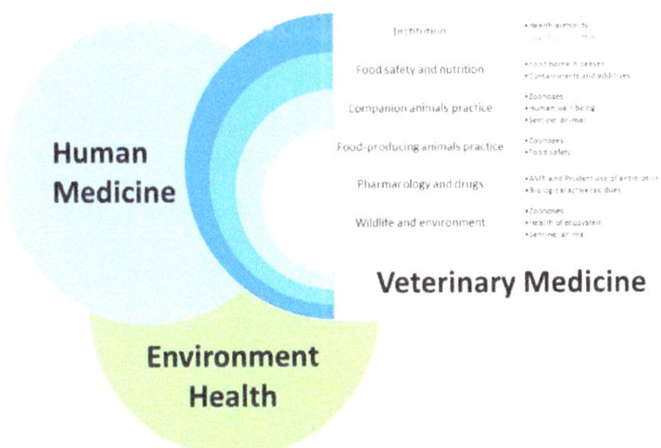

Figure 1: Potential contributes of veterinary medicine to public health in a One Health and One Communication perspective.

Institutions

Health care authorities and systems have the responsibility to manage health system, and communication is part of the management. Therefore, the role of communication is related to the institutional setting. We reported, as example, one European health system. In the Italian health system, communication for human and veterinary medicine is unique at the higher institutional level, because the Ministry of Health (Ministero della Salute) manages both. At lower regional and local institutional level, health authorities work separately on human and animal health, so the communication efforts often are uncoordinated. However, the institutional communication in veterinary medicine gives a high contribution to public health, because of the continuous overlapping between veterinary and human medicine in public health. This institutional activity includes, for example, health campaigns on zoonoses or food safety [39,40].

This organization of veterinary system has both pros and cons. The major benefit of the integration in the Ministry of Health is that the veterinary health system has a peculiar focus on health, and it is much less biased by production aspects, when compared to the systems under the Ministry of Agriculture. However, the focus on health, sometimes, put an excessive pressure on the production system, reducing its efficiency, by applying unnecessary barriers to the production process. At the local level, the system splits into the two components of human and veterinary medicine, and this disconnection gives to the veterinary medicine the opportunity to be more independent and effective in a given area, even if a coordination would be hopeful.

Moreover, the veterinary diseases surveillance networks have a key role in human surveillance and its utility would be increased through a better integration between the two systems, as happens through the joining of health service [41]. Likewise, a coordination also at the communicative level would produce more efficient efforts in enhancing public health. Also at policy and management levels, communication has a key role, as demonstrated by the example of Regional Veterinary Prevention Plan 2012–2014 (Piano Regionale della Prevenzione Veterinaria 2012–2014) of Regione Lombardia [42]. This was a new and powerful tool for public health, supporting veterinary health system at regional level, giving to all the operative units and officers an unique and coherent frame of reference [43]. Indeed, our research group developed a model (scorecard) to assess zoonoses and food safety issues. The scorecard supports daily practice setting priority in prevention and risk management, by assigning different scores to various risk and management aspects of each disease or food safety problem. Once this assignation has been done, the veterinary officers know the priority of each intervention and, also, if there is a lack of information about the specific disease. This model established a completely new approach to risk characterization in Italian public health authorities; it had to be understood and adopted by all the personnel involved in the regional veterinary system and, for this reason, communication was crucial. Both internal and external communication strategies were needed. All the members of the regional healthcare system were the audiences of internal communication: Regione Lombardia, local health authorities (Azienda Sanitaria Locale), regional diagnostic and surveillance laboratory (Istituto Zooprofilattico Sperimentale della Lombardia e dell'Emilia Romagna), research centers. At internal level, the aims of communication were to verify the outcomes of the plan application, to share information and to consolidate cooperation. External communication was addressed to stakeholders, with the aims to involve people, gather information and share results. All the initiatives, planned to inform and involve the target audience, were focused on objectives and results of the prevention plan application. However, the first communication need concerned the plan itself, and the understanding of the new risk characterization praxis. Indeed, the document was very articulated; it had many tables (the scorecards) and schemes for disease control plans, prevention protocols and risk characterization, each one concerning one of the veterinary areas. Indeed, in Italy the veterinary health system has three areas: A for animal health, B for food safety and C for herd management and animal welfare. One of the parameters considered for an effective communication of the plan was its graphic aspect. Due to the high amount and complexity of information delivered, we chose a simple and immediate graphic aspect, assigning a specific colour to each area. Every piece of information addressed to the animal health sector was green, to the food safety sector was red and to the herd management and animal welfare sector was yellow. Everything concerning the past or general topics was blue. This simple color code had a very useful function clarifying the whole document and making it more understandable. Moreover, this code made every local health authority having the same color for the same unit. All the veterinary officers recognized themselves in the color of their area, independently by the district of the local health authority. Therefore, the primary aim of the plan—to make uniform veterinary health system to improve public health—was achieved also with this simple communicative choice, and it was maintained also in the subsequent edition of the plan [44].]

Food Safety and Nutrition

Communication on food safety and nutrition frequently pertains to veterinary medicine, being related to food-borne disease, GMO, contaminants, additives and foods of animal origin.

Consumers receive much information about food, but often it is contradictory and conflicting. This includes alerts, recommendation on what is good for health and what could be dangerous, risks and benefits associate in the same food, food components to reduce, nutrients to increase, warning on different diets and eating styles. All this information provide a non-unique frame of reference, which is difficult to manage and to understand by consumers. Sometimes unfounded concerns may overlap reliable messages from health authorities, resulting in more confusion and uncertainty [45]; especially during an alert or an outbreak, this situation may lead to fear and distrust in the product involved. Examples are the recent European food scares on *E. coli* in vegetables, horsemeat scandal, blue mozzarella cheese, BSE and avian influenza.

The health and welfare of food-producing animals during breeding, transportation and slaughtering have consequences for human health and are responsibility of veterinarians. Therefore, due to the pivotal role of veterinary medicine in animal nutrition, animal health, food inspection and food safety, communication in this area is important for public health, contributing to consumers' protection from field to fork.

Communication about food is often risk communication. Accordingly with the

Codex Alimentarius Commission (CAC), risk communication is "an interactive exchange of information and opinions concerning risk among risk assessors, risk managers, consumers and other interested parties [46]. Therefore, food risk communication enables informed decision-making to promote health, fosters the understanding of both the real and the perceived food risk, and shares knowledge between government officials, health professionals, academicians, food producers, stakeholders, journalists and public. Misleading messages can have serious consequences not only on public health but also on the entire food supply chain. Thanks to a proper communication, authorities, experts and other stakeholders can communicate more successfully, making the public reacting properly [47].

To meet these needs, many local and international organizations, such as EFSA and FAO, promoted food risk communication [48,49].

Clinical Practice

Companion Animals

Companion animals, due to their close relationship with people, are important in the prevention of zoonoses and in their management. Moreover, pets have a role as sentinel animal and could be used to protect human health. For example, they are useful in cancer prevention and treatment in humans, because often they share the same risk and carcinogen factors, have many of the same types of cancer and are treated almost with the same drugs as humans [50]. Communication on such topics can contribute significantly to public health [51].

However, the focus of veterinary medicine in public health is not limited to zoonoses, because the One Health concept involves all of the aspects of health, including mental health via the human-animal bond phenomenon [52]. This latter aspect gives to the veterinary medicine a further role in public health, through disciplines centred on human-animal bond such as pet therapy. Moreover, the One Health statement amplifies the role of companion animals clinical practice in maintaining and improving human health, because it concerns not only zoonoses but also the owner-pet relationship.

The importance of communication in clinical practice has been widely recognized, even if only recently in veterinary medicine, where effective communication increases client satisfaction and compliance [53,54,55,56,57,58,59,60]. Therefore, this skill has become part of the veterinary education programs in many countries, being as important as other clinical skills [54,61,62,63].

However, in many European countries communication is still poorly considered. This situation may lead to communication errors, failures in meeting client expectations and, eventually, to complaint or malpractice claim as has been observed in human medicine [64]. Recent studies showed that in one of these countries, the large majority of pet owners consider the own pet as family member and this also affected owner responses and attitudes towards the veterinarian [65]. These results confirm the role of communication in improving veterinary practice and promoting clients' comfort, satisfaction and well-being.

Food-Producing Animals

Communication has a key role also in food-producing animals practice, improving management and animal health, as demonstrated for example in dairy farms [66,67,68].

Communication strategies are essential in promoting dairy herd health and are required to support diseases control programs [69,70]. Indeed, how consultant delivers information affects ideas, beliefs and motivation of the farmer, thus his/her behaviour and actions. [71,72,73]. Therefore, the leading role of communication in dairy herds is due to its power in influencing how farmers apply consultants' advice and, thus, in improving animal health and food safety. It is crucial for public health in a "from field to fork" perspective, because farmer's actions and management directly influence the quality of meat, milk and milk products.

All these aspects improve also herd sustainability. An effective communication in food-producing area supports development and improves health and innovation, also in emerging countries.

However, communication in veterinary practice is poorly considered in many countries including Italy. In this country, recent studies showed that dairy farmers are not satisfied with their consultants' communication [74]. This gap in veterinarians' skill represent a problem because an effective farmer-veterinarian communication is essential to improve farm management, herd health, food safety and herd sustainability.

Pharmacology and Drugs

The activity of veterinarians related to pharmacology and drugs is often cross-disciplinary, covering companion and food producing animal practice, food security, and official drugs residue controls. However, the rising importance of prudent use of antibiotics makes this topic suitable to become a specific area under the One Health approach. Indeed, the concern on antimicrobial resistance (AMR) increased in recent years; it is considered a major public health threat, due to misuse of antibiotics in both human and animal therapy. Therefore, it is a cross-disciplinary issue, engaging veterinarians to reduce and monitor antimicrobial usage in livestock [75,76].

Many veterinary organisations promote the responsible and prudent use of antimicrobial agents in animals, such as The World Organisation for Animal Health (OIE) [77]. Moreover, OIE developed standards and guidelines for OIE Member Countries to address the risk of the emergence or spread of resistant bacteria that result from the use of antimicrobial agents in food producing animals [78].

The European Medicines Agency (EMA) implemented the European Surveillance of Veterinary Antimicrobial Consumption (ESVAC) project, to identify possible risk factors that could lead to the development and spread of antimicrobial resistance in animals. The aim was to develop a harmonised approach for the collection and reporting of data on the use of antimicrobial agents in animals from EU Member States. Thus, EMA published reports on sales of veterinary antimicrobial agents in EU/EEA countries [79]. The International Dairy Federation (FIL-IDF) published a Guide to Prudent Use of Antimicrobial Agents in Dairy Production [80] and also the Federation of Veterinarians of Europe (FVE) developed a document on AMR and prudent use of antibiotics in Veterinary Medicine [81]. A specific interest on this topic was shown by U.S. Food and Drug Administration (FDA) and the U.S. Centers for Disease Control and Prevention (CDC) [82,83]. The latter one funded the development of the Antimicrobial Resistance Learning Site (AMRLS), which is a suite of educational materials promoting the prudent use of antimicrobial agents in veterinary practice [84]. Despite the large interest of veterinary sector on AMR, the communication was poorly considered. However, communication in veterinary medicine can promote the prudent use of antimicrobials, being synergic with the initiatives in human medicine. To highlight the problem and to support a rational antimicrobial use, the European Union promoted the European Awareness Day, an health initiative marked annually on 18 November and coordinated by European Center for Diseases Prevention and Control (ECDC). For this event, ECDC provides campaign communication materials for the European national health authorities in order to develop a consistent communication campaign on the prudent use of antibiotics. National campaigns use several communication tools, such as leaflets, poster, videos, websites and social media, that are aimed to both prescribers and the general public. Many communication initiatives take place across Europe, to disseminate messages on risks related to the antibiotic misuse and explaining how to take antibiotics responsibly [85,86,87]. Similar campaigns are promoted also in the United States, Canada and Australia [88,89].

All these programs show the importance of communication in human medicine to contain AMR, but communication in veterinary medicine is equally indispensable to promote a rational use of antibiotics and enhance the collaboration of veterinary organisations with the public health sector to reduce the antimicrobial resistance.

Wildlife Fauna and Environment

The One Health concept considers also the health of ecosystem, being health of humans, animals and environment interrelated. Indeed, both animals and humans live in the same environment, sharing air, water and food. If there is a poor health for the environment, there is a poor health for people and animals. The environmental pollution is a health hazards but it is not the only threat, because the health of plants is indispensable for having food [90]. Through an effective and responsible management of the natural resources, the One Health approach protects human and animal health and ensures a safe food supply [36,37]. Veterinary medicine can contribute to the health of the ecosystem, because agricultural contamination may lead to contamination of foods of animal origin. Moreover, these foods can be used as sentinel for monitoring contamination in the environment. For example, pesticide contamination of honey can be related to the contamination source and could reflect the specific pollution of an environment [91]. The use of animal sentinel for health hazards is very helpful to detect and manage more quickly and efficiently shared health risks [92]. Also when considering toxic risk, as shown by the potentials of "One Toxicology", the protection of domestic and wild animals' health is relevant to protecting humans [93].

In recent years the emerging diseases gained a leading role in epidemics on a global scale, and zoonoses were dominant [94]. These diseases are currently the main and global threat for human health, and are related to both domestic and wildlife fauna. Therefore, the synergy between medicine and veterinary medicine is indispensable for the research, the surveillance, the control and the communication of global health challenges at the animal-human-ecosystem interface [95]. The result of this cooperation is well known in developing countries, where it already resulted in an improved health care for the local populations [96]. Also in this area of veterinary medicine, coordinated communication efforts make an important contribution to public health.

CONCLUSIONS

In almost all the areas of veterinary activity communication can contribute to human health. It takes many forms and employs several channels, and this variety of communication opportunities represent a challenge for veterinarians. For this reason, communication courses should be included in the curricula of Veterinary Medicine Schools, as it happened in some already in North America.

Veterinarians should improve their communication skills because human and animal health are interrelated, as is health communication in human and veterinary sectors. Both of them cover the same issue (zoonoses, food safety *etc.*) and use the same channels. For example, it is not possible to differentiate between food risk communication in human and veterinary areas, having the same target, using the same strategies and considering the same risks.

Despite the fact that health communication is a recent matter, it has a growing importance in human medicine but it is less considered in veterinary medicine. However, because of the role of veterinary medicine in public health, communication in veterinary area also has the potential to improve public health. Therefore, a One Health approach applies to communication as well, leading to the "One Communication" concept, which is the result of the synergy in communicative efforts both in human and in veterinary medicine. As One Health, One Communication is a strategy for expanding collaborations in health communication and it will enhance health care.

AUTHOR CONTRIBUTIONS

Micaela Cipolla conceived and designed the study, wrote the paper; Luigi Bonizzi designed the study, revised the paper; Alfonso Zecconi designed the study, revised the paper.

REFERENCES

1. Harvard School of Public Health. The Field of Health Communication. Available online: http://www.hsph.harvard.edu/health-communication/ (accessed on 17 May 2015).
2. Hornik, R.C. *Public Health Communication—Evidence for Behavior Change*; Routledge-Lawrence Erlbaum Associates: Mahwah, NJ, USA, 2002.
3. CDC. What is Health Communications? Available online: http://www.cdc.gov/healthcommunication/healthbasics/whatishc.html (accessed on 17 May 2015).

4. National Cancer Institute; Public Health Service; National Institutes of Health. *Making Health Communication Programs Work (Pink Book)*; U.S. Department of Health & Human Services: Washington, DC, USA, 2002.
5. Wickremasinghe, D. What makes for good health communication? In *Global Health Communication—Global Health Histories*; WHO: Geneve, Switzerland, 2013.
6. Rajiv, N.; Rimal, M.; Lapinski, K. Why health communication is important in public health. *Bull. WHO* 2009, *87*, 247–247.
7. WHO. Special theme issue: Public health communication. *Bull. WHO* 2009, *87*, 565–644.
8. *Afghanistan Report—Health Communication*; WHO: Geneve, Switzerland, 2003; p. 19.
9. Obregón, R.; Chitnis, K.; Morry, C.; Feek, W.; Bates, J.; Galway, M.; Ogden, E. Achieving polio eradication: A review of health communication evidence and lessons learned in India and Pakistan. *Bull. WHO* 2009, *87*, 624–630.
10. WHO. Create HPV vaccination communication strategies. Available online: http://www.who.int/immunization/hpv/communicate/en/ (accessed on 17 May 2015).
11. WHO. *HPV Vaccine Communication—Special Considerations for A Unique Vaccine*; WHO: Geneve, Switzerland, 2013.
12. Parks, W.; Lloyd, L. *Planning Social Mobilization and Communication for Dengue Fever Prevention and Control*; WHO: Geneve, Switzerland, 2004.
13. *Effective Media Communication During Public Health Emergencies*; WHO: Geneve, Switzerland, 2005.
14. WHO. *World Health Organization Outbreak Communication Planning Guide*; WHO: Geneve, Switzerland, 2008.
15. WHO. *Outbreak Communication Guidelines*; WHO: Geneve, Switzerland, 2005.
16. UNICEF. Communication for development. Available online: http://www.unicef.org/cbsc (accessed on 17 May 2015).
17. Waisbord, S.; Larson, H.J. Why Invest in Communication for Immunization? Evidence and Lessons Learned. A Joint Publication the Health Communication Partnership Based at Johns Hopkins Bloomberg School of Public Health/Center for Communication Programs (Baltimore) and the United Nations Children's Fund (New York). 2005. Available online: http://www.who.int/immunization/hpv/communicate/why_invest_in_communication_for_immunization_unicef_healthcommunicationspartnership_path_usaid.pdf (accessed on 10 July 2015).
18. O'Sullivan, G.A.; Yonkler, J.A.; Morgan, W.; Merritt, A.P. *A Field Guide to Designing a Health Communication Strategy*; Johns Hopkins Bloomberg School of Public Health/Center for Communication Programs: Baltimore, MD, USA, 2003.
19. United Nations Children's Fund Regional Office for South Asia. *Strategic Communication for Behaviour and Social Change in South Asia*; UNICEF: Kathmandu, Nepal, 2005.

20. Wittet, S. *Hepatitis B Vaccine Introduction—Lessons Learned in Advocacy,Communication and Training*; PATH: Seattle, WA, USA, 2001.

21. WHO; UNICEF; FAO. *Communication for Behavioural Impact—A Toolkit for Behavioural and Social Communication in Outbreak Response*; WHO: Geneve, Switzerland, 2012.

22. Feig, C. WHO: Communicating for health. In *Global Health Communication—Global Health Histories*; WHO: Geneve, Switzerland, 2013.

23. Zaman, F.; Underwood, C. *The Gender Guide for Health Communication Programmes*; Johns Hopkins Bloomberg School of Public Health, Center for Communication Programs: Baltimore, MD, USA, 2003.

24. U.S. Department of Health and Human Services Office of Disease Prevention and Health Promotion. *A Quick Guide to Health Literacy: Fact Sheets, Strategies, Resources*; U.S. Department of Health and Human Services, Office of Disease Prevention and Health Promotion: Washington, DC, USA, 2005.

25. Department for International Development. *Radio Broadcasting for Health—A Decision Makers Guide*; Information and Communication for Development, UK Department for International Development: London, UK, 2004.

26. CDC. Gateway to Health Communication & Social Marketing Practice. Available online: http://www.cdc.gov/healthcommunication/about.html (accessed on 17 May 2015).

27. US Department of Health and Human Services. Health Communication, Health Literacy, and E-Health. Available online: http://www.health.gov/communication/Default.asp (accessed on 17 May 2015).

28. FAO; OIE. *Global Animal Health Communication Strategy to Support Prevention and Control of H5N1*; HPAI FAO/OIE International Animal Health Communicators' Roundtable in Support of the FAO/OIE Global Strategy for the Prevention and Control of HPAI: Rome, Italy; Paris, France, 2007.

29. One Health Initiative. About the One Health Initiative. Available online: http://www.onehealthinitiative.com/about.php (accessed on 17 May 2015).

30. CDC. History of One Health. Available online: http://www.cdc.gov/onehealth/people-events.html (accessed on 16 June 2015).

31. Schwabe, C. *Veterinary Medicine and Human Health*; Williams & Wilkins Co.: Baltimore, MD, USA, 1964.

32. The Manhattan Principles. Available online: http://www.cdc.gov/onehealth/pdf/manhattan/twelve_manhattan_principles.pdf (accessed on 16 June 2015).

33. CDC. One Health. Available online: http://www.cdc.gov/onehealth/ (accessed on 17 May 2015).

34. EFSA. *Programming Document 2015-2017*; EFSA: Parma, Italy, 2014.

35. OIE. One Health. Available online: http://www.oie.int/for-the-media/onehealth/oie-involvement/ (accessed on 17 May 2015).

36. FAO. *One Health: Food and Agriculture Organization of the United Nations*

Strategic Action Plan; FAO: Rome, Italy, 2011.

37. FAO. FAO workshop leverages country case studies for stronger collaboration on One Health. Available online: http://www.fao.org/ag/againfo/programmes/en/empres/news_041013.html (accessed on 17 May 2015).
38. OIE. One Health at a Glance. Available online: http://www.oie.int/for-the-media/onehealth/ (accessed on 17 May 2015).
39. Ministero della Salute. Influenza Aviaria. Available online: http://www.salute.gov.it/portale/temi/p2_6.jsp?lingua=italiano&id=816&area=Malattie%20infettive&menu=altremalattie (accessed on 17 May 2015).
40. Ministero della Salute. Infezione da Virus West Nile. Available online: http://www.salute.gov.it/portale/temi/p2_6.jsp?lingua=italiano&id=1201&area=Malattie%20infettive&menu=altremalattie (accessed on 17 May 2015).
41. Zinsstag, J.; Schelling, E.; Bonfoh, B.; Fooks, A.R.; Kasymbekov, J.; Toews, D.W.; Tanner, M. Towards a One Health research and application tool box. *Vet. Ita.* 2009, *45*, 121–133.
42. Bonizzi, L.; Cipolla, M.; Grieco, V.; Grilli, G.; Lanfranchi, P.; Mortarino, M.; Zecconi, A. *Piano regionale della prevenzione veterinaria 2012-2014*; Regione Lombardia: Milano, Italy, 2011.
43. Scali, F.; Bonizzi, L.; Ferrero, F.; Frazzi, P.; Grilli, G.; Lanfranchi, P.; Mortarino, M.; Sala, V.; Taloni, D.; Zecconi, A. Risk prioritization as a tool to guide veterinary public health activities at regional level. *Vet.Ita.* 2014. in press.
44. Alfonso Zecconi, U.O.V.R. *Piano regionale integrato della sanità pubblica veterinaria 2015-2018*; Regione Lombardia DG Sanità: Milano, Italy, 2014.
45. EFSA. Risk Communication. Available online: http://www.efsa.europa.eu/en/efsawhat/riskcommunication.htm(accessed on 17 May 2015).
46. FAO; WHO. *Codex Alimentarius Commission Report of the Twenty-Second Session*; FAO: Rome, Italy, 1997.
47. EFSA. Risk communication: Making it clear, timely and relevant. Available online: http://www.efsa.europa.eu/en/press/news/120711e.htm (accessed on 17 May 2015).
48. FAO. *The Application of Risk Communication to Food Standards and Safety Matters*; FAO: Rome, Italy, 1998.
49. EFSA. *When Food is Cooking Up a Storm—Proven Recipes for Risk Communications*; EFSA: Parma, Italy, 2012.
50. Thamm, D.; Dow, S. How companion animals contribute to the fight against cancer in humans. *Vet. Ita.* 2009, *45*, 111–120.
51. Ministero della Salute. *Rabbia—conoscere per prevenire*; Istituto Zooprofilattico Sperimentale delle Venezie: Legnaro, Italy, 2010.
52. One Health Initiative. Mission Statement. Available online: http://www.onehealthinitiative.com/mission.php (accessed on 17 May 2015).
53. Grant, C.H.; Cissna, K.N.; Rosenfeld, L.B. Patients' perceptions of physicians

communication and outcomes of the accrual to trial process. *Health Commun.* 2000, *12*, 23–39.

54. Shaw, J.R.; Adams, C.L.; Bonnett, B.N. What can veterinarians learn from studies of physician-patient communication about veterinarian-client-patient communication? *J. Am. Vet. Med. Assoc.* 2004, *224*, 676–684.
55. Kurtz, S.M. *Teaching and Learning Communication Skills in Medicine*, 2nd ed.; Radcliffe Publishing: Oxford, UK, 2005.
56. Kanji, N.; Coe, J.B.; Adams, C.L.; Shaw, J.R. Effect of veterinarian-client-patient interactions on client adherence to dentistry and surgery recommendations in companion-animal practice. *J. Am. Vet. Med. Assoc.* 2012, *240*, 427–436.
57. Chadderdon, L.M.; King, L.J.; Lloyd, J.W. The skills, knowledge, aptitudes, and attitudes of successful veterinarians: A summary of presentations to the NCVEI subgroup (Brook Lodge, Augusta, Michigan, December 4–6, 2000). *J. Vet. Med. Educ.* 2001, *28*, 28–30.
58. Coe, J.B.; Adams, C.L.; Bonnett, B.N. A focus group study of veterinarians' and pet owners' perceptions of veterinarian-client communication in companion animal practice. *J. Am. Vet. Med. Assoc.* 2008, *233*, 1072–1080.
59. Shaw, J.R.; Bonnett, B.N.; Roter, D.L.; Adams, C.L.; Larson, S. Gender differences in veterinarian-client-patient communication in companion animal practice. *J. Am. Vet. Med. Assoc.* 2012, *241*, 81–88.
60. Shaw, J.R.; Adams, C.L.; Bonnett, B.N.; Larson, S.; Roter, D.L. Veterinarian satisfaction with companion animal visits.*J. Am. Vet. Med. Assoc.* 2012, *240*, 832–841.
61. Adams, C.L.; Kurtz, S.M. Building on existing models from human medical education to develop a communication curriculum in veterinary medicine. *J. Vet. Med. Educ.* 2006, *33*, 28–37.
62. Latham, C.E.; Morris, A. Effects of formal training in communication skills on the ability of veterinary students to communicate with clients. *Vet. Rec.* 2007, *160*, 181–186.
63. Martin, F.; Ruby, K.L.; Deking, T.M.; Taunton, A.E. Factors associated with client, staff, and student satisfaction regarding small animal euthanasia procedures at a veterinary teaching hospital. *J. Am. Vet. Med. Assoc.* 2004, *224*, 1774–1779.
64. Beckman, H.B.; Markakis, K.M.; Suchman, A.L.; Frankel, R.M. The doctor-patient relationship and malpractice. Lessons from plaintiff depositions. *Arch. Intern. Med.* 1994, *154*, 1365–1370.
65. Cipolla, M.; Bonizzi, L.; Zecconi, A. Attitude toward companion animals and breaking bad news: The role of caretakers' attitude and other factors on client-veterinarian communication. *Soc. Anim.* 2015. submitted.
66. Kleen, J.L.; Atkinson, O.; Noordhuizen, J.P. Communication in production animal medicine: Modelling a complex interaction with the example of dairy herd health medicine. *Ir. Vet. J.* 2011, *64*, 8.
67. Jansen, J.; Steuten, C.D.; Renes, R.J.; Aarts, N.; Lam, T.J. Debunking the myth

of the hard-to-reach farmer: Effective communication on udder health. *J. Dairy Sci.* 2010, *93*, 1296–1306.

68. Jansen, J.; Lam, T.J. The role of communication in improving udder health. *Vet. Clin. North Am. Food Anim. Pract.* 2012,*28*, 363–379.
69. Jansen, J.; Renes, R.J.; Lam, T.J. Evaluation of two communication strategies to improve udder health management. *J. Dairy Sci.* 2010, *93*, 604–612.
70. Lievaart, J.J.; Noordhuizen, J.P.T.M.; Buckley, D.; Van Winden, S.C.L. The marketing of herd health and production management services on dutch dairy farms: Perceptions of dairy farmers and their veterinary surgeons. *Ir. Vet. J.* 2008,*61*, 668–676.
71. Jansen, J.; van den Borne, B.H.P.; Renes, R.J.; van Schaik, G.; Lam, T.J.G.M.; Leeuwis, C. Explaining mastitis incidence in dutch dairy farming: The influence of farmers' attitudes and behaviour. *Prev. Vet. Med.* 2009, *92*, 210–223.
72. Valeeva, N.I.; Lam, T.J.G.M.; Hogeveen, H. Motivation of dairy farmers to improve mastitis management. *J. Dairy Sci.*2007, *90*, 4466–4477.
73. Kristensen, E.; Jakobsen, E.B. Challenging the myth of the irrational dairy farmer; understanding decision-making related to herd health. *N. Z. Vet. J.* 2011, *59*, 1–7.
74. Cipolla, M.; Zecconi, A. Short communication: Study on veterinarian communication skills preferred and perceived by dairy farmers. *Res. Vet. Sci.* 2015, *99*, 60–62.
75. WHO. Antimicrobial Resistance. Available online: http://www.euro.who.int/en/health-topics/disease-prevention/antimicrobial-resistance (accessed on 17 May 2015).
76. WHO Regional Office for Europe. Tackling antibiotic resistance from a food safety perspective in europe. WHO Regional Office for Europe: Copenhagen, 2011.
77. OIE. Antimicrobial agents and antimicrobial resistance. Available online: http://www.oie.int/our-scientific-expertise/veterinary-products/antimicrobials/ (accessed on 17 May 2015).
78. OIE. Antimicrobial Resistance (AMR). Available online: http://www.oie.int/en/for-the-media/amr/ (accessed on 17 May 2015).
79. EMA. European surveillance of veterinary antimicrobial consumption (ESVAC). Available online: http://www.ema.europa.eu/ema/index.jsp?curl=pages/regulation/document_listing/document_listing_000302.jsp (accessed on 17 May 2015).
80. International Dairy Federation. *Guide to Prudent Use of Antimicrobial Agents in Dairy Production*; International Dairy Federation: Brussels, Belgium, 2013.
81. Federation of Veterinarians of Europe. *Antibiotic Resistance & Prudent Use of Antibiotics in Veterinary Medicine*; FVE: Brussels, Belgium, 2012.
82. FDA. Antimicrobial Resistance. Available online: http://www.fda.gov/AnimalVeterinary/SafetyHealth/AntimicrobialResistance/default.htm (accessed on 17 May 2015).

83. CDC. Antibiotic use in food-producing animals. Available online: http://www.cdc.gov/narms/animals.html (accessed on 17 May 2015).

84. College of Veterinary Medicine, Michigan State University; College of Veterinary Medicine, University of Minnesota. Antimicrobial resistance learning site. Available online: http://amrls.cvm.msu.edu/ (accessed on 17 May 2015).

85. ECDC. European antibiotics awareness day. Available online: http://ecdc.europa.eu/en/eaad/Pages/Home.aspx(accessed on 17 May 2015).

86. ECDC. Antimicrobial resistance. Available online: http://www.ecdc.europa.eu/en/healthtopics/antimicrobial_resistance/Pages/index.aspx (accessed on 17 May 2015).

87. AIFA. Campagne di comunicazione. Available online: http://www.agenziafarmaco.gov.it/it/content/campagne-di-comunicazione-0 (accessed on 17 May 2015).

88. CDC. Get smart about antibiotics week. Available online: http://www.cdc.gov/getsmart/campaign-materials/week/index.html (accessed on 17 May 2015).

89. NPS MedicineWise. Join the fight against antibiotic resistance. Available online: http://www.nps.org.au/about-us/what-we-do/campaigns-events/antibiotic-resistance-fighter (accessed on 17 May 2015).

90. Fletcher, J.; Franz, D.; LeClerc, E. Healthy plants: Necessary for a balanced One Health concept. *Vet. Ita.* 2009, *45*, 79–95.

91. Panseri, S.; Catalano, A.; Giorgi, A.; Arioli, F.; Procopio, A.; Britti, D.; Chiesa, L. Occurrence of pesticide residues in italian honey from different areas in relation to its potential contamination sources. *Food Control* 2014, *38*, 150–156. [CrossRef]

92. Rabinowitz, P.; Scotch, M.; Conti, L. Human and animal sentinels for shared health risks. *Vet. Ita.* 2009, *45*, 23–24.

93. Beasley, V. One Toxicology, ecosystem health and One Health. *Vet. Ita.* 2009, *45*, 97–110.

94. Gibbs, E.P.; Anderson, T.C. One World—One Health' and the global challenge of epidemic diseases of viral aetiology.*Vet. Ita.* 2009, *45*, 35–44.

95. FAO; OIE; WHO; UN System Influenza Coordination; UNICEF; The World Bank. *Contributing to One World, One Health—A Strategic Framework for Reducing Risks of Infectious Diseases at the Animal–Human–Ecosystems Interface*; FAO: Rome, Italy, 2008.

96. FAO. *FAO's Support to the One Health Regional Approach—Towards Integrated and Effective Animal Health—Food Safety Surveillance Capacity Development in Eastern Africa*; FAO: Rome, Italy, 2013.

13

CHAPTER

A REVIEW ON THE PUBLIC HEALTH IMPORTANCE OF BOVINE SALMONELLOSIS

Jelalu Kemal

Keywords: Cattle, Foodborne, Human, Salmonella, Zoonosis

INTRODUCTION

The genus *Salmonella* was named after Daniel E. Salmon who first reported the isolation of *Salmonella* from a pig in 1885 and named the organism Bacterium choleraesuis (currently known as *Salmonella enterica* serovar Choleraesuis) [1,2]. *Salmonella* causes gastroenteritis and typhoid fever and is one of the major foodborne pathogens of significant public health concern [3]. *Salmonella* is considered as one of the most wide spread foodborne zoonosis in industrialized as well as developing countries even though the incidences seems to vary [4]. Salmonellosis is a disease caused by many serotypes of *Salmonella* and characterized clinically by one or more of the three major syndromes; septicemia, acute and chronic enteritis [5].

*Salmonella*e are common in cattle. They are often concern due to disease of cattle and the potential to infect human that come in contact with cattle or consume dairy product or bovine meat product. Meat processing and packaging at the whole sale or retail level contribute to higher levels of contamination in minced beef product compared to beef carcass. The presences of even small number of *Salmonella* in carcass meat and edible offal may lead to heavy contamination of minced meat. When meat is cut in to pieces more microorganisms are added and increased surface area of exposed tissue from the contaminated equipment. Raw meat particularly, minced meat has a

Citation: Kemal J (2014) A Review on the Public Health Importance of Bovine Salmonellosis. J Veterinar Sci Technol 5: 175. doi:10.4172/2157-7579.1000175.

very high total count of microorganisms of which *Salmonella* are likely to present large number [6].

Bovine salmonelosis usually manifest clinically as a syndrome of septicemia, acute or chronic enteritis and abortion [7]. There are few serotypes that are associated with cattle and of this *Salmonella enterica* subspecies *enterica* serotype Dublin (*S. dublin*) and *Salmonellaenterica* subspecies *enterica* serotype Typhimurium (*S. typhimurium*) is the most common [8]. The presence of *S. typhimurium* in cattle and the cross contamination of beef carcass tissue is one of the most common cause of *Salmonella* infection in developed countries [9].

In addition to causing infection many *Salmonella* isolates particularly *S. typhimurium* definitive type (DT) 104 have developed resistance to multiple antibiotics. Many isolate of this phage type are resistance to ampicillin, chloramphinicol, streptomycin, sulfonamides and tetracycline (ACSUT) with increasing number of isolate showing resistance to trimethoprim and fluoroquinolones [10,11].

The resistance organism may act as donor of resistant determinant to another facultative pathogen of the human commensal flora of intestinal tract which may later be associated with disease and, in turn, supply the resistances gene to other pathogen [12].

There are more than 2500 different *Salmonella* serotypes and all are considered potentially pathogenic to human [13]. In human *Salmonella*is one of the most common causes of bacterial gastroenteritis. Death from *Salmonella* food poisoning estimated 1,000 deaths each year in USA [14]. The economic loss associated in human salmonellosis is due to investigation, treatment and prevention of illness [15]. Therefore, the objective of this review paper is to show the effect of eating of raw or undercooked meat, drinking of unpasteurized milk from the perspective of public health and to forward recommendation based on conclusion.

GENERAL OVERVIEW OF BOVINE SALMONELLOSIS

Classification

The current nomenclature of the genus *Salmonella* adopted worldwide through different publications is the one used by CDC is based on the recommendations from the WHO collaborating centre and it adequately addresses the concern and requirements of clinical and public health microbiologists (Table 1) [16]. Scientifically *Salmonella* classification is described under:

- Domain: Bacteria
- Phylum: Protobacteria
- Class: Gamma Protobacteria
- Order: Enterobacteriales
- Family: Enterobacteriaceae

- Genus: Salmonella, and

Species: *Salmonella enterica* and *Salmonella bongori* [17]. The species *Salmonella enterica* being divided into six subspecies (I–VI); S.*enterica* subsp. *enterica* (I), S. *enterica* subsp. salamae (II), S. enteric subsp. arizonae (IIIa), S. *enterica* subsp. diarizonae (IIIb), S. *enterica*subsp. houtenae (IV) and S. *enterica* subsp. indica (VI) [18] on the basis of biochemical characteristics (biotype), differences observed in multilocus enzyme electrophoresis (MLEE), phylogenetic analysis using 16S rRNA or other sequences, or analyses using other molecular techniques such as amplified-fragment length polymorphism (AFLP). Members of *Salmonella enterica* subspecies I account for 99% of all human infections [19].

Etiology and characteristics

Strains of genus *Salmonella* obey the definition of the family *Enterobacteriaceae*, they are straight rod usually motile with peritrichous flagella (except *S. pullorum* and *S. gallinarum*), facultative anaerobe, ferment glucose usually with production of gas (except *S. typhi* and *S. dublin*), but failed to ferment lactose, sucrose, salicin and urea, reduce nitrate to nitrite and most are phototropic [20,21]. *Salmonella* multiply optimally at a temperature of 35°C to 37°C, pH about 6.5-7.5 and water activity between 0.94-0.84. They are chemo-organotrophic organisms [22]. They are also able to multiply in the environment with low level or no oxygen [23]. The bacteria are sensitive to heat and will not survive a temperature above 70°C; so it is sensitive to pasteurization, but resist to drying even for years. Especially in dried feces, dust and other dry materials such as feed and certain food [24].

Table 1: Currently recognized number of Salmonella serovars [62]

Salmonella species and subspecies	No. of serovars within subspecies	Usual habitat
S. enterica	2557	
S.e. ssp. *enterica*	1531	Warm blooded animal
S.e. ssp. *salamae*	505	Cold blooded animals and environment
S.e. ssp. *arizonae*	99	Cold blooded animals and environment
S.e. ssp. *diarizonae*	336	Cold blooded animals and environment
S.e. ssp. *houtenae*	73	Cold blooded animals and environment
S.e. ssp. *Indica*	13	Cold blooded animals and environment
S. bongori	22	Cold blooded animals and environment
Total (genus *Salmonella*	**2579**	

Salmonella strains are serologically classified using Kauffmann- White scheme, and at the present the genus contains more than 2500 serotypes [13,25,26]. However, a report from the Centre for Infectious Disease Research and Policy (CIDRAP) classifies members of the*Salmonella* species into more than 2541 serotypes (serovars) according to their somatic lipopolysaccharide (O), flagellar (H) antigens and at times capsular (Vi) antigen and most strains show diphasic variation of the flagellar antigns

[27,28]. Recently, Dignostic Services of Monitoba (DSM) suggested the number of *Salmonella* serotypes that causes disease in human now approaches 3000 and new serotypes are identified continuously [29] (Table 2).

Table 2: The most common serovars of Salmonella that infect livestock and syndrome they induce [63]

Species	Serovars	Common syndrome
Cattle	*S. dublin* and *S. typhimurium*	Septicimia, acute and chronic enteritis and abortion
Sheep	*S. typhimurium*	Septicemia, typhocolitis and abortion
Pig	*S. choleraesuis S. typhimurium, S. typhisuis*	Septicemia
Horses	*S.typhimurium*	Septicemia, acute colititus and abortion
Chicken	*S. pullorum, S. gallinarum*	Septicemia, acute and chronic enteritis
Human	*S. enteritidis, S. typhi, S. paratyphi*	Gastroenteritis, bacteremia

Epidemiology

The epidemiology of *Salmonella* is complex which often makes control of disease difficult. Epidemiological pattern of prevalence of infection and incidences of disease differ greatly between geographical area depending on climate, population density, land use farming practice, food harvesting and processing technologies and consumer habits. In addition, the biology of serovar differs so widely that *Salmonella* infection or*Salmonella* contamination are inevitably complex [24].

Geographical distribution:

S. entritidis is the most prevalent species followed by *S. typhimurium* which are a worldwide distribution. Change in the relative frequency of serotypes can be observed over a short period of time. Some times within one or two years only limited number of serotypes is isolated from man or animals in a single region or country and the predominance of one or other can vary over a time. Some serotypes like S. entritidis and *S. typhimurium* are found worldwide in contrast to S. weltevreden which seems to be confined to Asia [30]. Sibhat et al. [31] found the serovars Newport, Anatum and Eastbourne to be the most prevalent in Ethiopia.

Occurrences:

The rate of infection in domestic animal has been estimated from 1-3%. In 1980, 16274 strains of 183 serotypes of*Salmonella* were isolated in USA from samples of meat obtained from slaughter house. In other examination of animals positive culture was obtained from 4.59% of 141, 827 bovine fecal samples. Epidemiological surveillance of animals including bird is of the most important since source of large majority of non-typhoidal salmonellosis cases are of food animal origin. There is scarce of data from developing countries in this regard [30].

Morbidity and mortality:

In a case control study of *S. typhimurium* DT 104 infection in cattle in Great Britain, Evans and Davies [32] reported an overall case fatality rate of 44%. In the herd with outbreak of *S. typhimurium* DT 104 the case fatality rate was 51.2% in calves, 37.4% in adult cattle and 26.2% in fattening cattle [32]. In dairy sucker and mixed herd the case fatality rate was found 44% where in calf rearing unit and dealer herd was found 50%-100% [33]. However modern antibiotic therapy may have reduced this rate. In an outbreak of *S. dublin* in calf rearing unit 29 (13.5%) of 214 calves died [34]. Mortality was significantly higher in group reared calves (19.25%) than in calves in single pens (9.2%). Mortality and morbidity is usually highest in calves under 12 week of age. In all species case fatality rate often reach 100% if treatment is not provided [24].

Economic importance:

Salmonellosis is a significant cause of economic loss in farm animals because of the cost of clinical disease, which include death, diagnosis and treatment of clinical cases, diagnostic laboratory cost, the cost of cleaning and disinfection and cost of control and prevention. In addition when the disease is diagnosed in the herd, it can create a considerable apprehension in the producer because of difficulty on identifying infected animals. An estimation of economic impact of an outbreak of *S. dublin* infection in calf rearing unit indicate that the cost of disease represented a substantial proportion of gross margin of rearing calves [24]. Estimated annual costs for salmonellosis have ranged from billions of dollars in United States to hundreds to millions of dollars in Canada and millions of pounds in United Kingdom. Analysis of five *Salmonella* outbreak due to manufactured food in North America gave direct cost with range from $36,400-$62 million, there have been few studies in to the cost and benefit of preventing *Salmonella* infection, but it has been suggested that for every £1 spent on investigation and curtailment of the outbreak there is a saving of £5 [35].

Source of infection and transmission :

Most *Salmonella* infection in farm animals are likely to acquire from animals of the same species, especially in the case of the host adapted serovars. In adult cattle there are important differences in the behavior of *S. dublin* and *S. typhimurium*. Those animals which recover from clinical *S. dublin* infection may become persistent excreters, shedding up to 106 organisms per gram of feaces daily. Other herd may harbor infection and excrete the organisms only when stressed particularly at parturition. Aerosol transmission has long been suggested as a means by which *Salmonella* may be transmitted and experimental infection of calves by aerosol has been reported recently. In addition pasture contamination results when flooding occurs and there are many reports of clinical case in adult cattle arising from grazing recently flooded pasture [35] (Figure 1).

Pathogenesis

The outcome of infection with *Salmonella* depends essentially on three factors: the infective dose, predisposing factor influencing the host and the level of immunity [7]. In cattle the common route of infection is ingestion of the bacteria through contaminated feed and water. It may disseminate to the rest body part of the host via the lymph fluid or blood and usually also lead to faecal excretion of bacteria. *Salmonella*e are normally inhibited by the high concentrations of volatile fatty acids and the normal pH below 7 in the rumen [36]. These bacteria have developed mechanisms to survive and cope with the host inhibiting factors, but the normal inhibition of *Salmonella* is primarily disrupted in the rumen and small intestine when (i) starvation or reduced feed intake occur [37], (ii) the feeding strategy leads to an increased pH in the abomasum, and (iii) antibiotic treatment kills the normal competing microflora of the intestine [38]. The bacteria adhere to and invade intestinal cells in the mucosa mainly associated with the Peyer's patches in the terminal jejunum and ileum through the columnar enterocytes and specialized microfold enterocytes (M cells). Once the bacteria have crossed the intestinal epithelium they enter macrophages in the underlying lymphoid tissue from where they are drained to the local lymph nodes, which are important barriers for further dissemination. If this barrier is overcome, the bacteria reach the reticuloendothelial tissue containing organs while surviving and replicating inside the macrophages [39].

The virulence of *Salmonella* is related to their ability to invade host cell and resist both digestion by phagocytes and destruction by complement system [40].The specific O antigen is important for the virulence strain of *Salmonella* (specific antigen) by decreasing the susceptibility of phagocytosis and ability to activate the alternative complement pathway [41]. Three toxins namely endotoxin, enterotoxin and cytotoxin play an important role in the pathogenesis of *Salmonella*. The endotoxin produce fever, the enterotoxin produce mucosal damage in the cell culture and cytotoxin inhibit protein synthesis [42] (Figure 2).

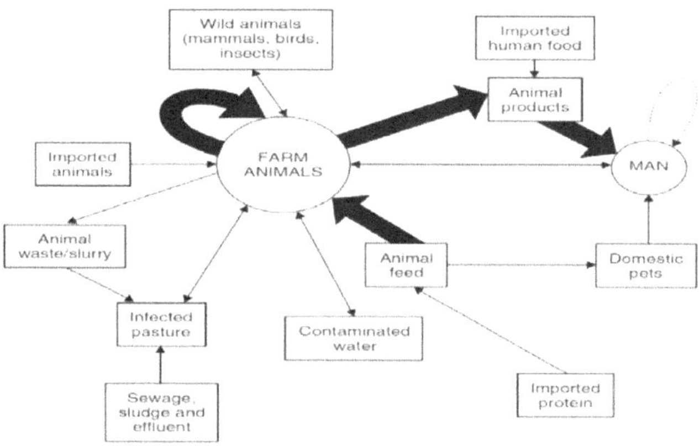

Figure 1: Figurative representation of Salmonella spp. indicating source of infection and transmission [53]. Feed, water, pasture, wastes; wild animals etc can serve for the transmission of the pathogen Salmonella into farm animals which in turn serve as a source for human.

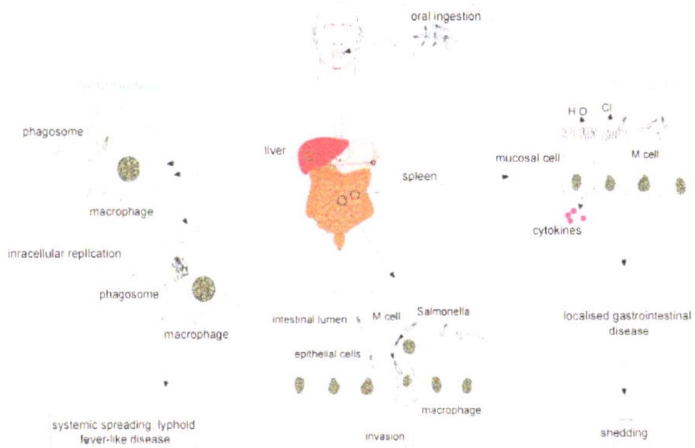

Figure 2: Schematic representation of host-pathogen interactions during pathogenesis of Salmonella infections in human. For the first stages of salmonellosis, Salmonella Pathogenicity Island (SPI1) function is required, i.e. the entry of Salmonella into nonphagocytic cells by triggering invasion and the penetration of the gastrointestinal epithelium and also for the onset of diarrhoeal symptoms. The function of SPI2 is required for later stages of the infection, i.e. systemic spread and the colonization of host organs [43].

In human the bacteria travel to the stomach and pass to the intestine, where they invade the cells, causing diarrhoea to their infected host body. *Salmonella* Pathogenicity Island (SPI1) function is required for the initial stages of salmonellosis, i.e. the entry of *Salmonella* into nonphagocytic cells by triggering invasion and the penetration of the gastrointestinal epithelium. Furthermore, SPI1 function is required for the onset of diarrheal symptoms during localized gastrointestinal infections. The function of SPI2 is required for later stages of the infection, i.e. systemic spread and the colonization of host organs. The role of SPI2 for survival and replication in host phagocytes appears to be essential for this phase of pathogenesis [43] (Figures 2 and 3).

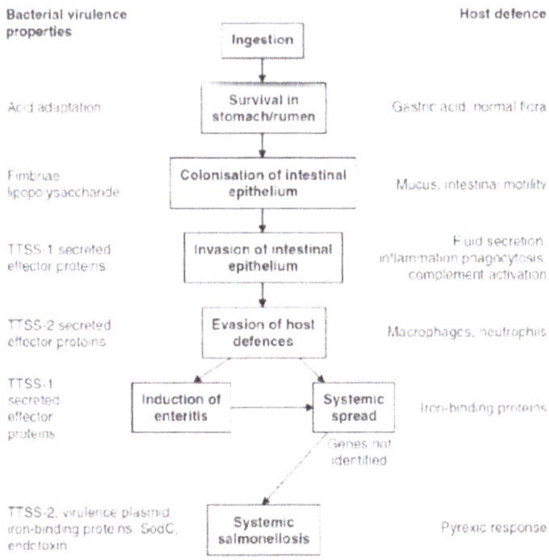

Figure 3: The attachment, colonization, invasion, virulence property and host defence mecha-

nism of Salmonella once ingested from food and pathogenecity island function [53].

Post mortem findings:

There may be no gross lesion in animals that have died peracutely but extensive submucosal and subserosal petechial heamorrhage are usually evident [24]. In adult cattle, a typical case reveals acute muco/necrotic enteritis, especially of the ileum and large intestine. The wall is thickened and covered with yellow-grey necrotic material overlying a red, granular surface. The mesenteric lymph nodes and spleen may be enlarged. In calves, the small intestine typically shows a diffuse mucoid or mucohaemorrhagic enteritis and the mesenteric lymph nodes are oedematous, congested and greatly enlarged [44].

Pathological findings :

In adult cattle acute heamorrhagic entritis with necrotic change usually most pronounced in the mucosa of large intestine is commonly found at postmortem examination and similar change may be seen in the small intestine. The mesenteric lymph node are in variably swollen, edematous and in many case heamorrhagic. The liver may show degenerative change and the wall of gall bladder may be thickened. In calves, the clinical sign are those of septicemia which resemble those described for adult cattle i.e. congestion and heamorrhagic areas in the intestine, enlarged lymph node and congested spleen. Petechial heamorrhages may be seen in the cortex of the kidney and epicardium [35].

The chronic form is manifested by discrete areas of necrosis of the wall of the cecum and colon. The wall is thickened and covered with yellow gray necrotic material overlying a red granular mucosal surfaces. Salmonealla are present in the heart, blood, spleen, liver, bile, mesenteric lymph node and intestinal contents in both septicemic and acute forms. In the chronic form the bacteria may be isolated from the intestinal lesions and less commonly from other viscera [24].

Clinical Sign

Adult cattle generally contract either acute or subacute enteric salmonellosis and pregnant animal may abort during the early stage of acute enteric disease. Severely affected animals show fever, depression, inappetence and drop in milk yield. These sign are followed by diarrhea which is fowl smelling, the faces being mucoid and usually containing a clot of blood and shred of necrotic intestinal mucosa. Sign of colonic congestion of mucus membrane and dehydration may be evident. The acute disease last for about a week. *S. dublin* in particular but also other serovars may cause abortion in cows at any stage of pregnancy (Table 3). Abortion may either precede the onset of dysentery or follow it within two or four weeks. Alternatively abortion may occur in cows that show no sign of illness, septicemia and/or placentitis being the case of death of fetus. Retention of the placenta occurs in approximately 70% of cases that abort but subsequent fertility is not usually affected [7].

In calves clinical disease is most common 2-6 week of age. Clinical sign vary but typically the enteric form of diseases predominate which is characterized by pyrexia, dullness and anorexia, followed by diarrhea that may contain fibrin and mucus. The feaces may become blood stained and "stringy" due to the presences of necrotic intestinal mucosa. Calves rapidly become weak and dehydrated unless treated. Infected calves usually die 5-7 days after the onset of disease. At this stage the organisms has become systemic as a result of reduced innate immunity and may be isolated from variety of tissue including blood. Calves that recover from infection do not typically remain carrier. Salmonellosis is very variable and in some animals particularly in very young animals rapid multiplication occur both in intestine and systemically associated with poor absorption of specific immunoglobulin G from colostrums or with calves receiving in sufficient or no colostrums [45].

DISEASE IN HUMAN

Distribution

Worldwide there are 16 million annual cases of typhoid fever, 1.3 billion cases of gastroenteritis and 3 million deaths due to *Salmonella*. In the US annually there are 2-4 million cases with a death rate of 500-1,000 and an economic loss of about 3 billion dollars. A recent CDC report indicates that the incidence of *S. typhimurium* decreased significantly (42% decline) from 1996–1998 to 2005; however, the incidence of other serotypes are on the rise such as S. enteritidis and S. heidelberg, each of which increased by 25% and S. *enterica* serovar Javiana increased by 82% [46].

Physiology

The *Salmonella*, in the family Enterobacteriaceae, are facultatively anaerobic, gram negative and rod-shaped bacteria. Given the close relationship with E. coli and the many years devoted to its study, the overall metabolism of *Salmonella* is well understood. The cells are typically 0.7-1.5 μm by 2-5 μm. They grow at 7-48°C with an optimum growth at 37°C (mesophile) and at pH 4.05-9.5 with an optimal growth at pH 6.5-7.5 (neutrophile). *Salmonella* grows optimally at a water activity of 0.995 and are chemo-organotrophs. They have both fermentative and oxidative metabolism. The primary route for metabolism of carbohydrates is the Embden-Meyerhof pathway (glycolysis). They ferment glucose to formate (with the production of gas) and to ethanol, acetate, or lactate [19].

Transmission to human

Human salmonellosis is generally foodborne and is contracted through consumption of contaminated food of animal origin such as meat, milk, poultry and eggs. Dairy products including cheese and ice cream were also implicated in the outbreak. However, fruits and vegetables such as lettuce, tomatoes, cilantro, alfalfa-sprouts and almonds have also been implicated in recent out-break [35]. Acute gastroenteritis is usually acquired from consumption of food which may be directly or indirectly contaminated with *Salmonella*.

A wide variety of animal species have been shown to be capable of harboring the organisms and in the developed world turkey, chicken, swine and cattle are found to be infected carriers in the studies conducted in the abattoirs. These carriers may readily shed *Salmonella* during transportation to the abattoir and contaminate abattoir workers or equipment during slaughter. The progressive trend forwards mass processing and distribution of food products has been an important factor in the increase incidences of *Salmonella* foodborne diseases. Person to person spread has been demonstrated on many occasions and may take place in young children and group living under poor socioeconomic condition where effective sanitation is lacking. Person to person spread also may occur in hospitals, nursing homes, mental institution in which large number of outbreak has occurred. Amplification of infection in these institutions may occur from contaminated food or asymptomatic carrier's babies being at special risk [35]. Direct or indirect contact with animals colonized with *Salmonella* is another source of infection, including contact during visits to petting zoos and farms [47].

Table 3: Important epidemiological and clinical difference between S. dublin and S. typhimurium infection in cattle [7]

S. *dublin*	S. *typhimurium*
Bovine specific usually endemic herd problem	Not host-specific usually sporadic disease outbreaks
Bovine carriers important as a source of infection	Various animal species and their product are important sources of infection
Carriers excrete organism for long times or sometimes (long life)	Carrier excrete organism for short period usually 3-4 months
Septicemia is common	Septicemia is uncommon: enteritis is common
Abortion relatively common	Abortion uncommon

Fecal oral route and vehicle born infection may result from ingestion of food or water that have been contaminated with human or animal feaces or from direct exposure to animals or their waste. A lower infectious dose of organism is usually required in the elderly, the immunocompromised, antibiotic users and those with achlorhydria or regular use of antacid and related medication. The commonly recognized vehicle of transmission includes inadequate cooked or raw meat, unpasteurized milk or milk product, contaminated and inadequately treated drinking water. www.dol.gov.

Contamination of milk may occur by a variety of route. Animal may occasionally, excrete the organisms in milk during the febrile stage of the disease or more likely infected feaces, from either a clinically infected cow or healthy carrier may contaminate the milk during the milking process. Milk also may be contaminated from use of polluted water from dirty equipment or from dairy workers. Indirect contamination also has been described when cattle have become contaminated with *Salmonella*. Contamination of food also may occur directly from *Salmonella*infected food handlers or indirectly from sewage polluted water [48].

Clinical Sign in Human

The incubation period depends on the number of bacteria ingested and varies from 5-72 hours. Affected individual's experience sudden nausea, vomiting and watery fowl smelling diarrhea which is in most case last only a few hours. If the colon is affected, the stool may also contain blood and or mucus. Fever up to 39°C is not uncommon. Convalescences within 1-2 days but the illness may last for 5-7 days [49].

More severe symptom may occur in people who are at high risk like those extreme age groups (the young because their immune system are immature and the elderly because the immune system are declining), person with decreased gastric acidity (because gastric acid is the first line of defense for the ingested *Salmonella*), person with altered gastric intestinal bacteria (including those taking broad spectrum antibiotics, purgatives or who have had bowl surgery) and person taking opiate drug in which the bowl movement is decreased. In these highest risk groups of people *Salmonella* may invade beyond the gastrointestinal tract (GIT) to cause severe systematic illness.

Salmonella gastroenteritis is usually a self-limiting illness and fatality is uncommon. Biopsy and endoscopic examination have demonstrated the colon to be a major site of infection. The change in the colon ranges from edema of lamina propria with a focal or diffuse inflammatory infiltrate to a more intensive inflammation with disruption of the surface epithelium and multi-focal micro abscesses. In more severe cases, vascular congestion, infiltration of the lamina proporia with polymorphonuclear leucocytes and abscess formation has been recorded [35].

PUBLIC HEALTH ASPECT OF BOVINE SALMONELLOSIS

Salmonellosis is an important global public health problem causing substantial morbidity and thus also has a significant economic impact. Although most infections cause mild to moderate self-limited disease, serious infections leading to deaths do occur [50]. In spite of the improvement in hygiene, food processing, education of food handlers and information to the consumers, foodborne diseases still dominate as the most important public health problem in most countries [51].

A salmonellosis incidence is defined as the identification of *Salmonella* from animals or group of animal's product or surrounding which can be specifically related to identifiable animals or from animals feed. On the human side, a registered medical practitioner in the US required under the Public Health (Control of Disease) act to notify the local authority, if the patient is suffering from or suspected of having foodborne disease [35].

Studies provide increasing evidence of adverse human health consequences due to the occurrence of resistant microorganisms. Use of antimicrobial agents in human and animal affects the intestinal tract placing those concerned at increased risk of certain infection. This is defined as the proportion of *Salmonella* that would not have occurred if the *Salmonella* were not resistant. In addition antimicrobial agent used in animal can result in increased transmission of resistant microorganisms between animal and therefore would results in case of transmission of such microorganisms to human through food. Increased frequency of treatment failure and increase severity of infection may be manifested by prolonged duration of illness. www.who.int.mediacenter.

Salmonella dublin is largely but not entirely specific to cattle with average 10 human case reported in each year in Ireland. Apart from its pathogenicity two other characteristics of *S. dublin* make it particularly important for Ireland from a public health viewpoints. First, it is very prevalent on Irish farms and secondly in evolutionary terms, it is only one step away from S. enteritidis, a common *Salmonella* serotype in poultry and the main case of clinical salmonellosis in humans. In genetic terms, difference between the serovars *S. dublin* and S. enteritidis are no greater than those found within each serotypes. This indicates that, *S. dublin* and S. enteritidis share a common ancestor. One branch evolved in to a poultry adapted serotype capable of causing disease in human, the other in to host specific cattle pathogen. If *S. dublin* has been confirmed in breeding herd there is a significant risk of persistent infection in carrier cows for as long as animal which were present at the time of the outbreak remain in the herd [53].

DIAGNOSIS OF SALMONELLOSIS

The clinical sign and finding at postmortem examination are not unique to salmonellosis although a tentative diagnosis may be made. They should confirm either in diseased animal or at necropsy by isolation of organisms in their feces and determination of viable counts. Fecal samples rather than swabs should be taken and these should obviously be obtained before administration of antibiotics. It may be also possible to isolate organism from oral secretion and by blood culture although these are less reliable than feces culture and must be taken with care to avoid contamination. Animal that died of salmonellosis usually have large number of *Salmonella* distributed throughout their tissue and sample of spleen, liver, hepatic, mediastinal and bronchial lymph nodes may yield count in excretion of 106 organisms/gram. Similar concentration may be present in the wall and content of the ileum, cecum, colon and associated lymph nodes. Sample should be taken from internal organs in order to distinguish animal that have died of enteritis without septicemia [53].

CULTURE METHODS

The traditional *Salmonella* culture method involves pre-enrichment, selective enrichment, isolation of pure culture, biochemical screening and serological confirmation, which requires 5-7 days to complete. The USDA and FDA recommended method involves a 6-24 h preenrichment step in a nonselective broth such as lactose broth, tryptic soy broth, nutrient broth, skim milk, or buffered peptone water with a recommended incubation temperature of 37°C. The selective enrichment step requires additional 24 hours incubation in Rappaport- Vassiliadis (RV) broth, selenite cystine (SC) broth, or Muller Kauffmann tetrathionate broth. The inoculation temperature of 41.5°C ± 1°C for RV broth and 37°C ± 1°C for SC and MKTT broth is used. Bacterial cells are isolated from selective agar plates such as Hektoen enteric agar (HEA), xylose lysine deoxy-cholate (XLD), and/or brilliant green agar (BGA). Biochemical testing is done using triple sugar iron agar and lysine iron agar, which requires an additional 4–24 hours [54,55].

Rapid detection methods

Detection of antibodies to Salmonella by enzyme immunoassay (EIA):

The detection of antibodies to *Salmonella* by EIA offers a sensitive and cost-effective method for mass screening of animal flocks/herds for indications of a past/

present *Salmonella* infection. The limitation of the method is that the immune response of the individual animal is not elicited before 1-2 weeks after infection takes place. A number of commercial kits are available for testing poultry, cattle and pigs. An obvious advantage of this method is that it can be automated and no incubation is required to increase the numbers of bacterial cells [56].

The EIA is a well-established technique for assaying antigens. Antibodies labeled with an enzyme are bound to *Salmonella* antigens, and the level of antigen present is determined by enzymatic conversion of a substrate, usually resulting in a color change which can be read visually or by a spectrophotometer. The EIAs rely on the standard cultural procedures for pre-enrichment and selective enrichment to provide enough*Salmonella* cells for detection. EIA technology that enables detection at an earlier stage of resuscitation and/or culture can provide even more rapid results. Serological test, such as ELISA, serum agglutination and complement fixation can be used for the retrospective diagnosis of salmonellosis or the detection of carriers [55].

Nucleic acid-based assays:

Real-time quantitative polymerase chain reaction using PCR (Q-PCR), reverse transcriptase PCR (RTPCR), and nucleic acid sequence-based amplification (NASBA) have been used for detection of *Salmonella* from various food matrices. *Salmonellaenterica* was detected at 1 cfu ml−1 after a culture enrichment of 8-12 h in the TaqMan-based Q-PCR using invA gene as target. NASBA method has been used for detection of viable *Salmonella* cells and it has been demonstrated to be more sensitive than RT-PCR, and moreover, it requires fewer amplification cycles than the conventional PCR methods [46].

Differential diagnosis

The differential diagnosis of *Salmonella* enterocolitis in humans include viral gastroenteritis and bacterial enteric infections including those caused by Shigella, Enterotoxigenic E-coli, Campylobacter species, Vibrio species and Yersinia enterocoliticia. The disorder must also be differentiated from toxin-mediated foodborne illness including those caused by Staphylococcus aureus, Bacillus cereus and Clostridium perfringens. Compared to the patient with toxin mediated disorder person with salmonellosis usually have less prominent vomiting and are the more likely have prolonged diarrhea and fever. The shorter incubation period of toxin mediated foodborne illness can be important to distinguish them from salmonellosis. A recent history of ingestion of raw milk, undercooked meat and contact with farm animals 48 hours before the onset of illness suggests the diagnosis of salmonellosis [49].

Treatment

Treatment of non-typhoidal *Salmonella* infection is different from typhoidal infection. In treatment of non-typhoidal *Salmonella* infection antibiotics should not be used routinely, as used in typhoid. Antibiotic should be only used if required as most infection with non-typhoidal*Salmonella* is self-limiting type and duration of diarrhea and fever are not much affected by use of antibiotics. Additionally antibiotic therapy can increase relapse of infection and also prolong the duration of gastrointestinal carrier states. The main treatment should be aimed at correcting dehydration that may arise due to prolonged diarrhea by fluid and electrolyte replacement. www.webcan.gogleuserconten.com.

Although *Salmonella*e are usually sensitive in vitro to many antibiotics, their use for treatment of uncomplicated gastroenteritis until recently has been generally contraindicated by their lack of favorable effect on the course of the disease and by prolongation of *Salmonella* shedding. Following the introduction of fluoroquinolones a number of clinicians have advocated their use for treatment of only on enteric fever but also of *Salmonella* gastroenteritis because of their efficacy in reducing the duration of illness and of *Salmonella* shedding. In case of patient with bacteremia and other complication antimicrobials are used. Likewise the treatment of enteric fever necessitates the use of antimicrobial drugs with chloramphinicol, ampicillin, amoxicillin, trimethoprimsulfamethoxazole and newer fluoroquinoazoles being drug of choice against sensitive *Salmonella*. Proper management of fluid and electrolyte balance is impotant in all patients with *Salmonella* gastroenteritis but is crucial in young children and elder individuals [35].

In animal treatment supportive treatment with intravenous fluid is necessary for patients that have anorexia, depression, significant dehydration. Individual patient may be treated aggressively following acid base and electrolyte assessment. Oral fluid and electrolyte may be somewhat helpful and much cheaper than IV fluid for cattle demand to be mildly or moderately dehydrated. The effectiveness of oral fluid may be somewhat compromised by malabsorption and maldigestion in salmonellosis patient but still should be considered useful. Cattle that are willing to drink can have specific electrolyte (NaCl, KCl) added to drinking water to help correcting electrolyte [57].

The implementation of broad prophylactic strategies that are efficacious for all *Salmonella*e may be required in order to overcome the diversity of *Salmonella* serovars present on farms, and the potential for different serovars to possess different virulence factors [58]. Early treatment is essential for septicemic salmonellosis but there is controversy regarding the use of antimicrobial agent for intestinal salmonellosis. Oral antibiotic may alter the intestinal micro flora and interfere with competitive antagonism and prolong shading of the organism. There is also a concern that antibiotic resistance strain of *Salmonella* selected by oral antibiotic may subsequently infect human. Antibiotic such as ampicillin or cephalosporin lead to lyses of bacteria with release of endotoxin. NSAID may be used to reduce the effect of endotoxemia [5].

PREVENTION AND CONTROL

Prevention and control in animals

Condition that contribute to an increasing incidence of epidemic salmonellosis include large herd size, more intensive and crowded husbandry and the trend of free-stall barn with loose housing, which contribute to the feacal contamination of the entire premise. When salmonellosis has been confirmed in a herd, the following control measure should be considered; isolate obviously affected animals to one group if possible, treat severely affected animals, affected animals institute measure to minimize public health concern like (no raw milk should be consumed) physically clean the environment and disinfect the premise following resolution of the outbreak or crises period. A mastitis survey should be conducted that include bulk tank surveillance. Prevention is best accompanied by maintaining a cross herd and culturing new feed additives and components before using the entire ration [57].

It is generally agreed that supportive therapy and good nursing are important. These include oral or parentral re-hydration, correction of electrolyte balance and stabilization of acid base equilibrium [7].

Salmonella vaccinology:

Calves vaccinated at 1-3 weeks of age with a modified aromatic dependant *S. dublin* bacteria have detectable anti-lipoplisaccharide immunoglobins after immunization. Safe live oral vaccine against *S. typhimurium* and *S. dublin* has been constructed and shown to control protection against experimental infection with virulent wide type strain of the organisms. A virulent S. choleraesuis vaccine is efficacies experimentally against salmonellosis due to *S. dublin* in calves to protect young calves. The best program is to vaccinate the cow during pregnancy which will give passive protection to calves for 6 weeks [24].

Generally, both live and attenuated vaccines produced from rough strain in bacteria commercially. There is some evidence that inactivated bacterins can induce a lower level of protection [59]. The veterinarian research institute produced vaccine against bovine salmonellosis in activated bacteria prepared from isolate of *S. dublin*, S. typhomurium and S. bovismorbificans and a live attenuated vaccine containing a virulent rough mutant of *S. dublin* [7].

Prevention and control in human

There is no vaccine to prevent salmonellosis in human whereas, vaccine against *Salmonella* typhi has been developed, especially in children, but is only 60% effective. A person given this vaccine would still have a strong chance of developing salmonellosis. It is not expected that there will be a single vaccine that is effective against all the different forms of *Salmonella* soon. Ongoing research is investigating what can be done to produce a useful human vaccine for *Salmonella* [59]. People should not eat raw or uncooked meat, they should not drink raw milk or unpasteurized dairy product, cross contamination of food should be avoided. Uncooked meat should be kept separate from cooked food ready to eat. Hands, cutting boards or knifes and other utensils should be washed thoroughly after handling uncooked food. Hands should be washed before handling any food and in between handling different food items. People should have to wash their hands after contact with animal's feces [46].

Pasteurization of milk and treating municipals water supply for reducing risk of *Salmonella* infection, improvement in farm animal hygiene in slaughter process in food harvesting and in packaging operation have helped to prevent salmonellosis

[55]. A periodic surveillance of the level of *Salmonella* contamination in different food product and environment is necessary to control spread of the pathogen. Reducing*Salmonella* prevalence requires comprehensive control strategy in animal and animal foodstuff with restriction in the infected flock until they have been cleaned from infection. In addition mandatory testing before slaughter should be conducted like the one implemented in Sweden [60]. Ensuring safe food production requires knowledge on the nature and origin of animal, animal feed, the health status of animals at the farm, the use of veterinary medicinal data regarding antimortem and postmortem findings and the risk association with post harvests production strategies [61].

CONCLUSION AND RECOMMENDATION

Salmonella is a leading cause of foodborne disease in human and consumption of both meat and milk has been implicated in salmonellosis outbreaks of people. Having animals and raw products it is not possible to be free from zoonotic agent; however the occurrences can be minimized by applying high standard of hygiene in all steps of the food production. Infected animals can present with a great variety of clinical symptoms, and risk factors for transmission to humans clearly differ by animal species, age groups, animal purpose and geographic region. In addition, strains of *Salmonella* resistant to multiple antibiotics have been isolated from dairy cow during salmonellosis outbreak on dairy operation. The same strains have also been isolated from ill people. A high degree of interaction between medical and veterinarian surveillance is needed. Finally, implementing basic and applied research to the agent that cause foodborne salmonellosis will be a crucial point for new approaches to prevent and control the disease.

Based on the above facts the following recommendations are forwarded:

- Strict hygiene of the slaughter house and lairage
- People should not drink unpasteurized milk or milk products and should not eat raw meat.
- Establishment of HACCP
- Education of food handlers
- Vaccination of cattle
- Maintenance of cold chains
- Setting import standards
- Sanitary examination of the product
- Collaboration between government agencies, professional organizations and special interest groups.
- New legislations or public awareness campaigns have leads to dramatic decreases in Salmonella incidence.

REFERENCES

1. Rao PV (2004) Essential of Microbiology. Satish Kumar Jain for CBS publishers and Distributors, New Delhi. India. 146-148.
2. FDA/CFSAN (2008) Food Safety A to Z Reference Guide Salmonnella.
3. Fluit AC (2005) Towards more virulent and antibiotic-resistant *Salmonella*? FEMS Immunol Med Microbiol 43: 1-11.
4. BayleyegnM, Dainal A, Woubit S (2003) Source of *Salmonella* serotypes isolated from animals, slauther house personnel and retail meat product in Ethiopia 1997-2002. Ethio.J.Health.Dev.17: 63-70.
5. Davison, S. 2005. Salmonellosis. In: Merck veterinary manual 10th edition. Edited by Cynthia, M. kahn. Merik and Co.J (inc. White House Station, N.J U.S.A).
6. EjetaG, Molla B, Alemayehu D, Muckle A (2004) *Salmonella* serotypes isolated from mincied meat beef, mutton and pork in Addis Ababa, Ethiopia Reve.med. Vet 155: 547-551.
7. Venter BJ, Myburgh JG, Van der Walt ML (1994) Bovine Salmonellosis. In: Infectious diseases of Livestock with Special Reference to South Africa. Eds. Coetzer, J.W., Thomson, G.R. and Tustin, R.C. Oxford University Press, Cape Town, Pp: 1104-1112.
8. McEvoy JM, Doherty AM, Sheridan JJ, Blair IS, McDowell DA (2003) The prevalence of *Salmonella* spp. in bovine faecal, rumen and carcass samples at a commercial abattoir. J ApplMicrobiol 94: 693-700.
9. Gomez TM1, Motarjemi Y, Miyagawa S, Käferstein FK, Stöhr K (1997) Foodborne salmonellosis. World Health Stat Q 50: 81-89.
10. Threlfall EJ, Ward LR, Rowe B (1997) Increasing incidence of resistance to trimethoprim and ciprofloxacin in epidemic *Salmonella*typhimurium DT104 in England and Wales. Euro Surveill 2: 81-84.
11. Piddock LJ (2002) Fluoroquinolone resistance in *Salmonella* serovars isolated from humans and food animals. FEMS Microbiol Rev 26: 3-16.
12. SalycrsAA (1995) Antibiotic resistance transfer in the mammalian intestinal tract: Implication for human health, food safety and Biotechnology New York.
13. Popoff MY, Bockemühl J, Gheesling LL (2003) Supplement 2001 (no. 45) to the Kauffmann-White scheme. Res Microbiol 154: 173-174.
14. Mead PS, Slutsker L, Dietz V, McCaig LF, Bresee JS, et al. (1999) Food-related illness and death in the United States. Emerg Infect Dis 5: 607-625.
15. Wray C, Wray A(2000) *Salmonella* in domestic animals, Veterinary Microbiology 81: 281-282.
16. Deb M, Kapoor L (2005) *Salmonella* nomenclature seen in the literature. Indian J Med Microbiol 23: 204-205.
17. Hafez, H.M. 2005. Government regulation and control of some important poultry diseases. World's Poult. Sci. J. 61: 574-575.
18. Brenner FW, Villar RG, Angulo FJ, Tauxe R, Swaminathan B

(2000) *Salmonella* nomenclature. J ClinMicrobiol 38: 2465-2467.

19. Craig DE, James MS(2006)The genus *Salmonella* In: The Prokaryotes 3rd Edition. 6: 123-158.
20. Lund, Barbara, Baird-Parker, Anthony C, Gould et al.(2000) The Microbiology safety and quality of food (II). Gaithersburg, Malaysia. Food Microbiology 12: 3-8.
21. Johnson TJ, Wannemuehler YM, Johnson SJ, Logue CM, White DG, et al. (2007) Plasmid replicon typing of commensal and pathogenic Escherichia coli isolates. Appl Environ Microbiol 73: 1976-1983.
22. Food Research International (FRI) (2010) *Salmonella* in Foods. Evaluation, Strategies and Challenges 43:1557-1558.
23. European Commission(2000)An opinion of the scientific committee on veterinary measure relating to public health on foodborne zoonoses. Health and consumer protection directorate general, Directorate B, Scientific health opinions, Unit B3-Managements of Scientific committees II 24-27.
24. Radostitis OM, Gay CC, Hinchliff KW, Constable PD (2007) Veterinary Medicine: A text book of the disease of cattle, horses, sheep, pigs, and goats. 10th ed. Elsevier Ltd. 325-326.
25. Popoff MY, Bockemühl J, Brenner FW, Gheesling LL (2001) Supplement 2000 (no. 44) to the Kauffmann-White scheme. Res Microbiol 152: 907-909.
26. Tindall BJ, Grimont PA, Garrity GM, Euzéby JP (2005) Nomenclature and taxonomy of the genus *Salmonella*. Int J SystEvolMicrobiol 55: 521-524.
27. Centre for Infectious Disease Research and Policy (CIDRAP) (2006) Academic Health Centre, University of Minnesota.
28. Scott S (2010)The most probable number method and its use in Enumeration, Qualification and validation. J of Validation Technology 16: 35-38.
29. Diagnostic Services of Manitoba (DSM) (2009) *Salmonella* Nomenclature and the Reporting of Results on *Salmonella* Species: Memorandum.
30. Acha PN, Szyfres B (2001) Zoonosis and communicable disease common to man and animals 3rd ed. 233-245.
31. SibhatB, Molla B, Zerihun A, Muckle A, Cole L, et al. (2011) *Salmonella* Serovars and Antimicrobial Resistance Profiles in Beef Cattle, Slaughterhouse Personnel and Slaughterhouse Environment in Ethiopia. Zoonoses public health 58: 102-109.
32. Evans S, Davies R (1996) Case control study of multiple-resistant *Salmonella* typhimurium DT104 infection of cattle in Great Britain. Vet Rec 139: 557-558.
33. Richardson A (1975) Salmonellosis in cattle. Vet Rec 96: 329-331.
34. Peters AR (1985) An estimation of the economic impact of an outbreak of *Salmonella* dublin in a calf rearing unit. Vet Rec 117: 667-668.
35. Wray C (1994)Mamalian salmonellosis In: Hand book of zoonosis 2nd Edition.

Edited by BeranGW, New York, C.R.C, press: 291-300.

36. Mattila T, Frost AJ, O›Boyle D (1988) The growth of *Salmonella* in rumen fluid from cattle at slaughter. Epidemiol Infect 101: 337-345.

37. Morisse JP, Cotte JP (1994) Evaluation of some risks factors in bovine salmonellosis. Vet Res 25: 185-191.

38. BäumlerAJ, Tsolis RM, HeffronF(2000) Virulence Mechanisms of*Salmonella* and their Genetic Basis. In: Wray, C., Wray, A. (Eds.),*Salmonella* in Domestic Animals. CABI Publishing, New York, pp. 57-72.

39. Scherer CA, Miller SI (2001) Molecular Pathogenesis of *Salmonella*e. In: Groisman, E.A. (Ed). Principles of Bacterial Pathogenesis. Academic Press, New York, pp. 265-333.

40. Quinn J, MarkeyBK (2003) Concise Review of Veterinary Microbiology: Blackwell publishing.

41. Mekaloson JJ (1990) Microbiology 4th edition. Lippincotcompany New York.

42. Koo FC, Peterson JW, Houston CW, Molina NC (1984) Pathogenesis of experimental salmonellosis: inhibition of protein synthesis by cytotoxin. Infect Immun 43: 93-100.

43. Hansen-Wester I, Hensel M (2001) *Salmonella* pathogenicity islands encoding type III secretion systems. Microbes Infect 3: 549-559.

44. Wray C, Davies RH (2000) *Salmonella* Infections in Cattle. Veterinary Laboratories Agency (Weybridge), New Haw, Addlestone, Surrey KT15 3NB, UK.

45. Barrow PA, Jones MA, Thomson N (2010) Pathogenesis of bacterial infection in animals 4th edition. Edited by Gyles, C.L., Songer, G. Theon, C.O: Blackwell publishing 233.

46. ArunK Bhunia (2008) Mechanisms and Pathogenesis In: Foodborne Microbial Pathogens: pp. 201-215.

47. Friedman CR, Torigian C, Shillam PJ, Hoffman RE, Heltzel D, et al. (1998) An outbreak of salmonellosis among children attending a reptile exhibit at a zoo. J Pediatr 132: 802-807.

48. Jones BD (2005) *Salmonella* invasion gene regulation: a story of environmental awareness. J Microbiol 43 Spec No: 110-117.

49. Krauss HM, Albert W, Appel M, Henery B, Lesenberg D, et al. (2003) Zoonosis infectious disease from animals to humans. 3rd edition. American Society, for Microbiology: 234-236.

50. de Jong B, Ekdahl K (2006) The comparative burden of salmonellosis in the European Union member states, associated and candidate countries. BMC Public Health 6: 4.

51. Domínguez C, Gómez I, Zumalacárregui J (2002) Prevalence of *Salmonella* and Campylobacter in retail chicken meat in Spain. Int J Food Microbiol 72: 165-168.

52. Mee JF, Moyes T, Gleeson D, Brien B (2002)A questionnaire survey of fertility

management on dairy farms in the Republic of Ireland. Irish Veterinary Journal, 55: 122-128.

53. Jones PJ, Weston PR, SwailT (2007) Salmonellosis In: Bovine medicine, diseases and husbandry of cattle. Edited by Andrew, A.H. 2nd Edition: Blackwell publishing 215-230.
54. International Organization for Standardization (ISO) (2002) Microbiology of Food and Animal Feeding Stuff-Horizontal Method for the Detection of *Salmonella*. 4th ed. ISO 6579.
55. Hans PR, Dean OC, Morris P(2006) *Salmonella* infection In: Foodborne Infections and Intoxications 3rd Edition. Food Science and Technology International Series: 57-136.
56. Zamora BM, Hartung M (2002) Chemiluminescent immunoassay as a microtiter system for the detection of *Salmonella* antibodies in the meat juice of slaughter pigs. J Vet Med B Infect Dis Vet Public Health 49: 338-345.
57. Rebhun CW (1995) Disease of Dairy cattle: 1st Edition. Awa Verly Company.
58. Mohler VL, Izzo MM, House JK (2009) *Salmonella* in calves. Vet Clin North Am Food AnimPract 25: 37-54, vi.
59. Danielle AB (2006) Deadly Diseases and Epidemics: *Salmonella*. David Heymann; Communicable Diseases Section. World Health Organization, Geneva, Switzerland. CHELSEA HOUSE PUBLISHERS pp. 8-74.
60. Boqvist S, Vågsholm I (2005) Risk factors for hazard of release from *Salmonella*-control restriction on Swedish cattle farms from 1993 to 2002. Prev Vet Med 71: 35-44.
61. SnijdersJMA, Kanapen FV (2002) Prevention of human disease and integrated quality control system. Livestock production Science 76: 203-206.
62. GrimontPAD, Weill FX (2007)Antgenic formulae of the *Salmonella* serovars 9th edition. Paris: WHO.
63. CoetzerJA, Thomson GR, Tustin RC (1994) Disease of livestock (2): Oxford University Press.

14

CHAPTER

LABORATORY MANUAL AND REVIEW ON CLINICAL PATHOLOGY

INTRODUCTION

Clinical pathology is one of the two major divisions of pathology, the other being anatomical pathology. Clinical pathology is itself divided in to subspecialties, the main ones being clinical hematology/blood banking, clinical chemistry, hematopathology and clinical microbiology and emerging subspecialties such as molecular diagnostics. Hematology studies the blood and blood-forming tissues to evaluate presence of disease and assist in therapeutic interventions as clinically indicated. Clinical chemistry (also known as chemical pathology and clinical biochemistry) is the area of clinical pathology that is generally concerned with analysis of bodily fluids.

Blood parameters play a critical role in diagnosis, assessing progression, and in the characterization of disease and phenotypes in clinical and research situations. The accuracy and reliability of the whole blood parameter analysis depends on identification and control or elimination of variables that may affect these results. Different blood collection and handling strategies represent source of variability that can be controlled in many instances.

Basic hematological procedures such as the complete blood count are frequently conducted to help physicians and veterinarians arrive at a diagnosis and prognosis, also to evaluate treatment. Hematology testing includes, but is not limited to: Hematology Sample Processing, Hematology Research Services, Hematology Automated Testing, Lamellar Body Counts, Microscopic Cellular Analysis, Body Fluid Analysis and Specialized Stains. The outline of this laboratory manual deals with the basic hematological procedures and clinical chemistry analysis which is meant for students use. The study of hematology begins with proper sample collection and handling. Part one deals with hematology containing different sections. Part two covers clinical chemistry including functional tests. All of the procedures described in this manual are classical methods that are routinely performed in a standard clinical pathology laboratory. Detail procedures including preparation of reagents, solutions, stains and buffers are given. Calculations of blood indices and chemical analysis are also discussed in part one and part two respectively

OBJECTIVES OF CLINICAL PATHOLOGY PRACTICAL COURSE

At the end of Clinical Pathology practical course the students will be able to:

a. Identify the most important hematological and functional pathological tests of vet importance

b. Diagnose different animal diseases by confirming the pathological causes that constraint live stock production in general

c. Have knowledge more about clinical pathology

d. Write lab report pertaining the tests carried out

PART ONE: HEMATOLOGY

Equipments and reagents required for hematological blood examination.

a. Hematocrit centrifuge

b. Compound microscope

c. Sahlis instrument

d. Capillary tube

e. Hematocrit reader

f. Distilled water

g. Haemocytometer pipette

h. Haemocytometer counting chamber

i. WBC diluting fluid

j. RBC diluting fluid

k. Slides, cover slip, special cover slip

l. ESR stand, ESR tube

m. Filter paper, blood lancets, lead pencils, marker

n. Giemsa stain, Wright's stain

o. Vacutainer tubes(different type), vacutainer needles, syringes, needle holder

p. Gloves

q. Blood samples

r. Staining racks and others

BLOOD COLLECTION

Site: The following lists of veins are the most appropriate blood collection sites from different species of veterinary importance

Jagular vein: The most commonly used site in the horse, cattle, sheep, goat, camel and large wild mammals: used occasionally in small animals. Vacutainer tube, vacutainer needle, syringe, needle, needle holder, and disinfectant should be used for blood sample.

Procedure

- Placement of the thumb of the left hand in the jagular furrow to occlude and anchor the jagular vein, while manipulating the syringe and needle with the right hand
- Clipping the site of sampling especially in long haired animals is recommended
- The veins are more clearly out lined when the site is rubbed with alcohol

Cephalic Vein - The most commonly used site for collection of small amount of blood in the dog. By constricting the area on the dorsal aspects of the fore limb at the level of the elbow which can be raised beginning just above the carpal vein.

Ear Vein- can be used in small dog, pig, cat and small lab animals (small dog, rabbit, guinea pig, and monkey).

1. A marginal vein on the dorsal side of the ear is selected
2. Remove the hair by shaving, clipping, or other method
3. Swab the skin with alcohol or other
4. Place the left index finger under the ear at the point of applying stylet or syringe
5. Gentle aspiration is used when using a syringe in small animals like rabbit, to avoid collapse of the vein

Toe or Toe Nail – can be used in small dog, puppy, guinea pig etc

1. Clip the hair away

2. Disinfect the capillary bed of the nail
3. Cut in to just short of the base of the nail
4. Take 20-40 drops as well as 80 drops (4ml) of blood

Tail – can be used in pig, cattle, sheep, rat, and mouse

- Veinipuncture –of the coccygeal vein on the ventral side
- Amputation – commonest method used in the rat and mouse. A small transverse incision with a razor blade produce drops of blood

Heart – may be used in animals like bird, fish, and others

Femoral or Tibial vessels – used in dog, cat, small mammals, rat etc

Mammary vein – used for dairy cattle

The vein appears at the anterior border of the mammary gland lateral from the linea Alba and runs forward passing through a foramen in the abdominal wall posterior to ribs.

Anterior vena cava – used for the pig

A needle (41/2 – 6 in. and 17 to 20 gauge needle) is inserted just anterior and slightly lateral to the cariniform cartilage and a line from the cartilage to the base of the ear.

Retro orbital Venus plexus – used for the rat, mouse, guinea pig

1. A best method for obtaining a large quantity of blood (1ml) in mouse
2. This technique is reported to be less traumatic than others

Wing vein or comb – used for birds

1. After the feathers in the axillary region are plucked, the alar vein is seen running from beneath the pectoral muscle then along the ventral surface of the humerus

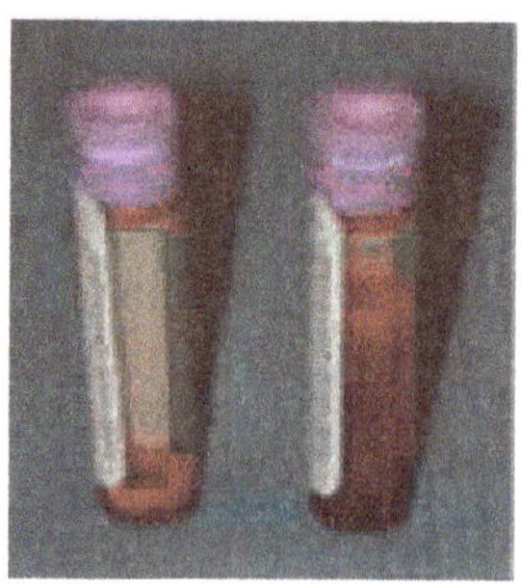

Figure 1: EDTA tubes should be filled to their labelled capacity. Short filled tube has an

excessive amount of EDTA relative to the blood volume. Short filled tubes cause a false increase in total plasma protein content and a false decrease in PCV and RBC count.

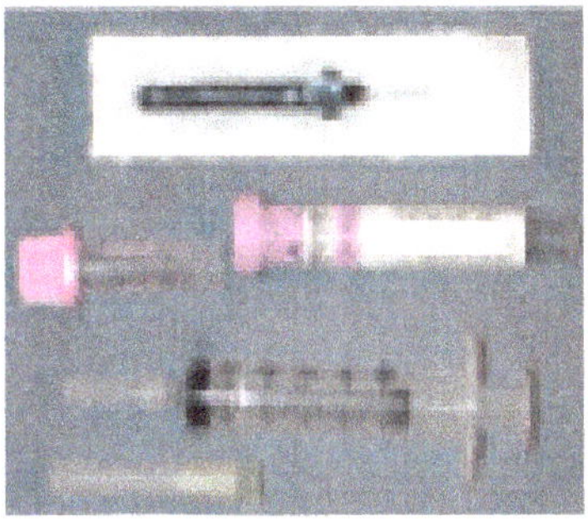

Figure 2: Collection materials for hematological assessment include syringe, needles, and purple topped collection tubes that contain EDTA.

In most animals up to 0.5 ml/kg blood collection has no any adverse effect. The total volume of blood collection differs in different animals.

Vacutainer Tubes

Red-stopper tubes – are for tests requiring clotted blood

Lavender stopper tubes – contain EDTA in concentrated liquid or desiccated powder form

Green stopper tubes – contain heparin and are used for blood gases, PH, (CO2, O2)....

Gray stopper tubes – contain oxalates, fluorides, or citrates

Yellow stopper tubes – available with Acid Citrate Dextrose (ACD) solution or physiological saline solution

Anticoagulants

The most important anticoagulants that can be used during blood collection with different mode of action are listed below.

Table 1: Commonly used anticoagulants, their mode of action and dose required

Anticoagulant / product	Mode of action	Amount required	Advantage	Disadvantage
EDTA/Ethylene diamine tetra acetic acid	Form insoluble Ca salts	10-20mg (1ml of 1 % solution dried at room temp. or at incubator	Recommended for routine hematological procedures, preserve cellular elements better	May shrinks cell because Na salt is less soluble
Heparin	Antithrombin and antithromboplastin	1-2mg (0.2ml of 1% solution)	Less effect on RBC hemolysis Used for blood gas analysis	May cause clumping of WBC, unsuitable for smears, as it interferes with stain ability of WBC expensive
Na citrate	Combine with Ca to form an insoluble Ca salt	10-20mg (1ml)	Can be used for blood transfusion	Interferes with many chemical tests, shrink cells
Potassium oxalate	Units with Ca to form insoluble calcium oxalate	20mg (2 drops of 20% solution dried in incubator	Very soluble	Causes shrinkage, it increase the volume of blood
Sodium oxalate	Units with Ca to form insoluble calcium oxalate	20mg	Used mainly for prothrombin time	Same as potassium oxalate

STAINING DYES

Wright's stain: Forms of dye available

- Dry powder as bulk and as preweighted vials, Capsule
- Readymade solution. Most convenient, but often deteriorated from long storage

Preparation of Stain

Conventional method

- Place 0.5gm of dry Wright's stain powder in a mortar
- Add 300ml of absolute methyl alcohol
- Grind the mixture and pour in dark bottle
- Shake the bottle each day for about two weeks, then filter
- Aging of the stain will take 2 to 4 before it will be satisfactory for use

Accelerated Method

- Place 0.3gm of dry Wright's stain powder in a mortar and over lay with 3ml of glycerol, grind thoroughly
- Rinse with 100ml of absolute methyl alcohol and place in dark container
- Mix with magnetic stirrer for about 1 wk without heat
- Filter before use

Giemsa Stain

General Consideration

- Giemsa stain has various azure compounds with eosin and methylene blue
- It is an excellent stain for blood parasites and for inclusion bodies
- It stains red granules well but neutrophilic granules and erythrocytes are poorly stained
- Commercial stock solution are recommended for purchase and are stable indefinitely

Preparation Method for Working Solution:

Take one part of giemsa stock solution and nine part distilled water and mix before one to two hours before use

Leishmen's Stain

Preparation

- Grind 0.15gm of Leishmen's stain powder with small amounts of absolute methyl alcohol until an even suspension is obtained. A total of 100ml methanol is added to produce complete solution
- Pour in to a dark bottle and age for a few weeks prior to use

Wright's-Giemsa stain (modified Wright's stain)

Preparation of Stain

- 500mg of dry Wright's stain powder and 50mg of Giemsa stain powder are ground in a mortar with 100ml of absolute methyl alcohol (acetone free)
- Allow to stand for 24-48 hrs before using
- Keep well stoppered to prevent evaporation of alcohol or absorption of water vapor

Commercial Wright's – Giemsa stain are available

- Wright – Leishmen stain
- May – Grunwald –Giemsa stain
- Methylene blue stain
- Field's stain
- Prussian blue stain and others

Buffered Distilled Water

Preparation: 5.47g monobasic potassium phosphate and 3.8g of dibasic sodium phosphate with 1000ml of distilled water

METHODS OF STAINING (STAINING PROCEDURE)

Wright's Stain

- Cover the dried blood smear completely with Wright's stain and allow to stand for 1 to 3 minute
- Add an equal amount of buffered distilled water or neutral water (pH 6.6 to 6.8 for most animals blood)
- Blow it gently and allow the mixture to stand for 3 to 5 minutes. A metallic scum should appears green

- Float off the metallic scum with a stream of water from a wash bottle or from the top. Use distilled water if tap water is too alkaline. Don't pour the stain off the slide before washing, as this will result in a precipitate forming on the slide
- Wipe the stain from the back of the slide with cleaning tissue
- Stand the slide on end, wave gently in the air, or blot gently with bibulous paper to dry
- Examine the preparation by placing a drop of oil on a slide
- If a permanent preparation is desired, the oil can be dissolved with xylene and a mounting medium like Canada balsam is applied.

Advantage: It conserves stain, Methyl alcohol, and time

Disadvantage: More precipitate is likely to be present

Table 2: Staining characteristics

Cell	Cytoplasm	Chromatin
Erythrocytes	Yellow to pinkish	Purple
Lymphocytes	Blue	Purplish red
Monocytes	Light blue	Purple
Eosinophils	Yellow to brownish red rods	Light purple
Basophils	Dark purple granules	
Hetrophils/Neutrophils	Yellow to brownish red rods	Light purple
Thrombocytes	Grey-blue	Purple

Giemsa Stain Method

- Place dried blood smear in a coplin jar containing absolute methyl alcohol for about 3 minute to fix the smear
- Drain off the alcohol and allow the slide to dry
- Transfer the slide to a second coplin jar containing fresh stain and allow staining for 16 to 60 minute. 60 minute staining period is used when blood parasite is suspected. 12 to 18 hrs for inclusion bodies
- Wash the stain with running/tap water, dry and examine under oil immersion microscope

Leishman's Stain Method

- Flood the air dried blood film with Leishman's stain and leave for 1 to 2 minute to fix
- Dilute the stain on the smear with double the volume of buffered distilled water and stain for 5 to 15 minute
- Blow on the mixture gently
- Wash with distilled water until the film has a pinkish tinge
- Wipe the back of the stain/the slide and allow to dry in upright position

SMEAR PREPARATION

- Wet smear
- Thin smear
- Thick smear

Procedures for Each Preparation

Wet Blood Smear/Film Preparation

- A drop of blood is placed at the centre of a clean slide
- Cover with a clean, dry cover slip
- Examine the film under the microscope (40 × objective)

The method does not require staining. It is rapid and simple to perform.

Extracellular blood parasites such as Trypanosomes and Microfilaria of filarial nematodes can be diagnosed. Note that you can see only the movement of Trypanosomes

Thin blood smears preparation

It can be made by spreading a drop of blood evenly across a clean grease free slide using a smooth edged spreader.

- Make a drop of blood on one end of glass slide
- Place the end of second glass slide /spreader slide / against the surface of the first slide, holding at an angle of 30-45 degrees
- Draw the spreader slide gently into the drop of blood and when the blood has along 2/3 of width of the spreader slide by capillary action, push the spreader slide forward with a steady even motion
- Dry by waving rapidly in the air

Thick Bloods Smear Preparation

- A large drop of blood is put at the centre of a clean dry slide
- The drop is spread with an applicator stick, needle or corner of another slide to cover an area of ½ an inch square
- The smear is thoroughly dried in a horizontal position so that the blood could not ooze to one edge to the film and protected from dust, insects and direct sunlight.

Causes of inadequately stained blood smears

Analysis of the poor results will determine what modification of technique is required to correct the problem

Entire smear is too blue - granules of neutrophil over stained and larger than normal, and granules of the eosinophil is deep gray

- Buffered water, wash water or stain too alkaline
- Excessive thickness of the smear
- Alkaline residue to the slide
- Insufficient washing
- Prolonged staining before diluting with buffered water

Nuclei of leukocytes are pale blue, and the erythrocytes and granules of eosinophils are usually red

- Buffered water, wash water or stain too acid
- Acid residue on slide

Entire Smear has a Pale Stain

- Under staining
- Weak stain
- Excessive washing or allowing water to stand on slide
- Using warm or hot water for washing slide

Variation in staining on different areas of the smear

- Buffered water un evenly applied and not thoroughly mixed with Wright's stain
- Acid or alkaline residue on the slide
- Water not properly drained from slide after washing

Precipitated Stain

- Lack of through washing
- Precipitate in Wright's stain not properly filtered
- Evaporation of alcoholic stain

HEMOGLOBIN DETERMINATION

Objective

To determine the amount of hemoglobin present in 100 ml of blood of a given sample.

Significance

a. It serves as an index of blood condition of the animal.

b. If the hemoglobin [Hb] content falls below the normal levels, it indicates anemia, or pregnancy (physiological).

c. If it increases to the normal value, it indicates polycythemia, decrease in O2 supply, heart disease, emphysema etc.

Method: Acid hematin method

Requirements: Sahlis instrument, blood sample

Procedure

- Take 0.1N HCl (1%) into central graduated tube up to mark 2.
- Suck the blood exactly up to mark 20 (20 μl) with the help of sahlis pipette.
- Transfer the blood from pipette to central graduated tube of the hemometer.
- Mix it well with the help of stirrer or rod and allow it to react for two minute.
- Make up with distilled water by adding drop by drop until the color matches with the Standard comparator tube and mix well.
- When the color matches take out and record the values on the side as gm/100ml and or in percentage.
- Repeat 5 to 6 times and take the average value

Normal value: Bovine 8 - 15gm/dl (11) Equine 11 -19gm/dl (14)

Ovine 9 – 15gm/dl (11.5) Feline 8 – 15gm/dl (12)

Caprine: 8-14gm/dl (11) Canine 12 – 18gm/dl (15)

HEMATOCRIT DETERMINATION (PCV)

Aim: To determine the hematocrit value for a given blood sample.

Principle: Blood compartment is separated into three parts using capillary tube in a hematocrit centrifuge.

Method: Wintrobe hematocrite method

Significance

- Packed Cell Volume (PCV) = erythrocyte mass; anemia when PCV falls dawn.
- Buffy coat; white to gray layer above PCV. It will give number of WBC (0.5mm to1.5mm).Leukopenia or leukocytosis.
- ***Plasma content***: usually about 55%, Yellowish in color. Degree of yellowness indicates icterus (jaundice).

Requirements: Hematocrit tube, hematocrite centrifuge, hematocrit reader and sealer.

Procedure

- The blood is filled in to a micro hematocrit tube (3/4th) and seals it with sealer.
- Centrifuge the filled hematocrit tube in a hematocrite centrifuge at 2000 rpm for 4-5 minutes.
- Read the value (the tube) with hematocrit reader and record the result.

Normal Value

- Bovine 37 - 55 % (45%)
- Ovine 24 - 50 % (38%)
- Caprine 24 - 50 % (40%)
- Equine 32 - 55 % (42%)
- Swine 32 - 50 % (42%)

TOTAL COUNT OF RBC

Objective: To enumerate the total count of RBC/cumm of a given blood sample.

Method: Hemocytometry method

Significance

- It performs some functions such as transportation of O2 and CO2
- A decrease in RBC accounts for less hemoglobin i.e., anemia

- An increase in RBC is referred as Polycythemia

Requirements: Hemocytometer, cover slip, microscope, RBC diluting fluid, Haeyem's solution or Physiological saline 0.85% Nacl.

Procedure:

- Take the blood in to RBC pipette up to 0.5 marks
- Immediately draw the RBC diluting fluid up to mark 101.
- Rotate the pipette between thumb and other fingers with finger eight (8) movements. This gives a dilution of 1:200.
- Clean the counting chamber of hemocytometer and cover slip
- Place the cover slip in position over the counting chamber by gentle pressure
- Expel a drop of blood on to the counting chamber by holding the pipette at an angle of 45°.
- Allow the hemocytometer for 2-3 min to settle down the RBC in counting chamber
- ***Counting***: Counting rules
    - Count less than 40 × microscope objective
    - Count cells touching the left and top side lines.
    - Don't count cells touching the bottom right side lines.
    - Count first left to right direction, then to vise verse.

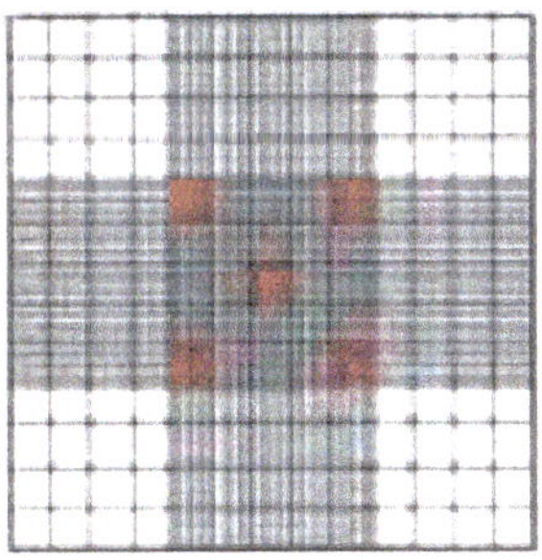

Figure 3: Hemocytometer grid lines. Erythrocyte and leukocyte count. Red = zones to be counted under high power for erythrocytes. White = zones to be counted under low power for leukocytes.

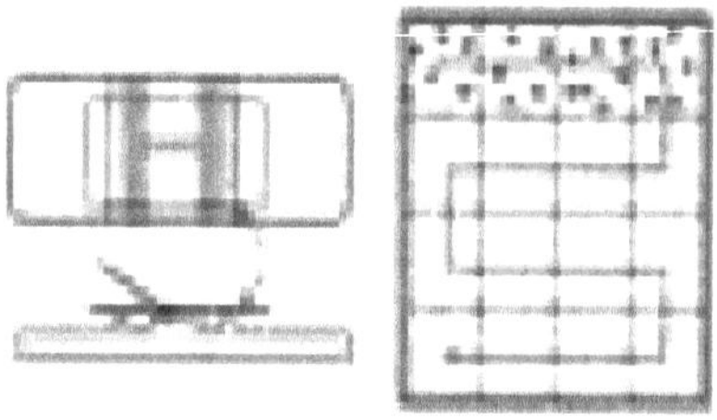

Figure 4: The hemocytometer and the direction in which the count should be made

Calculation

Volume of one small square = 1/20mm × 1/20mm × 1/10mm = 1/4000mm3

Volume of 80 small square = 80 × 1/4000mm3 = 1/50mm3

Total number of RBC = Cells counted (N)/Volume of all squares × dilution factor

Total RBC = N (cell counted)/1/50mm3 × 1/200 = N × 10,000

TOTAL COUNT OF WBC (WHITE BLOOD CELLS)

Objective: To enumerate the total number of WBC/cumm of blood.

Method: Hemocytometer method

Significance: The normal WBC performs some important physiological functions. The chief function of it is imparting immunity to the body. Therefore, the decrease or increase in circulating WBC indicates physiological condition i.e., increase in WBC indicates inflammation where as decrease in WBC may indicate AIDS.

Requirements: Hemocytometer, cover slip, microscope, WBC diluting fluid, or 1% HCl (1% Glacic Asetic Acid) i.e., 1ml GAA + 1 ml MB + 100ml dist.H2O.

Procedure

- Draw the blood in to WBC pipette up to 0.5 marks.
- Immediately draw the WBC diluting fluid up to 11 marks.
- Rotate the pipette between thumbs and finger horizontally. This will gives you a dilution of 1:20.
- Clean the counting chamber of hematometer and cover slip.
- Place the cover slip on the counting chamber with gentle pressure.
- Expel the fluid in the pipette by an angle of 45°.

- Allow the hemocytometer for 2 minute to settle down the WBC.
- Count the WBC in the 4 large squares in the corners of counting chamber (16 small squares).

Counting:

Count cells touching the left and top side lines

Don't count cells touching the right and bottom side lines

avoid duplication of cells

Calculation: Total WBC count = Cells counted × 50

Area of one smallest square = 1/4 × 1/4 = 1/16mm2

Depth of the counting chamber = 1/10mm

Volume of one smallest square = 1/10mm × 1/16mm2 = 1/160mm3

4 corners × 16 ss = 64 ss × 1/160mm3 = 64/160mm3 = 0.4mm3

Total volume = 64 ss × 1/160mm3 = 64/160mm3 = 0.4mm3

Dilution = 1:20

Therefore, Total WBC = cell counted/dilution × volume

= cell counted/1:20 × 0.4

= cell counted × 20/0.4

= cell counted × 50

DIFFERENTIAL LEUKOCYTE COUNT

Aim: To enumerate the different types of leucocytes namely neutrophil, eosinophil, basophil, monocyte, and lymphocyte.

Method: Blood film (smear) with Wright's or Giemsa stain

Significance

- They are responsible for the defense of the organism
- They are 5000-7000mm3
- Leucocytes divide in to granulocyte and agranulocyte

Neutrophils

- Very active in phagocyting bacteria

- Found in highly in pus
- Died after phagocyting pathogens
- High during inflammation

Eosinophils: Attack parasites and phagocyte antigen-antibody complexes

Basophils

- Secrete anticoagulant and vasodilatory substances (histamines, serotonin)
- Their chief function is secreting substances

Lymphocytes: The main constituents of immune system defense against viruses, bacteria, fungi and protista.

Monocytes: Precursors of macrophages. Have intense secretory activities (lysosomes, interferons)

Requirements: Clean glass slide, sterile needle, microscope, stains solution, oil immersion

Protocol

Making the Smear

- Place a small drop of blood near an end of the slide
- Bring another slide in contact with the drop and allow distributing at an angle of 30-40 degrees
- Push to the left in a smooth and quick motion
- Dry the slide with air

Fixing - Dip the smear in a vessel containing 95% containing ethyl or methyl alcohol for 3-5 minutes

Staining

- Stain the smear with Giemsa or Wright's stain for 16-60 or 1-3 minutes respectively
- Rinse the slide with distilled water at room temperature
- Drain off the water and leave the slide to dry

Cover Slipping

Place a drop of Canada balsam on the smear and then mount the cover slip

Observation

- examine under dry objective or oil immersion
- count about 100-200 cells and take average

Interpretation

Neutrophils

- Very tiny light staining granules
- Multi-lobed nucleus connected by thin strands of nuclear material
- Are most numerous, normally they account 50-70%
- If the count exceeds this amount, the cause is usually due to an acute infection (appendicitis, small pox, rheumatic fever)
- If the count is considerably less, it may be due to a viral infection (influenza, hepatitis, rubella)

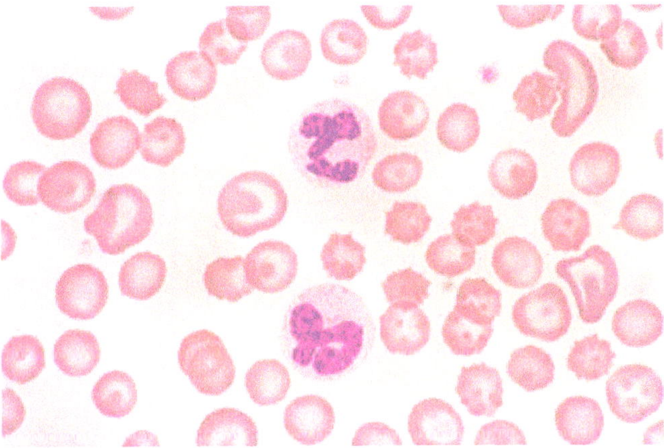

Figure 5: Normal canine neutrophils. Both neutrophils have a lobulated nucleus in a light pink finely granulated cytoplasm.

Eosinophils

- Has large granules (acidophilic), pink red
- The nucleus often has two lobes connected by a band of nuclear material, looks like telephone receiver which contains digestive enzymes against parasites.

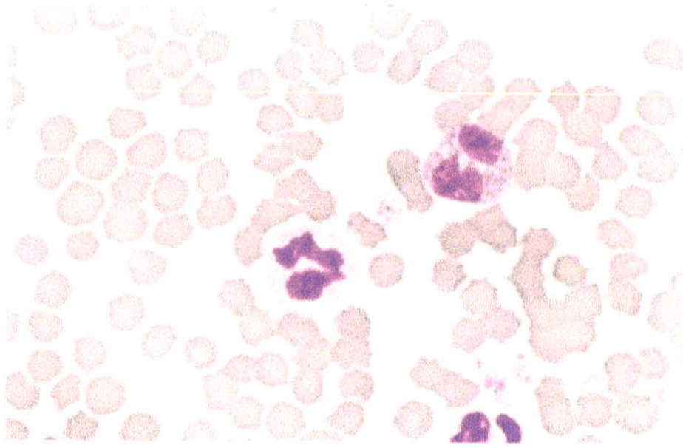

Figure 6: Feline eosinophils. Eosinophil (top) has granules that are pale pink and rod-shaped.

Lymphocytes

- An agranulocyte cell with very clear cytoplasm
- Very large nucleus which fills almost the cell with leaving thin rim of cytoplasm (Figure 5).
- Smaller than the three granulocytes (N,E,B)
- Play an important role in our immune response
- The T-lymphocytes act against virus infected cells and tumor cells
- The B-lymphocytes produce antibodies
- 2nd numerous leukocyte, accounting for 25-35% of the counted in differential WBC count
- When number of this cells exceeds the normal value, one would suspect parasites
- Patients with AIDS keep a careful watch on their T-cell level

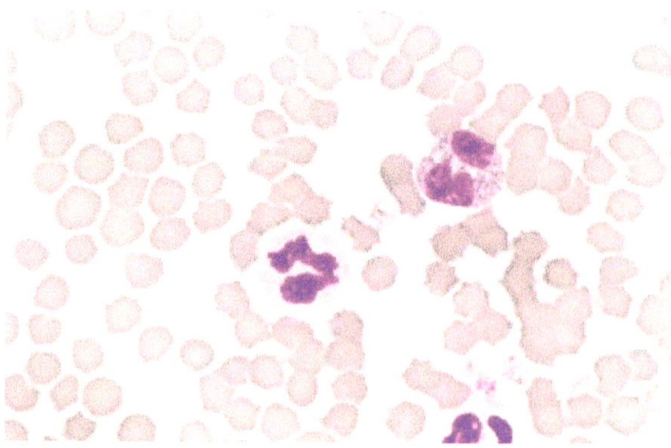

Figure 7: Normal lymphocytes. Lymphocytes in the dog and cat are the same size or

smaller than a neutrophil. Feline lymphocytes are similar to those in the dog (A and C 100x, B 120x).

Monocytes

- The largest of leucocytes and are agranular
- "U" or kidney bean shaped nucleus
- Abundant cytoplasm and light blue
- Account for 3-9% of the total leukocyte
- People with malaria, endocarditis, typhoid fever, and rocky mountain spotted fever, monocyte increases in number

Normal value

Neutrophil = 50-70%

Eosinophil = 2-4%

Basophil = 0-1%

Lymphocytes = 20-40%

Monocytes = 3-8%

DETERMINATION OF ERYTHROCYTE SEDIMENTATION RATE (ESR)

Purpose: To determine the ESR of a given blood sample

Principle: The distance (in mm) that the erythrocyte fall during a given period of time when blood to which anticoagulant has been added in a tube placed in a vertical position

Significance

- It is not a specific test, but reflects change in plasma protein accompanying most of acute and chronic infection
- Some pathological condition causes rouleax formation
- The greater the ESR reading, the more the severity of pathological condition
- During TB and rheumatic disease ESR increases

Method: Westergrens method

Requirements: ESR stand, ESR tube, blood sample

Protocol

- Take the anticoagulant blood in to ESR tubes exactly up to '0' mark.
- Place the tube vertically (upright position) in ESR stand.
- Take reading after 5min as 'zero' hour reading and again note the reading after 1 hour and 2 hours.

Normal value: 0-mm at 1hr, 2-3mm at 24hrs, but if above this value at 24 hrs, it indicates some pathological defect

Horse	10-30 min
Cattle	8-24hr
Sheep	24hr
Goat	24hr
Pig	8hr
Dog	1hr, because of large sized erythrocyte
Cat	1hr
Man	1hr

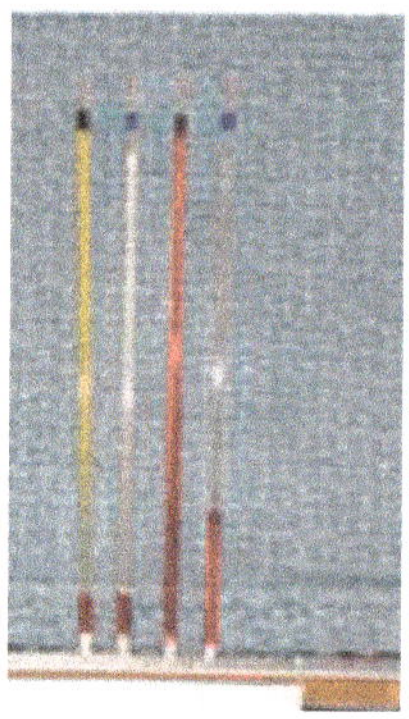

Figure 8: Erythrocyte sedimentation rate.

COAGULATION TIME DETERMINATION (WHOLE BLOOD CLOTTING TIME)

Lee-White Method

- Obtain at least 3ml of blood in a plastic syringe by careful vein puncture (start a stop watch)

- Place 1ml of blood into each of the three tubes
- Place the test tube in a water bath at 37°C
- After 2 minutes one of the three test tubes is tipped gently at one minute interval
- Test the third test tube in the same manner
- The time elapsed between the first appearance of the blood in the syringe and clot formation in the third tube is clotting time

Capillary Tube Method

Capillary tube, filter paper, clock watch should be used as requirements

- A skin puncture is made and wiping away the first drop, fill a special capillary tube with blood noting the time when the blood first appeared
- Holding the tube between the thumb and index finger of both hands, gently break the tube every second until a strand of thread fibrin is seen extending across the gap between the ends of the tube
- The interval between the appearance of the blood and the appearance of the fibrin stand is the coagulation time

Interpretation

Normal Value

- Lee- white method in glass tube --- 3-12 minutes
- Capillary tube method---3-15 minute in horse and cattle---1-5 minutes other animals

Prolonged

- Deficiency in coagulation factors
- Vitamin K deficiency
- Thrombocytopenia
- The presence of circulating anticoagulants

Table 3: Normal values of whole blood clotting time in various species of domestic animals (capillary tube method).

Species	Time in minutes
Bovine	3-5
Ovine	1-6
Caprine	2.5-11.5
Equine	3-15
Porcine	4
Canine	3-4
Feline	5

BLEEDING TIME

Determination of bleeding time is a simple and sometimes useful tool for evaluating the efficiency of the capillary – platelet aspect of homeostasis

Purpose: To determine the bleeding time

Method: Dukes method

Significance

The study helps in diagnosis, treatment, and study of hemorrhagic diseases

The prolonged time indicates coagulation defect

Requirements: Blood lancet, filter paper, clock (stop clock)

Protocol

- Make a moderately small, deep puncture in clean, sterile blood lancet or sterile needle, and note the time when blood first appears (nose is preferable)
- Remove the drops of blood with filter paper every 30 second being careful not to touch the skin. The use of highly absorbent paper such as cleaning tissue tends to prolong bleeding time due to more effective removal of surface blood
- Note the end point, when blood no longer appears from the puncture site

Interpretation

Normal values: 1- 5 min in domestic animals

Prolonged due to

- vascular lesions

- platelet defect
- severe liver disease, uremia
- anticoagulant drug administration

CALCULATING RED BLOOD CELL INDICES

Objectives

- To be able to calculate MCV, MCH, and MCHC from red blood cell count, hematocrit and hemoglobin concentration
- To compare with normal ranges of the blood indices of different domestic animals

Significance

Here one can classify red blood cells as normo, hypo, and hyperchromic anemia. Apart from these facts, the size of red blood cell as normo, micro, and macrocytosis can be classified.

Materials

The following formulas depict method of calculating the blood indices

- MCV indicates a change in the size of a single RBC
- Normocytosis means normal size
- Microcytosis indicates smaller size due to iron deficiency etc and thus lower hemoglobin concentration
- Macrocytosis indicates larger size and is usually caused by vit B12 and folic acid deficiencies
- MCH is mostly associated with hemoglobin concentration
- Decreased MCH causes hypochromic anemia because of a deficiency of iron in the diet
- Increased MCH may be caused during hemolysis where extracellular hemoglobin level increases
- MCHC is the most accurate of the indices , because it doesn't require RBC count s. decreased value indicates iron deficiency and reticulocytosis and increased value may be due to hemolysis

Discussion

Considering the size, the calculated RBC indices indicate what?

What differentiates MCHC from other two RBC indices?

Blood group and Rh-factor determination

Objective: To be able to perform ABO and Rh- blood grouping

The following table shows characteristics of the ABO blood group

Table 4: Blood group characteristics

Blood groups	Antigens (on blood cells)	Antibodies (in plasma/serum)
A	A	Anti - B
B	B	Anti - A
O	No antigen	Anti – A and anti – B
AB	A & B	No antibody

Materials

- Marked plastic plate or slide
- Sterile lancet
- Uncoagulated blood
- Sticks for mixing
- Antiserums

Method

- Place one drop anti – A anti body (blue) on the first bore of the plastic plate
- Place one drop anti – B anti body (yellow) on the second bore of the plastic plate
- Add a drop of blood in to each of the above anti-serums
- Using a separate clean stick for each bore , mix the blood and the antiserums
- Tilt the plate gently from side to side to enhance agglutination
- Observe for agglutination reactions following few minutes
- Similar steps follow for Rh blood , except you use anti – D antibody

Interpretation

Agglutination in a specific well therefore indicates the presence of specific antigen. If no agglutination is observed in anti – A and anti –B antibodies, then blood group is O. if agglutination is observed in both A & B antibodies, the blood group is AB.

For Rh factor, agglutination with anti –D serum indicates Rh+, and no agglutination indicates Rh- blood. Results

Identify if which blood groups and Rh factors show agglutination reaction with the corresponding antibodies, Mark (+) for agglutination and (-) for no agglutination reactions (Table 5).

Results 1: Identify if which blood groups and Rh factors show agglutination reaction with the corresponding antibodies, Mark (+) for agglutination and (-) for no agglutination reactions (Table 5).

Table 5: Blood groups and Rh factor characteristics

	Blood groups					
Serum	A	B	AB	O	Rh+	Rh-
Anti –A	+	-	+	-	+	-
Anti –B	-	+	+	-	+	-
Anti –D					+	-

Determine your Owen blood group and decide which member of your colleagues could denote or receive blood to each other

No	Your blood group	You can denote blood to	You can receive blood from	Remark
1	E.g. A	B ,AB	B ,O	
2	B	A, AB	A ,O	
3	O	A ,B,AB	O,A,B	
4	AB	-		

Discussion

Answer the following questions based on your results

- What is the cause of transfusion incompatibilities in ABO blood groups?
- What blood type is a universal donor and why is it said a universal donor?
- State two differences between the ABO and Rh blood type?
- What would happen if Rh- mother bears a child from Rh- father?
- What pathological consequences would arise if Rh+ father marries Rh- mother?

PART TWO: FUNCTION TESTS

The spectrophotometer

It is an instrument used to measure the amount of light absorbed by the solution. It includes

- Light source- gives steady white light
- Prisms- splits white light to visible colors (red, orange, yellow, green, violet)
- Monochromater (wavelength selector)- system for isolating radiant energy of a desired wave length and excluding others
- Cuvate – contains sample solution
- Detector (photoelectric tube)-converts the transmitted light energy into an equivalent amount of electrical energy.
- Meter (recording device)-displays the amount of transmitted light or provides numerical display of absorbance

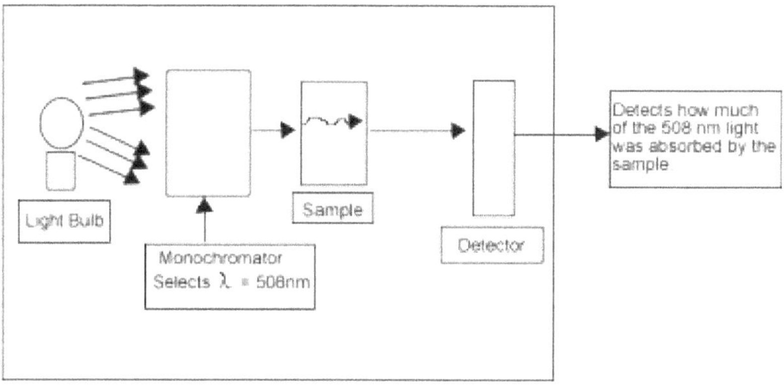

Figure 9: Spectrophotometer.

Beer lambert's law States that the light passing through colored medium is absorbed in direct proportion to the amount of the colored substance in the light path A = abC where A – Absorbance a – molar absorbitivity (constants) b – Length of light path (constants) C – Concentration Molar absorbitivity (a) – is the absorbance of molar concentration of substance with path length of 1cm determined at specific wave length under defined conditions of solvent , PH and temperature A = abC , a = A/ bC For standard solution and sample solution a - is the same For both solutions b (light path) is the same, so that 18. Determination of Aspartate Amino Transferase (AST) and) Glutamic Oxalacetate Transminase (GOT) Principle: Aspartate Amino Transferase catalyzes the transfer of the amino group from aspartate to oxoglutarate with the formation of glutamate and oxalacetate.

Reagent Composition

R1 – AST substrate: TRIS buffer 121mmol, L – aspartate 362mmol/l

Maltate dehydragenase > 460ul, lactate dehydragenase > 600ul

R2 – AST coenzyme: NADH Reagent preparation

Working reagent – mix 4ml of R1 + 1ml of R2 (stable for 4 weeks at +2 to 8°C)

Samples

Serum and EDTA or heparinized plasma

Procedure

- Pre incubate working reagent , samples and controls to reaction temperatures
- Set the photometer to "0" absorbance with distilled water
- Pipette in a cuvette

Reaction To	37°	30°
Working reagent	1ml	1ml
Sample or control	50ul	100ul

- Mix gently by inversion, insert the cuvette in to the cell holder and start stop watch
- Incubate for 1 minute and record the initial absorbance
- Repeat the absorbance reading exactly after 1, 2, and 3 minutes
- Calculate the difference between absorbance
- Calculate the mean of the results to obtain the average change in absorbance per minute (ΔA min)
- Calculation: ΔA min * 3333 (37°) or ΔA min * 1746 (30°)

DETERMINATION OF ALKALINE PHOSPHATASE (ALP)

Principle: Alkaline Phosphatase catalyzes the hydrolysis of 4 – nitrophenyl phosphate (4 – NPA) with the formation of free 4 – nitrophenol and in organic phosphate

Reagent Composition

R1 – ALP buffer: DEA buffer 1.25mol/l, MgCl 0.6mmol/l, biocides

R2 – ALP substrate: 4 – NPP 50mmol/l, biocides

Reagent Preparation

Working reagent – mix 4ml of R1 + 1ml of R2 (stable for 4wks at +2 to 8°)

Samples

Serum or heparinized plasma, or EDTA, oxalates, citrates inhibit enzyme

Procedures

- Preincubate working reagent , sample and controls to reaction temperatures
- Set the photometer to '0' absorbance with distilled water
- Pipette in a cuvettexc

Reaction temperature	37°C
Working reagent	1ml (ALP)
Sample control	20ul

- Mix gently by inversion , insert the cuvette in to the cell holder and start stop watch
- Incubate for 1min and record the initial absorbance
- Repeat the absorbance reading exactly after 1, 2, and 3 minutes
- Calculate the difference between absorbances
- Calculate the mean of the results to obtain the average change in absorbance per minute (ΔA/min)

Calculation: ΔA/min * 2746

DETERMINATION OF CREATININE

Principle: Creatinine in alkaline medium react with picrate ions to form yellow orange complex whose color intensity is measured at 492nm

Reagent composition

R1 (picric acid) – 35mmol/l

R2 (NaOH) – 0.32mmol

R4 (Creatinine standard) – 2mg/dl

Reagent Preparation

Mix equal volume of R1 and R2: Stable for 10 days at 4 to 8° or 1day at + 20 to 25°

Specimen

Serum, plasma, urine (diluted with distilled water)

Procedure

	Standard	Sample
Working solution	1000ul	1000ul (1ml)
Standard	100ul	-
Sample	-	100ul

Mix and pour into a cuvette after exactly 20seconds read A1 of sample and standard exactly 80sec after first reading, read A2 of sample and standard.

$$Ctest = \frac{\Delta Atest \times Cstd}{\Delta std}$$

Table 6: Normal values of creatinine

Normal values (mg/dl)	Dog	Cow	Horse	Sheep	Goat	Man
	0.1 – 0.8	0.6 – 1.8	0.9 – 2.0	0.9 -2.0	0.7 – 1.5	0.7 -1.2

Conversion of mg/100ml into mmol/l and vice versa

$$Mmol/l = \frac{mg/100ml \times 10}{Molecular\ wt}$$

$$Mg/100ml = \frac{mmol/l \times molecular\ wt}{10}$$

TOTAL PROTEIN DETERMINATION

Principle: In the biuret reaction, a chelate is formed between the Cu2+ ion and the peptide bonds in protein in alkaline solution to form a violet colored complex whose absorbance is measured to the concentration of protein in the sample

Reagent Composition

R1: Biuret reagent (cupric sulphate 6mmol/l, sodium – potassium tartrate 21mmol, potassium iodide 6mmol, sodium hydroxide 0.75mol/l, CAL protein standard [Bovine Serum Albumin 7g/dl (70g/l)]

Samples

Serum, EDTA or heparinized plasma and exudates. Total protein is stable in serum for one week at room temperature, for at least 1 month refrigerated at 2 – 8°C, for up to 2 months at -20°C

Interferences: Grossly haemolytic or lipemic samples result in positive interference

Materials Required

- Photometer or colorimeter capable of measuring absorbance at 540+ 20nm
- Constant temperature incubator set at 37°C
- Pipettes to measure reagent and samples

Procedure

- Pipette in to labeled tubes

Tubes	Blank	Sample	Standard
Biuret	1ml	1ml	1ml
Sample	-	20ul	-
Standard	-	-	20ul

- Mix and incubate the tubes for 10 min at 37°C
- Read the absorbance (A) of the sample and standard 540nm against the reagent blank

Calculation

$$\frac{\text{A sample}}{\text{A standard}} \times \text{Cstandard} = \text{g/dl total protein}$$

If the results are to expressed as SI units apply g/dl × g/l

UREA DETERMINATION

Use: enzymatic in vitro test for the quantitative determination of urea in serum, plasma and urine samples

Test principles

$$\text{Urea} + H_2O + 2H \xrightarrow{\text{Urease}} 2NH_4^+ + CO_2$$

The ammonium ions formed react with the salicylate and hydrochloride to give a green dye

Reagent Composition

R1: Phosphate buffer PH 6.7------------------------------------ 60mmol/l

EDTA--1.5mmol/l

Sodium salicylate-- 60mmol/l

Sodium nitroprusside --------------------------------------- 5.2mmol/l

R2: Urease-- >5000u/ml

R3: Sodium hydrochloride ------------------------------------- 18mmol/l

Sodium hydroxide --- 450mmol/l

R4: Urea --- 50mg/dl (8.325mmol/l)

Preparation and Stability

Working Reagent: Add one vial R2 to bottle of R1. It is stable up to 4 weeks at 2 to 8°C, 6days at 20 to 25°C. R3 and R4 are ready for use

For photometers, which need a minimum of 2ml, dilute R3 by 4 volume of distilled water, eg 10ml of R3 and 40ml of distilled water. The dilute reagent is stable for 6 months at 2 to 8°C.

Specimen

Serum, or heparinized plasma, urine diluted with 1:10 part with distilled water

Limitations

Interference, Icterus, hemolysis, Lipemia

Testing Procedure

Controls = 0.9% Nacl

Wave length = 580 – 600nm

Temperature = 20/25/37°C

Cuvette = 1cm light path

Zero adjustment = against reagent blank

	Reagent blank	Standard	Sample
Working solution	1000ul	1000ul	1000ul
R4(standard)	-	10ul	-
Sample	-	-	10
Incubate at +37°C for 5min , or for 10min at 20/25°C , then add			
R3 or diluted reagent /R3 (1:5)	200ul	200ul	200ul
	1000ul	1000ul	1000ul
Mix, incubate at +37°C for 5min or for 10min at 20/25°C and read absorbance against reagent blank (ΔA)			

Calculation

$$\text{Urea conc. (mg/dl)} = \frac{\Delta A \text{ sample}}{\Delta A \text{ standard}} \times \text{standard conc.}$$

Whereas, R4 /standard concentration = 50mg/dl (8.325mmol/l)

TOTAL AND DIRECT BILIRUBIN DETERMINATION

Use: Quantitative determination of direct bilirubin and total bilirubin in serum or heparinized/EDTA plasma

Test principle:

In the presence of caffeine accelerator, total bilirubin couples with sulphonlic acid to form a red azobilirubin dye

Reagents:

R1: Sulfonlic acid ---------------------------29mmol/l

Hcl ---------------------------------------0.17mmol/l

R2: Sodium nitrate ------------------------25mmol/l

R3: Caffeine ---------------------------------0.26mol/l

Sodium benzoate ---------------------0.52mol/l

R4: Tartrate --------------------------------0.93mol/l

NaOH ----------------------------------1.9mol/l

Preparation

R1 ready for use

Specimen: Fresh serum, heparinized /EDTA plasma. Hemolysis interferes with result

Testing Procedure: materials – working solution above, calibrators, controls (0.9% Nacl solution)

Wave length – Hg 578nm

Temperature – 20 to 25°C

Cuvette – 1cm

Zero adjustment – against sample blank

	Sample blank	Sample
R1	200ul	200ul
R2	-	50ul
R3	1000ul	1000ul
Sample	200ul	200ul
Mix and incubate at room temperature for 10 to 60 minutes, add		
R4	1000ul	1000ul
Mix and incubate at room temperature for 5 – 30 minutes, read absorbance of sample		

Calculation

$$\text{With calibrator Bilurubin} = \frac{\text{ÄA sample}}{\text{ÄA calibrator}} * \text{calibrator conc.}$$

With factors concentration in mg/dl = 10.8 * Δ Abilirubin total

N.B –Direct bilirubin determination should have its own procedure and calculation findings

Glucose

ENZYMATIC KINETIC COLORIMETER TEST (GOD – PAP)

Principle: Enzymatic colorimeter test on basis of Trinder-Reaction

$$\text{Glucose} + O_2 + H_2O \xrightarrow{\text{Glucose oxidase}} \text{Gluconate} + H_2O$$

$$2H_2O_2 + \text{phosphate} + 4\text{ - amino-antipyrine} \xrightarrow{\text{Peroxidase}} \text{Red chinonin} + 4H_2O$$

Reagent

R1: buffered enzyme reagent

Phosphate buffer, PH 7.5 ---------------------- 0.5mol/l

Phenol -- 7.5mmol/l

GOD (Glucose oxidase) ------------------------ 12000u/l

POD -- 660u/l

4-amino-antipyrine---------------------------0.4 mmol / l

R4: Standard

Glucose ---100mg/dl (5.55mmol/lit)

Preparation: the reagent is ready for use Sample: Serum or heparinized plasma Procedure

Wave length ---------------------Hg 546nm (492-550nm)

Temperature --------------------- +25 (+30) +37°C

Cuvette -------------------------- 1cm light path

Zero adjustment -------------- Reagent blank

	Blank	Standard	Sample
Working reagent	1000ul	1000ul	1000ul
Standard/R4	-	10ul	-
Sample	-	-	10ul

Mix, measure and incubate at 37°C for 15 minute or 30min at +25°C with in 60min, read absorbance

Calculation:

$$\text{Glucose (mg/dl)} = \frac{\ddot{A}\text{A sample}}{\ddot{A}\text{A standard}} \times \text{standard conc.}$$

Standard conc: 100mg/dl (5.56mmol/l)

LIVER FUNCTION TEST

Vander Bight's test

Principle of the test

Direct Reaction

- Bilirubin – in the serum from obstructive jaundice reacts immediately with

Ehrlich's Diazo reagent, while serum with hemolytic jaundice requires the addition of alcohol and a longer time interval for the reaction

- Measurement of direct 1-min bilirubin demonstrates the gulucronide compound while 30-min bilirubin represents total bilirubin. The quantity of free (indirect reaching) bilirubin is the difference between the total (30min) and direct (1min) values
- Qualitative method

Direct Reaction

- Place 1ml of non hemolized serum from a fasting animal in a graduated centrifuge tube
- Allow 0.5ml of Ehrlich's Diazo reagent must be prepared each day by mixing 10ml of solution A with 0.3ml solution B below (keep in brown bottle in refrigerator)

Solution A	Solution B
Sulfanlic acid ------1gm	Sodium nitrite --------0.5ml
Conc. HCl acid ------15ml	Dist H2O --------------- 100ml
Dist H2O-----------1000ml	

- The contact zone between the serum and the reagent is examined against a good back ground for the development of a reddish purple ring in 30sec

Indirect Reaction

After the determination of the direct reaction shake the tube containing the serum and diazo reagent and add 3ml of 95% alcohol and mix

If a definite pinkish color fails to appear in 15min and only a white turbidity occur, the reaction is recorded as Negative. If a color already presents from a positive direct test depends up on the addition of alcohol, the reaction is recorded as positive for the indirect test.

WALLACE-DIAMOND TEST

Principle: Depends up on the reaction of urobilinogen and other chromagens with Ehrilich's benzaldehyde reagent to form a red color

Reagents: Ehrlich's benzaldehyde reagent

Para – dimethyl amino benzal dehyde – 2gm

2% aqueous solution of conc. Hcl – 100ml

Procedure:

Take 5ml of urine in a test tube , add 0.5ml of Ehrlich's bengaldehyde reagent

It is essential that the urine be fresh since urobilinogen exposure to light and air is changed in to urobilin , which doesn't react

If large amount of bile are present in equal parts of urine and 110% aqueous solution of barium chloride should be mixed and filter to remove all precipitate as bilirubin interg-ers with reading the result of the urobilinogen reaction

Allow the tube to stand for 5minutes and observe for pink to red color development by viewing length wise through the tube against a white back ground

Result

Normal – pink to light red color

No urobilinogen – absent of pink or red color

Increased urobilinogen – cherry red color

KIDNEY FUNCTION TEST

Gross examination of urine /physical examination/

Urine volume: This is dependant normally up on fluid intake, environmental condition, diet and activity of the animal. The following data indicates the normal value of urine for different species

Dog ---------12 – 30ml/Ib body wt/24hrs

Cat ---------- 4.5 – 9ml/Ib body wt/24hrs

Horse ------ 2 – 8ml/Ib body wt/24hrs

Swine -----------2 – 14ml/Ib body wt/24hrs

Cattle ----------- 8 – 20ml/Ib body wt/24hrs

Shoat ----------- 4.5 – 14ml/Ib body wt/24hrs

Value above or below the normal value can be considered as pathological but it should be combined with clinical and laboratory examination

Color-Can be observed in a test tube or in a urinometer tube. The following designations are used to observe the sample and correlated to the following terms.

- ✓Colorless
- ✓Pale yellow
- ✓Yellow
- ✓Dark yellow
- ✓Yellow brown
- ✓Greenish yellow
- ✓Green
- ✓Red
- ✓Reddish brown
- ✓Brown
- ✓Blue
- ✓Milky

Interpretation

Yellow to amber – Normal

Colorless to pale yellow – dilute urine with low specific gravity and polyuria

Dark yellow or yellow brown – concentrated urine with a high specific gravity and small quantity

Yellow brown or greenish yellow – yellow green foam when urine is shaken

Urobilinoids – chromagon derived from heme green biliverdin yellow-brown-billirubin-and urobilin

Cloudy – hematuria (clearer after centrifugation)

Translucent – hemoglobinuria

Brown to brownish black – hemoglobin up on standing bile large amounts, Normal horse urine is a yellowish color when voided, but it turns a deep brown color up on standing for a time due to oxidation of pyrocatechian

Green – bile biliverdin

Red to pink – phenothiazine

Transparency Clear – freshly voided urine from normal animal is clear, except in the horse where it is normally thick and cloudy due to calcium carbonate ($CaCO_3$) crystals and mucus

Cloudy – not necessarily pathological as many samples may become cloudy

Epithelial cells – present in large numbers

Blood – red to brown color and smoky

Leukocytes – may produce milky, ropy appearance if large number

Bacteria – produce a uniform turbidity if in large number; the turbidity doesn't settle out and cannot be removed by filtration.

Mucus

Crystals $CaCO_3$ – in fresh horse urine

Amorphous urate – white or pink cloud in acid urine

Amorphous phosphate – white cloud in alkaline urine

Specific gravity - determined by refractometer and indicator paper stripes. Normal value in most species will be in the range of 1.015 – 1.050 but values as high as 1.060 – 1.080 can occur.

Table 7: Normal values of urine specific gravity in different species

Species	Range	Average
Horse	1.020 – 1.050	1.035
Cattle	1.025 – 1.045	1.035
Sheep and goat	1.025 – 1.045	1.030
Pig	1.010 – 1.030	1.015
Dog	1.015 – 1.045	1.025
Cat	1.020 – 1.040	1.030
Man	1.010 – 1.030	1.020

Average normal = 1.025

Odour

Normal odor – aromatic or acetone

Abnormal odor – aromatic odor of ketone bodies

Foam

Shake the sample and observe

- If the amount of foam produced is in excess and slow to disappear – proteinuria
- If the color of the foam great – yellow or brown – bile pigments
- If the color of the foam red to brown – hemoglobinuria

MICROSCOPIC EXAMINATION OF URINE SAMPLE

It is of great clinical importance and should never been omitted. Important structure to be include casts, erythrocytes, leukocytes, and bacteria Method

- Agitate the urine to suspend any sediment that may settled to bottom
- Fill the centrifuge tube with urine and centrifuge for 3min at low rate of speed
- Pour all the urine and there is sufficient urine on the slide to drain to the bottom and suspend the sediment
- Pour a drop of sediment on a glass slide, and cover with a cover glass that has been wiped clean of oil and lint
- Examine under microscope with the lower power objective
- Finding should be reported as few, many or abundant
- If necessary stain with new methylene blue
- Organized sediments, epithelial cells

Chemical Examination of Urine

pH of Urine

The normal hydrogen ion (pH) concentration, in the urine depends on the type of diet. Animals on vegetable diet produce alkaline urine while those on a high protein diet produce acidic urine.

Deep paper strip in to urine several times match the color of the paper strip with the chart 1min after welting with urine

Methods of Measuring pH using pH Meter

- Switch on the instrument and allow to "warm up" for a few minutes
- Rinse electrodes with distilled water and remove excess with soft paper, taking care not to touch the glass bulb
- Place electrodes into reference buffered solution
- Rinse as in "2" above
- Place in solution to be measured and take reading
- Rinse again and switch off instrument
- Keep electrodes wet, it should be not allowed to be dried

PROTEIN TEST

Method: Robert's test

Principle: Precipitation of protein by strong acid

Robert's reagent: Conc. Nitric acid – 1 part

Saturated Magnesium sulphate – 5 part (770gm to 1 litre)

Procedure

- Place 2ml of Robert's reagent in a test tube
- Layer 2ml of clear urine on the reagent by inclining the tube and allowing the urine to run slowly dawn the side from along dropped or pipette
- A positive test is indicated by a white ring at the zone of concentration, which should be read against a dark back ground and reported as

Negative - No ring at the zone of concentration

Trace - barely precipitate ring

+ Distinct narrow ring

++ Wider definite ring

+++ Very wide ring

++++ Thick, dense ring occupies most or all of urine layer

Note: In many clinical laboratories, Robert's test is routine method as it is simple, quick and easy to read even when only a small amount of protein presents.

GLUCOSE TEST

Quantitative Test of Benedicts

No glucose is present in the urine normally which passes glomerular filter, because it is completely absorbed in the tubules

Method: Qualitative method

Principle: Reducing sugars present in the urine react with the copper sulphate to reduce the copric ions to cuprous oxide giving a color change depending on the amount of reducing substances present

Reagent used

Benedict's reagent: Sodium sulphate --------------173g

Sodium carbonate ---------- 100g

Copper sulphate ------------- 17.3g

Distilled water ---------------- 1000liter

Procedure

Place 4ml of benedicts solution in a test tube

Add 1ml of urine and mix very well

Place the test tube in a boiling water for 5min and observe the color change

Result

Negative ------	blue
+ ---------------	trace light (light green)
++ --------------	green (significant)
+++ ------------	moderate orange to yellow
++++ ----------	brick red (high concentration, serious)

ACETONE (KETONE BODY)

Ross Test

Principle: Sodium nitroprusside decomposed to sodium ferrocyanide, sodium nitrite and ferric hydroxide in an alkaline solution. These products are oxidizing agents that form a complex having a purple color in the presence of di – acetic acid and acetone

Reagent

It consists of a powdered mixture of: Sodium nitroprusside ----------- 1 part

Ammonium sulphate ----------- 100 parts

Procedure:

- Place half of the powdered reagent in a dry test tube
- Add 5ml of urine to the tube and agitate
- Add 1ml to 2ml of conc ammonium hydroxide (NH_4OH) to form a layer above the mixture

In the field a flank of sodium hydroxide can substituted for the ammonium hydroxide solution and should be added before the tube is agitated

Result

Trace -------------- very slight purple color

+ ------------------- slight purple color

++ ----------------- moderate purple color

+++ --------------- dark purple color

++++ -------------- dark purple color or black

N.B: This test is also effective when applied to milk. The ketone bodies include acetone acetoacetic acid (diacetic acid) and beta-hydroxybutric acid. A state in which these substances are present in increased amount in the blood and urine is called ketosis. Aceto acetic acid and beta-hydroxybutric acid from which acetone is derived is normal intermediate product of fat metabolism. When greater amounts of fatty acids are utilized with the production of more acetoacetic acid and beta-hydroxybutric acid can be oxidized by the tissues. These bodies accumulate in the blood and are excreted in the urine.

RUMEN FUNCTION TEST

Rumen fluid is collected by stomach tube; keep it at room temperature for 9 hours before examination

Gross Examination

Color: Color of the rumen content fluid depends up on the type of the feed. The color should be from green to live to brownish green. It will be green in grazing animals and grey in those animals that feed fodder betts, yellow brown in those that feed on silage or straw. Abnormally it may be greenish black in decomposition

Consistency: It is slightly viscous under normal condition. This viscosity is pronounced if large amount of saliva is included under the condition; it is advisable to discard the first part of the rumen fluid. It will be watery in case of acidosis and foamy in foamy bloat.

Odor:

Under normal condition the odor of the rumen is aromatic odor and non replant

Penetrating odor in acidosis

Foul smelling in decomposition

Different smell in active rumen

Total Acidity of Rumen Contents

The pH of the rumen fluid varies from 5.5 – 7 which may be affected by saliva which contains bicarbonate. The PH of rumen fluid will be alkaline in active rumen during starvation and urea poisoning, the bacteria responsible for digestion and production of acid are weak and alkaline is predominates.

Urea poisoning, because of the breakdown of urea and formation of ammonia, the content of rumen becomes alkaline

Indicator or dip stick test

Insert an indicator /deep stick in to the fluid and observe the color change

Titrable Acidity Test

- 0.1N NaOH
- Phenotaline solution (indicator)
- 10ml of rumen fluid

Procedure

- Pour 0.1N NaOH in the blurrette, write down the volume of the solution
- Measure 10ml of rumen content in the beaker and add 1-2 drops of phenophtaline indicator and mix well
- Let 0.1N NaOH be in the beaker drop to neutralize and go on until fresh color fluid comes out

Result

Multiply total amount of NaOH by 10 i.e, NaOH /ml × 10 clinical units under normal condition the clinical units range from 8 – units but in abnormal conditions it could be 10 – 70 units

SEDIMENTATION ACTIVITY TIME

Procedure

- Directly use rumen fluid or filter the fluid allow to stand for a few minutes
- The fine particles and infusoria settle down while floatation flows due to the production of gas by micro flora of rumen.

The time required for the setting down of infusoria and fine particles and floating of the production of gas by the microorganisms is known as the sedimentation activity time.

Under normal condition the SAT will be very weak floatation, slow or absent due to the absent of active microorganism, example in starvation. In acidosis Lactobaccili are very active and there is large amount of gas production and floatation are very quick and large.

BACTERIA EXAMINATION

Purpose: To determine the dominate bacteria in the ruminal fluid

Method: Gram stain

Materials: Gram staining dyes (GV, iodine, safranin, methanol or acetone), slide, microscope

Procedure

- Take a rumen fluid on the slide and make a smear
- Dry and stain with gram stain
- Observe under oil immersion for the presence or absence of the microorganisms. The bacteria in the rumen is referred as leading bacteria
- Observe the gram negative and gram positive bacteria, write the dominate and the ratio
- Under normal condition gram negative bacteria are the dominate
- In the rumen of the animals feed on roughage, the large streptococci kidney shaped cocci, saracia are predominantly present
- Under acidosis condition Gram positive bacteria predominantly present

MICROSCOPIC EXAMINATION OF RUMEN CONTENT PROTOZOAN'S

There are two form of protozoa to be predominate in rumen fluid

- Ciliates
- Flagellates

The ciliates are important because massive in numbers than the flagellates. There are 10 – 20 millions species which inhibits in the rumen as far as the physiological significance of these protozoan are considered to be not use full. However they are important in stabilizing bacterial digestive process.

Procedure

- Take one or two drops of rumen fluid on the slide
- Cover with cover slip and warm around 13°C
- Observe under microscope
- Grade the number of protozoa

Result

- If it is abundant---------------- + + +
- If it is moderate --------------- + +
- If it is few ----------------------- +
- If no protozoa ------------------ ve

Interpretation

The size of the protozoa could be large or small and medium. The large protozoa are the first to die. There is no digestion in the rumen in the death of protozoa. Therefore, observe the proportion of death to alive one, in case of acidosis, No digestion i.e., no protozoa

CELLULOSE DIGESTION TEST

Procedure

- Take 10ml of rumen content in the test tube
- Add about 0.3ml of 10% glucose solution
- Suspend cotton thread to the solution and incubate in 37°C for 48 hrs
- The expected result is the action of microflora on the thread

Result: If the rumen is active, there will be break down of the thread

PANCREATIC FUNCTION TEST

Microscopic examination

Fat test

Purpose: To determine the presence of fat substance in the fecal sample

Reagent preparation: Sudan III or Sudan IV stain. Take equal parts of 70% alcohol and acetone with excess of Sudan III or Sudan IV stain

Sample required: Feces

Procedure

- Mix a small portion of feces with water or saline on the slide
- Combine the feces with equal parts of Sudan III or IV stain
- Examine under the low power objective (×10) after placing a cover glass on the mixture

Result

Neutral fat will appear as orange as red globules, which vary in size and shape and indicate deficiency of pancreatic lipase, i.e. undigested fat in feces indicates absence of pancreatic lipase which results pancreatic insufficiency

TRYPSIN

Film test

Test for proteolytic activity employing gelatin digestion (for small animals)

Procedure

Bring 9ml of 5% sodium bicarbonate to 19ml total volume by adding feces and mix well

Place ½ to ¼ of the mixture in a vial or test tube, place a narrow strip of radiographic film in the vial

Incubate at 37°C for half an hour

Wash the film under a gentle stream of tap water

Result

A cleared area on the submerged portion of the film indicates the presence of Trypsin. With a deficiency of tryipsin the emulsion will only be water marked or partially removed

GELATIN TEST METHOD

This test is more sensitive than the film test method

Preparation

Mix 7.5gm of gelatin powder with distilled water in a 100ml of volumetric flask, bring 199ml, boil it, and distribute 2ml in a test tube and keep it in the refrigerator

Procedure

- Warm two test tube each containing 2ml of 7.5% gelatin in 37°C to liquefy
- Bring 9ml of water to a total volume of 100ml by adding feces and mix well
- Add 2ml of the feces mixture as described above to one gelatin tube
- Add 2ml of 5% sodium bicarbonate (NaHCO3) to the other gelatin tube for the control, mix well
- Incubate both tubes at 37°C for 1hr

- Refrigerate or place in cold water (4°C) for 20 minutes

Result

Failure to gel formation indicates the presence of trypsin, which has digested the gelatin i.e No pancreatic insufficiency

Gel formation (coagulation) indicates the absence of trypsin. i.e pancreatic insufficiency if tests are repeatedly deficient.

REFERENCES

1. Benjamin MM (1978) Outline of Veterinary Clinical Pathology. (3rd Edn), Ames, IA, the Iowa State University Press.
2. Denny Meyer, John W Harvey, Ray Kersey (1997) Veterinary Laboratory Medicine: interpretation and Diagnosis, Second Edition: Elsevier Health Sciences.
3. Jiro Jerry Kaneko, John W Harvey, Michael I Bruss (2008) Clinical Biochemistry of Domestic Animals, Sixth Edition.
4. Kenneth S Latimer (2011) Duncan and Prasse's Veterinary Laboratory Medicine: Clinical Pathology, Fifth Edition
5. Krehl Ludolf von (1907) The principles of clinical pathology, a text-book for students and physicians; Philadelphia Lippincott
6. Marion L Jackson (2007) Veterinary Clinical Pathology: An Introduction, First Edition.
7. Marry Anna Thrall (2006) Clinical Case Presentations for Veterinary Hematology and Clinical Chemistry
8. Marry Anna Thrall (2006) Veterinary Hematology and Clinical Chemistry.
9. Robert J Duncan, Edward A Mahaffey, Keith W Prasse (1994) Veterinary Laboratory Medicine: Clinical Pathology, Third Edition.
10. Steven E Crow, Sally O Walshaw, Jennifer E Boyle (2009) Veterinary Clinical Pathology. Manual of Clinical Procedures in Dogs, Cats, Rabbits, and Rodents.
11. Steven L stockham, Michael A Scott (2002) Fundamentals of Veterinary Clinical Pathology, First edition.
12. Steven L Stockham, Michael A Scott (2008) Fundamentals of Veterinary Clinicaln Pathology Second Edition.

INDEX

A

Acid Citrate Dextrose (ACD) 207
Adjuvant chemotherapy 84, 87
Aloe vera (AV) 136
Amplified-fragment length polymorphism (AFLP) 185
Antimicrobial resistance (AMR) 173
Antimicrobial Resistance Learning Site (AMRLS) 174
Arachidonic acid (AA) 45
Argyrophilic nucleolar organizing region (AgNOR) 157

B

Bacillus Calmette–Guérin (BCG) 70
Bone marrow-derived cells (BMDC) 135
Bone mineral density (BMD) 116
Brilliant green agar (BGA) 194

C

Central nervous system (CNS) 35
Centre for Infectious Disease Research and Policy (CIDRAP) 185, 200
Cerebrospinal fluid (CSF) 37
Codex Alimentarius Commission (CAC) 172
Collagen antibody-induced arthritis (CAIA) 49
Connective tissue (CT) 138
Copy number aberrations (CNAs) 157
Cytotoxic T lymphocyte (CTL) 71

D

Definitive type (DT) 184
Dendritic cells (DCs) 70
Dignostic Services of Monitoba (DSM) 186
Distilled water (DW) 10

E

Enzyme immunoassay (EIA) 194
Enzyme-linked immuno sorbent assay (ELISA) 118
Ethylene diamine tetra acetic acid (EDTA) 118
European Center for Diseases Prevention and Control (ECDC) 174
European Medicines Agency (EMA) 173
European Surveillance of Veterinary Antimicrobial Consumption (ES-VAC) 173

F

Federation of Veterinarians of Europe (FVE) 174
Fluorescence in situ hybridization (FISH) 4, 155, 165
Folic acid (FA) 116
Food and Drug Administration (FDA) 174
Full thickness (FT) 136

G

Gastrointestinal tract (GIT) 193
Genome-wide association study (GWAS) 86
Glucocorticoid (GC) 36
Glutamic Oxalacetate Transminase (GOT) 228

H

Hektoen enteric agar (HEA) 194
Human breast carcinoma (HBC) 159
Human pediatric osteosarcoma 84

M

Magnetic resonance imaging (MRI) 35
Malignant transformation 83
Mesenchymal stem cell (MSC) 83

N

National Human Genome Research Institute (NHGRI) 154
Neuron-specific enolase (NSE) 60
Nucleic acid sequence-based amplification (NASBA) 195
Nucleolar organizing region (NOR) 157

O

Organisation for Animal Health (OIE) 173

P

Packed Cell Volume (PCV) 214
Periodic acid-Schiff (PAS) 2
Phosphate buffered saline (PBS) 10

R

Rheumatoid arthritis (RA) 49

S

Standard deviations (SD) 138

W

World Health Organization (WHO) 63, 167

X

Xylose lysine deoxy-cholate (XLD) 194